Ethics, Animals and Science

Ethics, Animals and Science

Kevin Dolan
SThL(JusCan), BD, DipLaw, FIAT

b

**Blackwell
Science**

© 1999 by
Blackwell Science Ltd
Editorial Offices:
Osney Mead, Oxford OX2 0EL
25 John Street, London WC1N 2BL
23 Ainslie Place, Edinburgh EH3 6AJ
350 Main Street, Malden
  MA 02148 5018, USA
54 University Street, Carlton
  Victoria 3053, Australia
10, rue Casimir Delavigne
  75006 Paris, France

Other Editorial Offices:

Blackwell Wissenschafts-Verlag GmbH
Kurfürstendamm 57
10707 Berlin, Germany

Blackwell Science KK
MG Kodenmacho Building
7–10 Kodenmacho Nihombashi
Chuo-ku, Tokyo 104, Japan

First published 1999

Set in 11/13pt Bembo
by DP Photosetting, Aylesbury, Bucks
Printed and bound in Great Britain by
MPG Books Ltd, Bodmin, Cornwall

The Blackwell Science logo is a trade mark of
Blackwell Science Ltd, registered at the United
Kingdom Trade Marks Registry

DISTRIBUTORS

Marston Book Services Ltd
PO Box 269
Abingdon
Oxon OX14 4YN
(*Orders:* Tel: 01235 465500
         Fax: 01235 465555)

USA
Blackwell Science, Inc.
Commerce Place
350 Main Street
Malden, MA 02148 5018
(*Orders:* Tel: 800 759 6102
           781 388 8250
       Fax: 781 388 8255)

Canada
Login Brothers Book Company
324 Saulteaux Crescent
Winnipeg, Manitoba R3J 3T2
(*Orders:* Tel: 204 837-2987
       Fax: 204 837-3116)

Australia
Blackwell Science Pty Ltd
54 University Street
Carlton, Victoria 3053
(*Orders:* Tel: 03 9347 0300
       Fax: 03 9347 5001)

A catalogue record for this title
is available from the British Library

ISBN 0-632-05277-5

Library of Congress
Cataloging-in-Publication Data

Dolan, Kevin.
    Ethics, animals, and science/Kevin Dolan.
        p.   cm.
    Includes bibliographical references and index.
    ISBN 0-632-05277-5 (pbk.)
    1. Animal welfare—Moral and ethical aspects.
    2. Animal rights—Moral and ethical aspects.
    3. Animal experimentation—Moral and ethical
    aspects.   I. Title.
    HV4708.D58   1999
    179′.3—dc21   99-12349
                                       CIP

For further information on Blackwell Science, visit our
website: www.blackwell-science.com

Contents

Preface   xi

Part I   Ethics   1

1   Exploring the moral maze   3
    General introduction   3
    Towards a definition of ethics   5
    Ethical look-a-likes   7
    The evolution of morality   10
    Moral systems   13
    Morality and religion   14
    The truth value of ethical statements   15
    Science, truth and certainty   17
    Science and ethics   19
    The subjectivity of ethical statements   20
    Ethical subjectivism and objective standards   22
    Objectivism in ethics   23
    Descriptivism   25
    Universalization in ethics   25
    The language of ethics   26
    The term 'good'   27
    The term 'ought'   30
    An 'institution' in the ethical sense   31
    The term 'right'   32
    The inadequacy of ethics   32
    Some redeeming features of ethics   34

2   Ethical theories   39
    Introduction   39
    Absolutism   40
    Relativism   43
    The deontological and teleological approaches in ethics   44
    Consequentialism   47
    Utilitarianism   48
    Scepticism   53
    Immanuel Kant   53

Intuitionism   54
Conscience   55
Emotivism   56
Some modern moral philosophers   58
Naturalism (the naturalistic fallacy)   60
Pragmatism   61
Situation ethics   61

3 Seeking a norm of morality   **66**
Introduction   66
The law as a norm of morality   68

4 The nature of freedom   **70**
Introduction   70
Free will   70
Determinism   72
Existentialism (the farthest reaches of freedom)   78
Liberty   78
Freedom of speech   79
Liberty and the commons   80
Ethics and pollution   80
Population and the commons   81
Liberty and rights   82
Slavery   83

5 Personal morality   **88**
Introduction   88
Coercion   89
'If I don't do it, someone else will'   90
Doing good by stealth   92

6 Society and ethics   **94**
Introduction   94
The social contract   96
Society and mores   97
Cultural relativity   100
Education   102
Ethics and law   103
Law and morality   104
What about justice?   107
Politics and morality   108

Part II   Ethics and animals   **111**

7 Human attitudes to animals   **113**
Applied ethics   113
All animals are equal   114

Attitudes to animals   122
Religious and legal attitudes to animals   124
Philosophical attitudes to animals   125
Personal attitudes to animals   126
More on speciesism   127
Species élitism   129
The biological continuum   129
Anthropomorphism   130
A summary of human attitudes to animals   132

8   Animal rights   **134**
Introduction   134
The nature of rights   135
What rights could animals have?   138
Arguments pertinent to animal rights   140

9   Benefits to animals from human activity   **144**
Domestication   144
Veterinary medicine   146
Transport   146
Conservation   147
Dependency of animals in general   147
The dependency of animals in research   148
The responsibility for some animals   149

10   Animal awareness and pain   **151**
Introduction   151
Doubts about animal consciousness   152
Acceptance of animal consciousness   153
Animal thought   154
The universality of pain   155
Animal pain   155
Measuring pain   157
Hedonism in practice   161
Acceptability of pain   161
Concluding words on the subject of pain   162

Part III   Ethics, animals and science   **165**

11   The controversy   **167**
Introduction   167
The involved   169
The concerned   172
Activists   173
Practical consequences (security)   174

Disadvantages of using animals in research   176
Obligatory use of animals in research   179
Sentiment   180
Public relations   181
The art of manipulation   184

12   The use of alternatives – the three Rs   188
Introduction   188
Inadequacies of alternatives   189
The three Rs and the law   189
Marshall Hall's principles   191
The three Rs   191
Replacement   193
Validation   201
Reduction   202
Refinement   205
A multiplicity of Rs   206

13   Cost–benefit – the balancing act   211
Introduction   211
Justification   212
The cost in animal suffering   214
Benefits   214
Trying to strike the balance   217
Various approaches to solving cost–benefit evaluation   218
Ethical scores for animal experiments   220
The Dutch system   224
A British ethical approach   233
A selection of other approaches   237

14   Ethics committees   244
Introduction   244
The Swedish experience   245
The Canadian system   246
The making of an ethics committee   248
The disadvantages of ethics committees   249
The advantages of ethics committees   250
The ethical review process   251
Authoritative source material   253
The text of the revised Annex (1/4/98)   256
A working model – human research ethics committees (HRECs)   258
Some examples of emerging ERPs   260
A final note on the 1997 report   262

15   Always there is a matter of degree   264
Introduction   264

Degrees of acceptability of the use of animals   265
Killing animals   272
Does a culture make a difference?   273
What animals matter?   274
Grading right and wrong   276
Concluding comments   278

Bibliography   **280**

Index   **285**

Preface

The main motive for writing this book has been to provide an introduction to ethics for those who work with animals in a scientific setting. It is an attempt to find common premises for discussions on animal use in research which has often proved difficult in the past.

There seems little doubt that in centuries past, the majority of the population, including scientists, regarded the use of animals for advancement of medical knowledge as justified. On the other hand, committed antivivisectionists have persistently and unequivocally opposed animal experimentation from a long way back. For this reason most of the literature on this subject is in the form of what in the past were referred to as 'apologies'. These apologies made a case; they were written to support a cause and often to defend an entrenched position. That is what they were intended to do and many did it well. Naturally, they selected the appropriate evidence for their side of the argument.

My intention is not to defend experiments on animals, though the direction from which I am coming, with over a quarter of a century in cancer research, indicates where my sympathies lie. My aim is to present the various arguments germane to this controversy. Prolonged contact with the animals has given me an awareness of their needs and concern for their welfare. I hope that an even longer period of over four decades lecturing in philosophical subjects for both A-levels and degree courses has given me an ability to view any dialectic with a certain amount of impartiality. The only other relevant qualification I can claim is 70 years of wondering at what there is to know, how little we can know and how much we depend on others for what we do know. Experience has taught me that the confession of ignorance is the beginning of wisdom. For that reason I am not intent on persuading others to accept my opinions and I am certainly not concerned in censuring the opinions of others. My purpose is to comment on various approaches: not to judge them.

I am aware that this may please few and disturb many. I wish to offend no one and I respect all who are sincere in their opinions and who try to be reasonable in their arguments. My intent is to provoke thought on the main issues in the polemics on animal experimentation. I have no authority on the subject, either from study or experience, to produce answers. However, I feel confident in being able to indicate where some of the problems lie. There are those more capable than I who will attempt to solve them.

In the heat of disputes, fundamentals tend to be buried in verbiage. So much is said about what actions are right and what are wrong that we tend to lose sight of what we mean by right or wrong. That is where ethics comes in.

It was the interest in my lectures on ethics and the accompanying notes on the importance of clarifying what we mean by ethics and its relevancy to discussions on animal use that tempted me to publish this book. I shall try to clarify what we are talking about when the term 'ethics' is used but I readily admit the variability of the connotation of the term 'ethics' in practice in ordinary conversation.

The text is divided into three parts so that readers who wish to avoid the more speculative portion on ethics can pass readily to the topics of interest to them. In the first part, the nature and function of ethics is considered. Other methods of assessing right and wrong conduct, for example religious morality and law, are discussed.

In the second part, the variety of relationships between humans and animals is explored. In the third part, the role of animals in science is discussed, special attention being paid to the casuistry appropriate to the justification of animal experimentation and the requirement to develop alternatives to animals in research. This book is not intended to be a treatise on ethics as such, nor is it strictly scientific in content, but is meant to be a general overall view of ethics, animals and science.

References to sources and quotations are given at the end of the chapters. References to dates, if before the first millennium, have BCE following them. Those belonging to the last two millennia are not followed by any initials. Unfortunately, no doubt to the discomfort of some serious academics, flippancy may creep into the text. This tendency may give the impression of going from the sublime to the ridiculous but often the ludicrous strikes a chord at a depth which the sublime just cannot reach. The references at the end of each chapter are clear indications of how much I have depended on others. To all authors of the various sources from which I gleaned valuable material, I am most deeply grateful.

In my class work I used as text books the works of J.L. Mackie, Peter Singer, Bernard Williams and Mary Warnock. I quoted them so often that their writings entwined with my own thoughts to such an extent that it has not been easy to separate out what they wrote and what I said. *Lives in the Balance* by J.A. Smyth and K.M. Boyd proved to be a fertile source on cost–benefit assessment. Among the publications which proved most useful were *Animal Welfare* (UFAW), *New Scientist* and *Nature*. TV programmes provided an abundance of topical information.

I appreciated the assistance provided by various institutes. The Imperial Cancer Research Institute helped me in many ways in this enterprise. The newsletters and bulletins of the Laboratory Animal Science Association, the Research Defence Society and the Institute of Animal Technology were a great help. The vast amount of literature on the subject published by the Universities Federation for Animal Welfare was of tremendous value to me in my research. The opportunity to lecture frequently on this subject for both Bioscientific Events and the City of Westminster College made this work possible.

Finally, the number of individuals who have helped me in this venture were numerous. To name some who, along with students in various classes and delegates at many seminars, encouraged me: Tim Betts, Sean Tobin, Steve Barnet, Ron

Raymond, Jasmine Barley, Roger Francis and Frasier Darling. My stepson Steven and my nephew John fed me valuable relevant snippets of information. I was able to devote myself completely to the task in hand because distracting domestic chores were ably handled by Vicky.

Part I

Ethics

Chapter 1

Exploring the Moral Maze

'There was a door to which I found no key:
There was a veil past which I could not see.'

The Ruba'iyat of Omar Khayyám, edn. 1, xxxii

General introduction

To those who are not philosophically inclined, confusion appears to be the salient feature of the speculative subject of ethics – a confusion unfortunately not always readily clarified by experts in the field. I cannot myself guarantee to elucidate the more obscure stretches of this subject but I hope to indicate the direction in which they lie. Suggested answers to the Socratic question 'How should one live?', was, we might say, the trigger mechanism for the emergence of a rational approach to morality – a movement away from the ready acceptance of authority, either divine or human, as a guide to the acceptability or unacceptability of human actions.

The answers suggested by such luminaries as Socrates (470–399 BCE), Plato (428–347 BCE) his student, and Aristotle (384–322 BCE) did not satisfy everyone. On the contrary, even two centuries of heated discussion could not produce even a hint of general agreement on ethics among the philosophers. Terence (185–159 BCE), the Roman moralist, could rightly state: 'Quot homines tot sententiae: suo quoque mos' (As many men as there are opinions and each has his own morals) (Terence c. 166).

The situation never changed. Ethics, if we may use a homely expression on such a serious and erudite topic, has ever lacked the healthy clout of the proffered morality of religious teachers or the attractive security of fundamentalism with its simple dispersion of any doubt. Over two millennia have passed without ethical speculation producing absolute answers. In ethics, speculation is the name of the game. Problems are the currency of ethics. They are revelled in as pregnant sources of proposed solutions. Down the centuries, however, the suggested philosophical answers have varied and reappeared in different guises. No one moral philosopher or school of philosophy has proved capable of attracting anything like universal acceptance of their theories. Credibility gaps have been endemic throughout the history of moral philosophy. The concern of the philosopher has often been not so much to seek to know the answer but rather to to try to understand the question.

In our own times, the difficulties within ethics have been exacerbated by the frequent occurrence of the term in strange contexts:

'I have always cared about ethics. When we started the Playboy Club in 1960, I was the guy who insisted on a Bunny Mother because I didn't want bunnies having to report simply to male management.'

(Hefner 1994)

Here, ethical concern may have been more aptly applied to the implied exploitation of women rather than to the minutiae of the delicacies to be maintained within the entertainment industry.

I came across the term 'an ethical thief' (Dalrymple 1994) used by a resident of one of Her Majesty's prisons in describing his own moral status. He never harmed anyone, unless they got in his way. He merely entered houses and took things. He did not accept the concept of private property except in respect to himself. He aspired to the ethical ideals of distributive justice attributed in legend to Robin Hood. Unfortunately, he claimed, he was called upon to assist the local constabulary in their enquiries before he had time to initiate the distributive feature supposedly associated with his enterprises.

On the various parts of the media, such as TV and radio, the term 'ethics' frequently occurs with varying degrees of clarity and correctness. In one such television discussion exploring the ethical problem associated with the suggestion, based on the detection of stress hormones that suggests fetuses could feel pain, one proponent made the statement: 'This is not about religion, morality or ethics'. One was left wondering if there may be some other form of judgemental technique transcending these three categories for assessing the righteousness of conduct.

In another television debate, a cleric, talking about his Christian colleagues, spoke of their moral ethics which he respected but did not share (BBC 1994a). Does this imply the existence of immoral ethics? There had been, on a previous programme (BBC 1994b), mention of the ethics of a parliamentary question. Is this the direction in which immoral ethics lie? Or is this merely a classical example of a contradiction in terms?

Perhaps the most contorted use of this much-abused term 'ethics' occurred in the expression 'ethical eggs', laid no doubt, by moral hens (BBC 1995). In fact, the word was being used as synonymous with 'free range'. Was this an intended innuendo that animal welfare and ethics are one and the same thing? Animal welfare is most desirable and, to my mind, a moral obligation upon anyone owning or in charge of animals; but it is not ethics. It is the proper result of an ethical approach to animal care.

All that I have so far written has presented nothing positive about ethics. It was not intended to. It was meant as a warning against being misled by spurious notions of what ethics is about and against being seduced by any assumption that ethics is capable of solving with ease the moral problems of the day. It is an attempt to draw attention to the lack of precision surrounding this now ubiquitous in-word. The word 'ethics' is in ordinary parlance by no means univocal but has varying connotations in differing circumstances.

Towards a definition of ethics

A good general definition of ethics is: 'The philosophical study of the moral value of human conduct and the rules and principles that ought to govern it.' In sound-bite mode, ethics could be described as the science of conduct, a phrase used by Henry Sidgwick (1838–1900) in his *Methods of Ethics*. In practical situations, ethics may be viewed as a code of behaviour considered correct, especially such codes as are associated with a group or profession.

A well-drafted and comprehensive definition of ethics is given in the *Fontana Dictionary of Modern Thought* (Fontana 1977):

> 'The branch of philosophy that investigates morality and, in particular, varieties of thinking by which human conduct is guided and may be appraised. It is concerned with the meaning and justification of utterances about the rightness and wrongness of actions, the virtue and vices of the motives that prompt them, the praiseworthiness or blameworthiness of the agents who perform them, and the goodness or badness of the consequences to which they give rise.'
>
> (Fontana 1977)

A crucial word in this definition is 'investigates'. This clearly indicates the subtle distinction between morality and ethics. This difference is not always apparent in usage. Often the terms 'ethics', and 'morals' or 'morality' (these two words have a similar connotation), are used indiscriminately. There is perhaps a popular notion that ethics is morality with a college education. As the definition implies, morality is concerned with what is right and what is wrong conduct whereas ethics is really concerned with why certain conduct is considered to be right or wrong.

Much of morality in the past had little to do with philosophy. It was based on authority, usually of a religious nature, the most primitive form appearing as taboos with a hint of the preternatural and carrying dire sanctions. Later, more sophisticated moral codes claiming divine authority backed by the *vox Dei* (the voice of God) appeared. Even in early civilizations, such as that of Sparta, there is evidence of morality being imposed by a dominant class on the basis of 'might is right'. Even the gentle, practical and almost mundane morals of Confucianism drew much of its force from authority – 'Confucius, he says'. Sustained authority of this type could develop a codified legal morality such as that attributed to Hammurabi (*c.* 1690 BCE) in Babylon. Plato, and much later Rousseau (1712–1778), suggested the feasibility of the development of morality within communities – a *vox populi* process (by public opinion) – that is to say, a morality by consensus, perhaps even a poll-produced morality.

In historical times, the first real evidence of a development of moral awareness based on dialectics (the question-and-answer mode of investigation associated with Socrates) was among the early Greek philosophers. From this rational approach to righteousness and justice, ethics, as we know it, emerged.

From the above definition of ethics, it follows that ethics is an exploration of theories about right and wrong. Morality tends to be prescriptive about what is right and wrong. Ethics elucidates the thinking about what is morally acceptable. It is essentially theoretical and is neither intended nor equipped to provide direct guidance on the correct niceties of specific acts. This is not to say that in the rough-and-tumble of debate the terms 'ethics' and 'ethical' are not used as synonymous with morals, morality or right conduct. Often, in polemics, protagonists will instil into their ethical statements all the dogmatism of a preacher and apply their ethical ideas to any detail of daily life. In academia, however, ethics is much more reticent and deals more with questions than answers. Even a basic term associated with ethics such as 'good' is treated with caution and seems to defy definition. It is tentatively posited by some that it may merely indicate 'morally desirable'. It might rightly be asked: 'By whom?'. 'Conduct', around which controversy rages, is far from being a precise term. It refers to a whole range of human activities, from words to blows; from a personal remark to the detonation of bombs by terrorists or freedom-fighters. The term selected to describe the perpetrators will be in keeping with the ethical attitude of the speaker to the reason for the remark or for the explosion.

Ethics examines the acceptability of motives. It is concerned with the reason for carrying out an action rather than merely with the performance of the act. Guilt – the awareness of wrong behaviour in the past – comes within the scope of ethics. Finally, it assesses the desirability of consequences and goes beyond present events to evaluate future results. The application of ethics can take the form of ethical justification which appraises consequences and applies ethical opinions to actual moral problems. However, once this pursuit of ethical justification moves into specifics, for example in the appraisal of proposed animal experiments, it becomes involved with casuistry.

The art of casuistry is the practice of attempting to present valid moral statements about particular situations which have a moral dimension. Such decisions are based on authoritative conclusions in previous similar cases. In law, the decisive authority is usually named and will be of a defined rank in the judicial hierarchy. In ethics, no such agreed authorities exist but reliance may be put on accepted moral principles or a known acceptable consensus.

The term 'ethic', which is occasionally encountered, is often used to convey the concept of a specific ethical stance or attitude. Sociologists talk of the 'Protestant work ethic'. A like-sounding word, 'ethos', applies to the pervading moral outlook or the ideals of a group, institution or establishment.

There are various levels of ethical speculation. An ethical statement may assert that some particular action is right or wrong; or that actions of certain kinds are right or wrong. It may offer a distinction between good and bad characters or dispositions; or it may propound some broad principle from which many more detailed judgements of this type might be inferred, for example that we ought always to aim at the greatest general happiness, or try to minimize the total suffering of all sentient beings, or devote ourselves to relieving poverty, or mind our own business and get on with our own lives. These propositions each express first-order ethical judgements of different degrees of generality.

By contrast with such statements, an ethical statement of the second order would be an attempt to describe what is involved in formulating the first-order statement;

that is, whether the first-order statement expresses a discovery or a decision. A second-order statement may indicate how we think about ethical matters or attempt to define ethical terms. Second-order statements deal with the thinking process behind a first-order statement. First-order statements are the expressions used by most people when they are talking about ethics in general. Second-order statements are the domain of the moral philosophers when they probe behind general ethical statements of the first order. Second-order statements are the result of this probing analysis of terms such as 'right', 'wrong' and 'good'.

The words 'moral philosophy' are applied to ethics within philosophy in order to distinguish it from other forms of philosophy. Philosophy *per se* is concerned with reality in general and various aspects of reality. It deals with the causes of all things and so speculates on material in both the physical and the metaphysical sphere. It is concerned with both empirical and transcendental knowledge, readily discussing both *a priori* or *a posteriori* data (that is, information of which we are aware by deduction as in mathematics, or objective information gained by experience). Philosophy, we may say, is thinking about thoughts.

Ethical look-a-likes

Moral theology

Moral theology, unlike moral philosophy, deals more with answers than questions and depends, by its very nature and definition, on revelation – coming from God, rather than on rational speculation. The dicta of moral theology will vary according to the religion of the theologian or even the school of thought to which the theologian belongs.

A particular moral theology may provide the believer with an acceptable code of conduct. In some expressions of religious teaching these dictates were backed by horrific sanctions in the afterlife. It is difficult to find in Christian moral theology any clear direct association of sin (this is the most prevalent term used traditionally for nearly two millennia in the moral context) with normal human–animal relationships. The term 'normal' has been used here with intent. One expression of the normal relationship has been the eating of meat, less restricted in Christian than in Old Testament regulations. Although the eating of meat obviously involved the killing, not always humanely, of animals, no censure of such activity is evident. In fact the very word 'carnival' implied a delight and rejoicing in carnivorous pursuits. It must be granted that 'carnival' implied the 'goodbye to meat' for the period of Lent. The abstinence from flesh, but not fish, was intended, however, for the good of the soul of the consumer, not for the integrity of the body of the animal. Anathemas only appear in this area when some effect damaging to humans, such as an increased propensity to cruelty to other humans, may result or if there is some extra factor unacceptable to the pious sensitivity of the moralist. The Puritans condemned bear-baiting, not because it diminished ursine happiness, but because it gave pleasure to the onlookers.

In recent times, due to the heightened popular interest in the use and abuse of animals, theological speculation has appeared which tends to run counter to the accepted Christian attitude down the ages. As a theologian having lectured in church history and patrology, I do not consider that statement unfair in the light of traditional theology.

The leading exponent of a more modern approach in theological thinking is Professor Linzey (Linzey 1994). His theological thinking may seem to be slightly at variance with ecclesiastical attitudes in the past which had remained unquestioned since apostolic times and throughout the high centuries of scholasticism. Linzey argues valiantly and makes a good case for a new theology on animal–human relations. He may recall, however, the good advice from high authority, not to try to put new wine into old bottles. Of course, I do not think anyone could argue with a theologian presenting the notion of a theocentric view of creation. That notion does occur in church history. His innovation is the introduction of theos-rights for animals expressed in practice by the 'Generosity Paradigm'. This approach seems to imply a form of sacrificial morality – not to be confused with animal sacrifice – a practice that loomed large in biblical customs in both Testaments. The parts of this sacrificial morality can be broken down into topics such as: reverence, responsibility and rights, the moral priority of the weak, humans as the servant species, liberation theology for animals and animal rights.

No doubt these are lines along which we can progress to greater consideration for animals and therefore the better provision of welfare for them. It is difficult, however, to find strong roots for this approach in basic theology. It is reminiscent of the guide's advice to the bewildered traveller: 'Well if that is where you want to go I would not start from here.' Linzey expresses his high moral stance in the phrase: 'Hunting constitutes nothing less than an offence to God.' A little out of tune with 'Hence came a proverb: even as Nimrod the stout hunter before the Lord' (Genesis 10:9).

It may be noted in passing that Dr Habgood, Archbishop of York, the best scientifically qualified English Primate since the renaissance, suggested at a scientific conference at Loughborough (summer 1994) that apes and other primates could have souls. That sounds more dubious theologically than it does scientifically.

Morality

In the past, moral theology had been the mainspring of accepted morality. Morality consisted in laid-down sets of principles of right conduct. It indicated how one should behave. Ethics was insulated from influencing behaviour in the real world, isolated in the realms of philosphy, concerned with theoretical discussions on morality. Ethics only began to influence opinion and enter general parlance on morality as the authority of religion began to wane. Moral philosophy, like all philosophy, had been seen by the Church or Churches, that set the standards of morality, merely as, at best *ancilla theologiae* (the handmaid of theology). Theology itself was the *ars artis* (the art of arts).

Some purely ethical theories do stand out as having some effect on popular morality, for example Stoicism, Epicurianism and Utilitarianism. Machiavelli's consequentialism no doubt influenced political morality in practice. The immediate attempt to suppress it, at least in theory, illustrated the diverse approach of moral theology and philosophy to underlying principles of morality. No doubt new ecological movements and nature groups are having a marked effect on popular notions of right and wrong in respect to the environment and animal rights. There may be some who think Thatcherism changed moral attitudes within our culture, creating a new more selfish morality. This is mentioned merely to illustrate the extent to which accepted morality is now exposed to a multiplicity of influences divergent from the more monolithic religious morality of the past.

In fairness, it should be stated that 'greed' and 'self' are old words known to moralists throughout the ages. Indeed, the moral ideal 'Love your neighbour as yourself' implies the standard of that love derives from love of self. Moral maxims are, in a loose sense, prescriptive sound bites. They sum up the various concepts associated with the prevailing morality: 'Thou shalt not kill'; or 'Honesty is the best policy'; or 'It is wrong to tell a lie'. The sum total of such maxims form the 'mores' (simply the Latin for morals) or the ethical mind-set of a group, community or even a nation. It is a function of ethics to rationally assess such mores.

Mores are the popular attitudes on acceptable and unacceptable conduct within a community. They are endemic in the ambient culture in which they are expressed. This does not necessarily mean that they are observed or even accepted by everyone within the group but they are regarded as a standard of behaviour by the majority. An example of the operation of differing mores was the reaction of the public in the different nations of Europe during the controversy on animal transport in 1995. Spectacular demonstrations occurred in this country, while in countries to which the calves were exported, no such disturbances were reported. Often, national legislation, such as our own, will reflect such mores.

We might consider that this apparent, or at least supposed, sensitivity to animal suffering, or suffering in general, is a national trait of which we may be truly proud. Mores, however, not only vary from place to place but also vary from time to time. In this country, seemingly concerned about cruelty, there was a time, not too long ago, when the puritanical Victorians could have cynically parodied the saying of St Ignatius of Loyola: 'Give me a lad of eight and I will give you the man' into 'Give me a lad of eight and I will have your chimney swept in half an hour'.

Sometimes mores, seemingly openly espoused by the public at large, are not always aligned with practice. There will be those within a community who merely pay lip-service to the current trends. The ideals of the mores may be blatantly contradicted by actions. Samuel Johnson cynically pointed out that the louder the Americans talked of freedom, the harder they beat their slaves.

One modern moral philosopher, John Rawls (Rawls 1971), introduced into his exposition of ethics the notion of a 'theory of justice'. In this form of speculation we may perceive a closeness between ethics and morality. There is an attempt to describe systematically our own moral consciousness or some part of it, such as our 'sense of justice', and to find some acts or principles which are fairly acceptable and with which, along with their practical consequences and applications, our intuitive (but really subjective) detailed moral judgements would be in 'reflective equilibrium'. That is, we might start with some *prima facie* acceptable general principles, together with the mass of *prima facie* acceptable detailed moral judgements, and where they do not fully agree adjust either or both until the most satisfactory coherent compromise is reached. This is a legitimate line of speculation; however, it must not be confused with the superficially similar, but in purpose fundamentally different, attempt of thinkers like Sidgwick to advance by way of various intuitions to an objective moral truth, to a science of conduct.

This is just one example of the speculations of modern moral philosophers on morality. There are many widely differing theories. G.J. Warnock, for example, is more concerned with the purpose of morality, than its object. For him morality is a species of evaluation, a kind of appraisal of human conduct. Some regard morality as a particular sort of constraint on conduct. A constraint which was needed for the flourishing of human life – shades of the social contract of Hobbes.

There is a distinction between the activity of a moralist who sets out to elaborate a moral code or encourage its observance, and that of a moral philosopher whose concern is not primarily to make moral judgements but to analyse their nature.

The evolution of morality

History bears ample testimony to changing moral opinions. Plato's defence of infanticide within an established society is hardly acceptable today. In the future, as in the past, changing conditions may call for new ethical approaches. The flexibility of morality has been essential because of contingent features of the human condition. From their contingent nature these features have changed and continue to change. The contrast between Protagoras (*c.* 490–420 BCE) and Hobbes (1588–1679) points to a change through time in the scale of a problem. Protagoras was looking for the ordering principles of a city, or *polis*. In ancient Greece a *polis* could be quite small, as low as a few thousand in population. His concern was how men could form social units large enough to compete with the wild beasts. For Hobbes the problem was how to maintain a stable nation state. Nowadays we can no longer share Hobbes' assumption that only civil wars were a menace and that international wars, in those days, only involving professional armies, were of little consequence.

Changes in the human situation which may well be relevant to morality have occurred in the last 100 years. The rapid development of worldwide mutual dependence has affected relationships between nations. The universal availability of instant information has, for example, altered attitudes to world poverty in the form of quicker responses to famine in distant places. Medical advances have increased the opportunity of doctors to do apparent good.

Developments in the means of communication have given some people increased powers over the minds of others. In the not too distant future there will be possibilities of genetic engineering applied to the human race.

New powers raise moral questions about their exercise. If we can keep people hardly alive at immense cost, the question whether we should do so is not irrelevant to the economic welfare of the whole community. With the progress of genetics, the relative claims of the present and the future generations are no longer purely academic. Present-day activities not only directly affect the environment of the future but also the prospects of future generations. The control of the numbers of inhabitants of particular countries, and eventually of the world as a whole, is becoming a conceivable political objective.

These increased powers are not at the disposal of mankind. Mankind is not an agent; it has no unity of decision. The powers will be exercised by individuals, probably within a political context, but need to be decided within some moral framework, perhaps as yet unformed.

Morality may need to be remade in part. Hobbes pointed out that it is a law of nature that men should perform their covenants. He presented this proposition with justification as an immutable fragment of morality. Some less general obligations not created by contract may be regarded by some as dispensable. There are those who suggest that, for example, patriotism may have outlived its usefulness and moral worth.

The appearance of new problems in morals needs little proof but a reflection on the varied expression of morality down the ages may be instructive. In the past, most moral codes stemmed from religion depending on revelation for their authority. There were, of course, other more earthy sources of morality; a prime example is the taboo.

The taboo

In primitive societies conduct was ruled not by the abstract principles of ethics but by taboo. This phenomenon did often have a quasi-preternatural character and was frequently associated with worship. It consisted of a complex collection of detailed and seemingly arbitrary prohibitions affecting every facet of daily life. These rules were usually sanctioned by the most horrific penalties, or dire consequences were supposed to inevitably follow the flouting of a taboo. There are still vestiges of this type of behaviour in the stringent dietary laws of some religions (Freud 1913). The consciousness of guilt, the questioning of one's own status, is linked to the lingering of the taboo. Taboos may have dissolved into a pervading religion since their awareness of evil was associated with worship.

The shadow of the taboo may not have disappeared from the psyche of modern man. There is a hint of operation of taboo in the emphasis on political correctness. It has been suggested that communities without taboos may lose cohesion. Without some taboos there is a closing of the distance between desire and action; this idea could be expressed as 'culture is repression'. Etiquette, the oil of social intercourse, is a faint echo of the taboo. There are still adults who will meticulously perform rituals demanded by popular superstitions. Taboos, however, were not merely superstitions; some had a rationale directly associated with danger to life or to the community, based on, perhaps misunderstood, past tribal experiences. The taboo had a survival value.

The influence of the Greeks

It was Socrates and Plato (*c.* 400 BCE) who first sought to define such notions as honesty, justice, and morality as objective concepts. They assessed these notions, not in reference to any divine revelation, but in respect to the nature of man. For the early Greeks, the pioneers of intellectual exploration, 'man was the measure of all things' (Protagoras). Plato claimed that we cannot know if a man is just until we know exactly what we mean by justice. *The Republic*, his seminal work on ethics, was a lengthy attempt to define 'justice' in order to provide a rational basis for good behaviour. Plato's adversaries were the Sophists, such as Thrasymarchus who taught pure relativism in morals. For him 'justice' was merely the interest of the strongest – whoever conquers makes his interest prevail and declares it to be right. According to Thucydides, the Greeks argued thus:

> 'In the discussion of human affairs, the question of justice only enters where there is equal power to enforce it. The powerful exact what they can and the weak grant what they must.'

To the fervent appeals for justice from the conquered men of the island of Melos, the victorious Athenians cynically replied, while slaying them all: 'If you were as strong as we are, you would do as we do.' That was a long time ago but this text was written on 14 July 1995 – remember Srebrnica.

In reponse to such blatant callousness Plato proposed a much more acceptable morality. Plato's 'just' man expressed his justice by his harmonious nature arising from the practice of justice, prudence, temperance and fortitude. In a take-over bid by Christianity, these four qualities became the cardinal virtues.

Plato's most illustrious pupil, Aristotle (384–322 BCE), was the author of the first works on ethics. In his *Ethics* he presented the subject in a more systematic and practical style than his predecessors. Aristotle assessed the moral worth of an action in relation to its capability to produce true happiness – a variable concept.

Other schools of thought followed in the wake of the great philosophers. The Epicureans, the first of a long line of hedonists, presented the norm of morality as pleasure. Epicurus, himself, lived a sober life and in no way advocated the pursuit of debauchery. The Stoics and the early Christian Fathers produced a much more demanding type of morality – the pursuit of virtue for virtue's sake. They were the harbingers of the cult of the stiff upper lip. Their views developed later into the grim goodness of the Puritan.

Development of morality from the Greeks to modern times

With the dominance of religion as the guide to life, both here and hereafter, ethics as a basis for good conduct became redundant. In the Christian era, philosophy came under the auspices of theology. Augustine sanitized Plato in the *City of God* and Aquinas sanctified Aristotle in his *Contra Gentiles*. Among the few independent thinkers on ethics during the Middle Ages were Moses Maimonides and Peter

Abelard. To the fury of the Scholastics, Abelard speculated on the relativity of morality.

The Renaissance gave room for speculation in every field, even regarding morality. Machiavelli defied ecclesiastical authority with his consequential ethics. The strict commitment to virtue reinforced by an autocratic religious authority was ill-suited to the freedom-loving neo-pagan man of the flourishing commercial cities of Italy. The moral philosophy expounded in *Il Principe* was consequentialism for real. 'The end justifies the means' brought the morality of the palazzo into the piazza.

Inhibitions were removed from the ambitions of the powerful. This more accommodating morality was more lax than the modest latitude developed by traditional moralists in the form of the doctrine of the 'double effect' – the acceptability of permitting but not intending an evil result to occur from one's action alongside the primary intended good effect. This latter concept is not to be confused with a choice between two evils which will be discussed in full later in connection with the use of animals in research. Examples will then be given.

After Machiavelli (1469–1527), moral philosophers tended to concentrate more on expounding ethical theories rather than pontificating on morality. The views of these later philosophers will be duly considered. One modern philosopher merits mention: Nietzsche (1844–1900). He reinstated power as a deciding factor in morality – a might is right approach, the natural morality of the jungle. He expressed his contempt for conventional standards: 'Morality in Europe today is herd morality' (see his work *Beyond Good and Evil*). The maxim of Protagoras (490–420 BCE), 'Man is the measure of all things' had shaken the orthodoxy of his day. Nietzsche went further with his proclamation: 'I teach you the superman, man is something to be surpassed' (Nietzsche 1885). Unacceptable though his opinions might be, his frank approach reflected an intellectual sincerity not overabundant among the cant and half-truths which can occur in ethical polemics. His stark aphorism is worth recalling: 'There are few who have the courage to think what they know.'

Moral systems

It is important to distinguish between a moral system and an ethical theory. A moral system is a set of moral maxims of varying generality. An ethical theory is a theory about morals and about a moral system or systems. It consists of reasoned answers to such questions as: 'Is there a single set of moral maxims or are there several possible moral systems?'; or, 'Is it possible to evaluate rationally and choose from among them?'.

A moral system should have at least three properties:

(1) No part of the morals within a moral system may be incompatible with any other part; that is, the morals should be consistent with each other.
(2) The set should be comprehensive; it should be a system that contains maxims covering every moral situation, for example nuclear warfare or environmental protection, and should provide a way of generating whatever morals might be needed in future circumstances.

(3)   The set should be integrated; every part of the system should be related to every other part, either directly or indirectly. Unless a set of morals is integrated, we will be unable to determine if the set is internally compatible.

One way of proceeding to construct a moral system is to maximize the use of generality. If we hypothesize that there is a set of morals of the lowest generality, say level one, then they might be grouped under another set of higher generality, say level two, and so forth, until finally there is a single maxim of the highest generality under which they all are grouped. They would be integrated because each would be indirectly related to every other because each is grouped finally under one and the same highest generality maxim. Moral philosophers have tried to construct moral systems with this technique. The classical example is the efforts of the Utilitarians. Utilitarianism proposes a single highest-level maxim – 'we ought to do that which will produce the greatest good for the greatest number'.

Morality and religion

In historic times, codes of conduct appeared, for example the Hammurabi Code in Babylon (*c.* 1690 BCE). Force was given to these laws by presenting them with the backing of divine authority, as in the case of the Decalogue. Other systems of morality, with religious associations, developed from the teachings of Zoroaster (Zarathustra) and Buddha. An acceptable system of social morals was derived from the sayings of K'ung-Fu-tzu (Confucius).

Prior to the blossoming of philosophy in the Eastern Mediterranean, morality was religiously based and continued for most people to be so based throughout history. At least subconsciously, religion still forms moral attitudes. To say an act is unchristian is often considered synonymous with saying it is morally reprehensible. Morality is not the same as religion, nor is religion simply morality. They are, however, so closely related that Dostoyevsky could proclaim with some amount of assent that 'If God is dead, everything is permitted' (Dostoyevsky 1880).

The decrease of the influence of religion on popular morality has been noted. The confident dogmatism and fiery sermon of former days has given way to the mild platitudes of the radio programme *Thought for the Day* and the liberal opinions of progressive clerics. Eternity does not seem to have the future it once appeared to have. Nietzsche's dire comment about churches, 'What are these buildings but the tombs and graves of God' has become more apt as time has passed. The united face of a certain and stable religious morality has become eroded due to the diverse responses of ecclesiastical authorities to moral questions in regard, for example, to marriage or birth control. Lack of agreement is even more obvious with regard to more modern issues such as nuclear warfare and genetic engineering. Past accepted attitudes to highly charged situations with problematic moral dimensions have begun to be called into question. The ethical features of the temptation of Eve, or Abraham's aborted attempt at human sacrifice, appear now to be a little tricky from a human point of view.

Unfortunately, religion, together with morality, does not always produce a moral person. Religious groups can on occasions display a wickedness that is more often associated with political or military groups. In life, kindliness and goodness, and their opposites, are the qualities of individuals. Group membership can blunt ethical perception and fetter moral imagination. The members of a group which supplies a comprehensive dogmatic code can easily become uncritical and let others do their thinking for them.

A function of the group ethic is to maintain the group. Thus, in the past, in meeting real tests of human concern, such as slavery and political oppression, religious bodies differed little in their attitudes from secular counterparts. They displayed hardly any more priority of perceptiveness. This is, of course, apart from some prophetic figures such as John Brown (1800–1859) and Bonhoeffer (1906–1945). The moral reformer often appeared as much an outcast from his own religious group as being presumed to be at variance with the heathen. Goodness may be even more a quality of the upright agnostic as of those who are unduly complacent in their conviction of automatic Godliness through membership of the chosen élite.

The Good Pagan's Failure (Ward *c.* 1940) by Barbara Ward argued strongly against the possibility of any divorce between proper morality and religion. She argued that any morality without religion would lack intrinsic validity and would be doomed to fail. Any residual morality within modern culture she regarded as still drawing its strength from a lingering religious force. In his book *Mere Christianity*, C.S. Lewis (Lewis 1963) also argues against the feasibility of an effective and comprehensive morality outside a religion setting.

Rudyard Kipling managed to present high moral ideals which were not overtly religious in his poem *If* and expounded on a common-sense approach to conduct in *The God of the Copybook Headings*.

The truth value of ethical statements

Ethical language is not scientific and moral views, being often intuitive, do tend to vary greatly. Feelings of guilt rather than awareness of truth reflect reactions to moral dicta. The consequences of empirical statements, for example 'alcoholism does the liver no good whatsoever' not only can be demonstrated empirically but is accepted as inevitable. On the other hand, an ethical statement such as 'temperance is good' is difficult to prove in every instance and seems a step removed from the material world. Consequently, modern philosophers such as A.J. Ayers (1910–1989) regarded ethical statements as expressions of the speaker's emotions.

According to the verification principle current in modern philosophy, ethical statements cannot be verified by empirical means. Contents of emotions are regarded as falling entirely outside the category of truth. The practical impact of this attitude is that looking for absolute, universally acceptable answers in this area is akin to looking for shadows in the dark. Even if they were present, it would be impossible to demonstrate their existence.

Verification

The positive aspect of the need for testability to establish the truth value of a statement was stressed by the Logical Positivists (The Vienna Circle). Alfred J. Ayer puts it this way: 'A sentence is only significant – conveying new and certain knowledge – if its position, can by observation, be accepted as true or rejected as false' (Ayer 1936). This is not to deny other statements any value, particularly as value judgements.

Statements lacking significance, in Ayer's sense, may be:

(1) analytical, in which the subject contains the predicate and so they are tauto-logical and give us no new knowledge; for example, 'bachelors are unmarried men';
(2) not literally meaningful but may be emotionally significant. Ethical propositions are consigned to this genre as value judgements.

Falsification

The falsification theory is the extreme and negative aspect of the proposition that some statements such as 'value judgements' are untestable. Anthony Flew describes the falsification principle in this way:

> 'A statement can only be held to be factually significant if we can specify some possible state or event which would, if it occurred, falsify it.'

Karl Popper (1902–1994), the Philosopher of Science, stressed the importance of the falsification principle to honesty and integrity in science. He defied researchers to test their findings to the full by positing the 'risky prediction' which, if it were not fulfilled, would undermine the credibility of the hypothesis. Popper stressed that scientific theories only have significance until the time when, if it comes, they are disproved. They must always be testable. On the other hand, he regarded value judgements as untestable, not only unverifiable but even unfalsifiable and conse-quently lacking the possibility of objective proof (Popper 1959, 1972).

A venture into epistemology

A salient feature of epistemology, the study of truth and certainty, since the time of the first sceptics such as Pyrrho of Elis (*c.* 270 BCE), has been concern about finding an absolute basis for the validity of our knowledge of reality. Truth and certainty are the essential elements of this validity. They are by no means the same thing. If you think they are, you have never had to console a ne'er-do-well who has lost his shirt on a 'dead cert' in the 2.30 at Aintree. Truth, as opposed to certainty, became starkly apparent as the horse fell at the second jump.

Truth we may describe as the conformity of our ideas or concepts with reality. Certainty is simply the complete lack of doubt. Being so sure, as in the previous, perhaps flippant example, to be ready to hazard the currency on the certainty that our concept truly reflects reality. Doubt can be distressing, but sometimes, certainty can be ludricous.

The only statement Descartes (1596–1650) could be certain of was 'Cogito ergo sum' (I think therefore I am). To his mind this was the only fact he could not doubt. Kant (1724–1804) having, as he said, been awakened from his philosophical slumbers by the ultimate scepticism of Hume (1711–1776), attempted to find a rational basis for certainty. Kant finally abandoned his search to know the *ding an sich* (the thing in itself). He settled for a merely phenomenal knowledge of reality. The numenon (reality itself) was beyond our ken. For the human intellect 'perception is reality' because what we perceive is all we can really know, and then only in and through the Kantian categories of our thought processes.

Cardinal Newman (1801–1890) was not overenamoured with logic. This attitude was reflected in his comment: 'I recollect an acquaintance saying to me that "the Oriel Common Room stank of Logic"' (*History of my Religious Opinions*). Perceiving that the proof of logical principles involves a *petitio principii* (a vicious circle), Newman posited an illative sense. This he saw as a sort of instinctive perception, an unconscious process of reasoning, acting as an arbiter of the truth value of statements in areas like ethics.

Science, truth and certainty

Hume pointed out the tendency of philosophers to break up reality into separate compartments, to divorce their subject from the intricacies and complexities of real life. The same may be true of scientists. The paediatrician who in his clinic sees illnesses as defects in a biological organism could not so view his own sick child. The billiard-playing microphysicist forswears in this activity the principle of indeterminacy. The erotically infatuated neuro-endocrinologist experiences the same vivid emotional changes as the rest of us, unaffected by his greater understanding of their biochemical underpinning. Few experimental physiologists see their own pets as animal models. Behaviourists cannot avoid mentalistic attributions in their daily dealing with friends and family, although such presumptions are against their puristic scientific feelings. The ultimate in compartmentalization can happen in science, for example in medicine – 'the kidney in room 306'. The archetypal behaviourist, Watson, at his most extreme, in his desire to deny objective reality to anything that could not be experimentally measured, claimed: 'We don't have thoughts, we only think we have.'

The supremacy of the proper controlled and recorded experiment as the sole foundation of truth may not be so apparent in the world of real life. No controlled experiment will provide me with better evidence that one of my friends is trustworthy or that people will cut corners to make money, than does my ordinary experience. Laboratory experiments on animal behaviour tend to focus on abnormal animals under abnormal conditions. Though the laboratory rat and cat are among the most highly studied subjects in psychological research, much of the data pertains to their behaviour under the most unlikely conditions, far removed from their home sewer or their fireside mat. Laboratory examination is, by definition, extraordinary and thus likely to be misleading.

Study of normal behaviour implies a natural environment, without human interference or manipulation. Such type of study, by its very nature, is uncontrolled and consequently usually anecdotal (the really dirty word in science). Some of the pioneering work of Lorenz and Tinbergen has been thus derided by ethologists and psychologists (real scientists) for being anecdotal – mere natural history. Darwin's pursuits on the Galapagos Islands were not quite controlled textbook experiments. They did, however, give rise to a dominant theory in biology, hardly proved under laboratory conditions. Scientists rightly claim that controlled conditions are needed for replicability, the shibboleth of scientific certainty. Is it not possible that data of a similar nature from diverse unconnected sources scattered over space and time could be a form of replication? Can truth only be found on the laboratory bench? If science insisted on data obtained under laboratory conditions, Newton could not have explained the movement of the tides and astronomy would not be a science.

These comments are not intended, in any way, to denigrate the most praiseworthy efforts, or truth value, of the results of scientific research. No facile philosophical speculation can detract from the tremendous tangible benefits which have been produced from science. This is merely an attempt to indicate that science may not be so much in possession of the epistemological high ground as is sometimes assumed. Biology, physiology, anatomy, etc. deal with external objects which are the furniture of a material world. The ultimate basis of that claim cannot, however, be an empirical one. Empirically, any data gathered could equally be compatible with solipsistic phenomenalism. Solipsism is the theory that nothing really exists but I and my mental states. A hint of the haunting whimper of the maniac: 'Is there anyone out there?' Had not Descartes, however, claimed that the only certainty he had, was of his own thoughts? To escape such an outrageous alternative, science makes some common sense and practical assumptions. It must be stressed, however, that they are assumptions. It is assumed that other subjects exist whose access to these outside objects is more or less the same and who, as observers, see, for example, the same colour which each separately perceives and calls, for instance, red, although they have no empirical way of checking that their experience of this external stimulation is identical. It is assumed that these other subjects can understand meanings, correctly manipulate symbols to convey information and can be trusted not to cheat. Science needs to assume that there is a past about which we can make judgements despite our inability, by definition, to experience it. Bertrand Russell, no ardent believer, pointed out that we have no scientific way of knowing that God did not create the whole universe *in toto* a few seconds ago, complete with fossils and us with all our memories.

It has become increasingly clear since Kant that there is no good reason for believing that facts can be gathered or even observations made independently of a theoretical base or even given significance without a linguistic matrix. Kant had pointed out that sensory information must be 'boxed' before it becomes an object of experience. Even the notions of 'object' and 'event' are brought to sensation rather than emerging from it. We, ourselves, decide the focus of our attention. We can edit our awareness and that can mean editing out most of the sensations which bombard us. I can go most of my life, for example, unaware that I have socks on until this moment when I consciously avert to the sensation on the surface of my feet.

Theory has a major role in perception. To see a fracture or a lesion on a radiograph requires theoretical equipment – to know what you are looking for – and a good deal of training. Although we might get the same sensation on our retina as the radiologist does, we do not see the same thing as she does. The same principle applies to the skill of the tracker recognizing the trail of an animal. The skilful painter sees dozens of hues in a model's face where we are merely aware of flesh colour. What we perceive in the standard ambivalent figures such as the vase and two faces (some see the shape of the vase as a face, some see the boundary of the vase as forming a face), the duck–rabbit picture (some see a large-billed duck, some see a large-eared rabbit) or the aged young girl (some see a pretty belle, some see an old hag), depends on what we are thinking about or what we are expecting to see.

Thomas Kuhn (b. 1922), the contemporary philosopher of science, moved the epistemological problem of the validity of human knowledge even into the heart of science itself. For him, as for many who think in depth in this matter, the experimenter is as important a factor in the experiment as any other statistically evaluated element. That means, of course also, all her/his beliefs, opinions and attitudes. Even the professional statistician may easily be influenced in her/his calculation by her/his view of the role of statistics.

Kuhn, although an admirer of Aristotle, could not ignore the errors in Aristotle's view of reality, especially his cosmology. Earlier philosophers had accepted that the earth went around the sun, yet Aristotle remained convinced that the earth was the centre of the universe. This long-lasting falsehood, accepted, by many including Christian philosophers, on Aristotle's authority, warped astronomy for one-and-a-half millennia. Scientific progress was also handicapped by Aristotle's belief that the world was made up of the four primary elements: earth, air, fire and water. According to Kuhn, Aristotle was led into error because of the way he and other philosophers in the past viewed the world: the paradigm of their thought. The Ancient Greeks saw the world as consisting essentially of qualities – shape, purpose, etc. Viewing the world in this way, they could not help making the mistakes springing from their view of the world. The obvious conclusion to be drawn from Kuhn's notion of paradigms is that there can be no single true way of viewing the world, either scientifically or philosophically. It can only be seen from the angle of the viewer. The conclusions we reach depend on the paradigms we adopt, i.e. our viewpoint, or in other words, the way we decide to think about the world. Following this line of thought, there is no such thing as ultimate truth (Kuhn 1997).

Science and ethics

It is in the applications of the results of scientific research, decided upon by politicians as in the case of the use of atomic weaponry or the development of xenotransplants from animals or the cloning of mammals, that value judgements become relevant.

Some claim that such decisions are no concern of the scientist, as a scientist *per se* only as a citizen. Oppenheimer, Director of Los Alamos laboratory in association with the atom bomb project, broke ranks from some of his scientific colleagues with their entrenched modes of thought, when he uttered: 'The physicist has known sin' (Oppenheimer 1995). A very old-fashioned phrase implying deep personal involvement with value judgements.

There are those who consider that if science itself is rooted in values then it can not be purely empirical or objective. If this were so, it would lose its right to claim superiority as a way of knowing about the real world.

The belief that science has nothing to do with values is closely connected with the notion that only what can be confirmed by experiment or observation is a legitimate object of scientific study. Some scientists are quick to distance themselves from philosophical concerns – be they ethical, metaphysical or epistemological – in their discipline. Yet to say that philosophical assumptions and questions are irrelevant to science is to make a highly questionable philosophical assumption.

Sometimes topics that might at first sight appear to belong to philosophy may, after redefinition, be espoused by science. Psychology might, for example, define evil out of existence since it is difficult to slot evil into physico-chemical terms. Thus if one has done something particularly heinous, one must be 'sick'. Consequently, treatment, not punishment, is appropriate. Moral problems which are regarded as not belonging to science are converted into scientific, i.e. medical, ones.

The subjectivity of ethical statements

Moral subjectivism claims that the statement 'This action is right' means 'I approve of this action.' This implies that moral judgements are equivalent to reports of the speaker's own feelings or attitudes. The implication of moral scepticism that there are no objective moral values is liable to provoke one of three different reactions.

First, there are those who would consider such a theory not only false but pernicious; perceiving it as a threat to the practice of morality, even as undermining the moral fibre of the community. This is the traditional cry of the Puritan.

Second, some may consider the statement of the essential subjectivity of moral statements as so obvious as hardly worth mentioning. For them the variation of moral attitudes and opinions about what is acceptable and what is unacceptable in human conduct is a patent fact. This was stated so well by Terence over 2000 years ago: 'Quot homines tot sententiae: suo quoque mos' (see page 1).

Third, other groups of moral philosophers may regard the statement that there are no objective values as meaningless. From their point of view no real issue is raised by the question of whether values are or are not part of the fabric of the world. They would not see the establishment of a logical connection between values and facts as relevant. For them, Hume's Law says all that needs to to be said: 'One cannot derive an "ought" from an "is".'

Because there can be such varying reactions to this theory of subjectivism, it is important to look more closely at what is involved in the arguments on this topic.

How could anyone possibly deny that there is a marked difference between a kind action and a cruel one? This is not the point. The kinds of behaviour to which moral values are ascribed are indeed part of the furniture of the world and so are the natural, descriptive differences between them; but not, perhaps, the differences in value. It is a fact that cruel actions differ from kind ones, and hence that we can learn to distinguish them in practice and to use the words 'cruel' and 'kind' with fairly clear descriptive meanings. The condemnation (a value judgement) of cruel actions may not appear so obviously a matter of fact. The same action may be considered as unjustified aggression or just retribution. The issue is with regard to the objectivity specifically of value, not with regard to the objectivity of those natural, factual differences on the basis of which differing values are assigned.

A strong argument favouring ethical subjectivism has as its premise the well-known variation in moral codes from one society to another and the differences in moral beliefs between different groups and classes within a complex community. It should, however, be realized that disagreement about moral codes seems to reflect people's adherence to and participation in different ways of life. The causal connection seems to be that way round: people approve of monogamy because they live in a monogamous society rather than that they participate in a monogamous way of life because they approve of monogamy. There have been moral rebels and reformers who, like Elizabeth Fry (1780–1845), turned against the established rules and practices of their own community. Sometimes they received belated approval. Often their reforms were grounded in the existing way of life. Frequently they merely highlighted inconsistencies within the accepted system. The argument for the subjectivity of ethics from the variation of morals from place to place, draws some support from the fact that the variations are more readily explained by the hypothesis that they reflect ways of life than by the hypothesis that they express perceptions of objective standards.

A counter-argument to the claim that variations of moral codes indicate the subjectivity of ethics is that objectivity is only being attributed by opponents of subjectivism to very general principles which are recognized, at least implicitly, to some extent in all societies. Such objective ethical principles would be, for example: the principle of universalization, i.e. that we should act in a way we would want everyone else to act; or the rule that one ought to conform to the rules of the life in which one takes part, from which one profits and on which one relies; or a utilitarian principle of doing what seems most likely to promote the general good. It is easy to show that such general principles will easily produce varying moral codes in differing circumstances and amidst different social patterns.

Further thoughts on subjectivism in ethics

If that which appears to each as right or good stands for that which is right or good, and if each one can make his own moral code or settle for none at all, then each could follow his own inclinations and even his caprice. Attempts to hinder anyone following their moral whim could then infringe personal rights.

To this argument it may first be objected that a theory is not invalidated because it is likely to cause mischief. It is true, however, that if we recognize as right everything that is held to be right by anybody, morality would indeed sink into chaos.

My moral judgements are my own judgements. They spring from my own moral consciousness. They judge the conduct of others from my, not from their, point of view. We may, when judging an act, take into consideration the moral conviction of the agent and the agreement or disagreement between his doing and his idea of what he ought to do. We may hold it wrong for a person to act against his conscience; we may at the same time blame him for having the sort of conscience he has developed.

Ethical subjectivists claim that they do not allow one to follow one's own idio-syncratic inclinations, nor do they lend sanction to arbitrariness and caprice. Our moral consciousness belongs to our mental constitution, which we cannot change as we please. Or can we? We approve or disapprove because we can not do otherwise. Really? Can we help feeling pain when burnt? Can we help sympathizing with our friends and under equal compulsion mock our enemies in the same predicament? Are these phenomena less necessary, less powerful in their consequences, because they fall within the subjective sphere of experience? Why, then, should the moral law command less obedience because it forms part of our own nature?

Ethical subjectivism and objective standards

The judging at dog shows, the grading of fruit, the awarding of prizes in various competitions and even the marking of examinations are carried out in relation to standards of quality or merit which are peculiar to each particular subject matter. The standards may be clearly set out but even if they are not codified in some way they are usually tacitly understood or in general agreed upon by those who are regarded as qualified judges or experts in the subject. We may note in passing that there do not seem to be such universally accepted specialists in the field of morals. Where such sufficiently defined standards exist, it will be an objective issue, a matter of how well any particular specimen measures up to those accepted criteria. It will be a factual question whether one competitor has performed better than another one.

The subjectivist does not deny that there can be objective evaluations relative to standards, even in the aesthetic and moral fields. Any award of marks or prizes would be unjust if it were at variance with the agreed standards for the specific contest in question. In this way the justice or injustice of decisions relative to standards can be objective, though there may still be a subjective element in the interpretation or application of standards. According to subjectivists, the statement that a certain decision is just or unjust will not be objectively prescriptive; that is, it cannot demand in every situation a specific line of action.

Recognizing the objectivity of evaluative judgements relative to standards merely shifts the question of the objectivity of values back to the standards themselves. The subjectivist may make this point by insisting that there is no objective validity involved in the choice of standards. No doubt the subjectivist would clearly be wrong if he said that the choice of even the most basic standards in any field was completely arbitrary. There will always be difficulty in deciding precisely where the subjective inner world of the self begins to intrude as a deciding factor in the making of judgements which seem to take the form of objective statements (Moore 1903). It eventually becomes obvious when no trace of objectivity is left, for example in a dream. Even though the dream is the product of the subject himself, it can seem very real to the dreamer. Indeed the dreamer has less control over this subjective phenomenon than over some events in the objective world when he is awake. Obviously, the vividness of an experience is no proof that it is not subjective.

An illustration of how subjective views may vary, even widely, yet still be essentially related to objective reality and so be kept within sensible bounds, can be taken from aesthetics. Various artists on various sides of a mountain will obviously produce a, sometimes very disparate, variety of images of the mountain. All the pictures could be accepted as reflecting the scene. If one eccentric painter, however, depicted the view in the form of a poached egg, he would be considered as totally out of order and utterly out of touch with reality.

Objectivism in ethics

Objectivism – the ready acceptance of the factual existence of all that we associate with outside reality – is a feature of traditional moral philosophy and a firm basis of ordinary thought. Claims to objectivity are ingrained in our language but that does not make it self-validating. There has been a trend in modern ethics, following from G.E. Moore (1813–1958), to regard the claim that moral values are objective as an 'error theory'. Consequently, strong arguments justifying objectivism in ethics had been demanded from some quarters. On the other hand, most users of moral language intend to make a definite statement about the morality of, for example, an action as it is in itself and not about their attitude to it. Moral statements are made to call for action or to refrain from action. The judgement is intended to be absolute, not contingent upon any desire, preference, policy or choice of the speaker or of any other individual. Someone in a state of moral perplexity, wondering, for example, if it was wrong to engage in research related to bacterial warfare, wants to arrive at a solid answer to this concrete case. His question is not whether he wants to do this work or whether it will satisfy him. He wants to know whether this course of action would be wrong in itself. He intends to be, and considers he is being, objective about the matter.

The denial of objective values can carry with it an extreme emotional reaction – that nothing matters at all, that life has lost its purpose. Although, as was pointed out previously, the fact that a theory may cause mischief does not prove it false, however desirable that might be.

The main tradition of European moral philosophy claims there are objective moral values and that ethical judgements are partly prescriptive, directive and action-guiding.

In Plato's theory, the Forms, and in particular the Form of the Good, are eternal, extra-mental realities (see The Myth of the Cave, an illustration used by Plato in *The Republic*). They are a central structural element of the fabric of the world. Plato holds that just knowing them will not merely tell men what to do but will ensure that they do it, overruling any contrary inclinations. The philosopher-kings in *The Republic* can, Plato thinks, be trusted with unchecked power because their education will give them knowledge of the Forms.

Aristotle begins his work the *Nicomachean Ethics* by saying that the 'good' is that at which all things aim and that ethics is a part of a science which he calls 'politics' whose goal is not knowledge but practice. He does not doubt that there can be knowledge of what is the 'good' for man. He claims that this 'good', which he considers to be happiness, can be known and that it can be rationally determined in what happiness consists of. He thinks this happiness is intrinsically desirable, not 'good' simply because it is desirable (desire has subjective overtones).

Kant introduced his 'categorical imperative' – the conscious demands of an inner moral faculty – as objective. Though he agreed a rational being gives the moral law to himself, the law that he thus makes is determinate and necessary. Thus it is independent from the individual.

Sidgwick (1838–1900) asumes there is a science of ethics – the science of conduct – and so argues that what ought to be 'must in another sense have objective existence'. 'What ought to be' must be an object of knowledge and as such must be the same for all minds. He says that the affirmations of this science 'are also precepts'. He talks in terms of happiness as 'an end absolutely prescribed by reason' (Sidgwick 1874).

A strong basis for traditional belief in the objectivity of ethics was the acceptance of the notion of 'natural law'. This was seen as binding precepts written into the heart of man. Simple convenient rules, for example driving on the left, could be easily seen as purely arbitrary, but more profound rules controlling intimate human relationships were seen as belonging to the same category as the rules of mathematics. Local differences in moral attitudes were regarded as mere varying expressions of immutable principles. It was argued that the fact that some forms of morality were considered superior to other forms implied the notion of an ideal morality – a real morality independent of what people think.

Frequently, the trump played by objectivists was the divine card. The 'natural law' was aligned with the divine law. So it was rendered not only objective but also eternal and supreme.

John Locke (1632–1704) pointed out that the truest teachers of moral philosophy are the outlaws and thieves who keep faith with one another and observe 'an honesty among thieves'. They abide by their rules of justice for mutual convenience with no pretence of receiving them as innate laws of nature. There was an objective basis for such an inviolable code of conduct: 'if they did not hang together they might hang separately'. Convenience is, indeed, the inspiration of many forms of moral behaviour. There is nothing more laudable in practice than the humble morality of the queue. I have seen many push to the front of the queue but have heard none condemn the principle.

Objections to objectivism in ethics

Pascal (1623–1662), the most devout of philosophers, admits that: 'We hardly know of anything, just or unjust, which does not change its character with a change of climate.'

Hume, a leading opponent of objectivism in ethics, insisted that moral judgements were neither necessary nor *a priori*, nor were they descriptions of any actual feature of the world. For Hume, all that there really was in the world was a series of sense impressions. Whereas, he admitted, we had sense impressions of the physical characteristics of things, he insisted that their moral value was not among those perceived characteristics. In keeping with his empiricism, he taught that when we use ethical or aesthetic terms we are not directly referring to things in the world but to our own attitude towards them.

Ayer (1910–1989) shares Hume's basic conviction that value is not part of the world. This is the fundmental feature of those theories of morals which have had the most powerful influence in the twentieth century.

Descriptivism

Associated with the controversy about the subjectivity of ethical statements is the doctrine of descriptivism. According to this school of thought, ethical terms and statements are purely descriptive and in no way prescriptive, emotive or evaluative. It is not an essential feature of ethical terms to commend or assert. Is that so?

Universalization in ethics

There are three advancing stages of universalization whereby moral tenets held by an individual are applied validly by that individual to similar modes of conduct of either himself or others.

First stage

The first stage of universalization implies the irrelevance of numerical differences. The fact that there are two or more similar cases necessarily implies they are different and not completely identical, otherwise there would only be one and the same case. So any factor associated with the cases being numerically distinct will be irrelevant to any moral judgement being made upon them. This means exactly the same moral stance should be taken in respect to each case. Anyone who says that a certain action (or person or state of affairs, etc.) is morally wrong, good or bad, and ought or ought not to be done (or imitated or pursued, etc.) is thereby committed to taking the same view about any other relevantly similar action (etc.). The attitude: 'Do as I say, not as I do' is unacceptable in ethical universalization.

Second stage

The second stage of universalization supposes that a person can put himself in the place of another. If one asserts that a moral maxim is really universalizable then one should be able to imagine oneself in the place of another person. Given that situation, one should be ready to accept the supposed maxim as a directive guiding the behaviour of others towards oneself. If one had a large income, no dependants, and an iron constitution, one may be inclined to believe that everyone should pay in full for any requisite medical attention. Would the same person, if on a low wage and having developed a chronic complaint, still endorse their previous moral stance?

Third stage

The third stage of universalization constitutes an even more stringent test of a moral commitment to the principle of universalization. At this stage it is required that one takes into account different tastes and rival ideals. This involves putting onself even more thoroughly in the other person's place. One must take on the desires, tastes, preferences, ideals and values as well as other qualities, abilities and external situation of the other. In the situation evoked by this extreme supposition, hardly any of one's own self is retained. One is trying to look at things from one's own and from another person's view at the same time and seeking action-guiding principles which one can accept from both points of view. In fact, it cannot realistically be a one-to-one affair. In real life it would need to involve a reconciliation of a multiplicity of divergent views. Could such an ideal be ever actually achieved in practice? Can one really see research from the rat's point of view? Should one perhaps lower one's sights a little? Should one look not for principles that can wholeheartedly be endorsed by everyone from every point of view but settle rather for principles which represent an acceptable compromise between sensible points of view?

The language of ethics

Since ethics pertains to philosophy rather than to law or science, the language in which it is couched is less precise than that in which the two other disciplines are expressed. It has few words which have universally accepted definitions. Even attempts at a definition of its central concept 'the good' are a source of involved controversy (Warnock 1963).

Some more traditional moral philosophers regarded ethical language as a sub-class of prescriptive language which is either directly imperative or logically related to an imperative. In plain words this means that ethical terminology is usually expressed in the form of orders. In extreme form, this surfaces as 'Thou shalt not'. On the other hand, most modern ethisists regard ethical statements as expressions of feelings, or as intended to arouse feelings. Ethical terms grade conduct as better or worse.

Nowell-Smith produced 'the Janus principle', namely the principle that any one statement or word may be expected to perform at least two functions on any one occasion of its use. Appealing to this principle, Nowell-Smith rejects the view that ethical expressions are just imperative or just emotive, or that they have any other single unique function. There are words which characteristically have, among other functions, that of suggesting a suitable reaction to something. An example of such a word would be 'horrible', which suggests that the object so described is apt to call forth horror. Nowell-Smith calls these words 'A words', short for aptness words, 'because they are words that indicate that an object has certain properties which are apt to arouse a certain emotion or range of emotions'. These A words are contrasted on the one hand with D words ('purely descriptive, according to the current distinction between descriptive and evaluative'), and on the other hand with G, or gerundive words, which suggest that an object has properties which ought to be regarded in a certain way. 'Praiseworthy' is an example of a G word. The distinction between A and G words would not be supposed by Nowell-Smith to be hard and fast. He concludes that A words are used to give explanations, make predictions and express emotions, not to give reasons. Their use is only proper if the user has in mind certain reasons which are not stated but contextually implied. Thus it will be proper to say of something that it is horrible, for example of an experiment, only if I have reasons for saying it, among which will be that I dislike the thing in question.

Hare, who describes his first book as a logical study of language, contends that prescriptive language is of two classes: the class of overt imperatives and the class of evaluative words or sentences. When this division is applied to ethics, it seems that 'ought', 'right' and 'you should' come into the first class, being genuine imperatives, according to Hare; while 'good', 'desirable', and so on, come into the second (Hare 1952).

The term 'good'

Nothing seems simpler than the words 'good' and 'bad'. We use them all the time. They have many synonyms such as 'worth' or 'value' and the less literary or more slangy terms we use so often, 'the goods', 'all right', 'OK', 'super', 'wrong'un'; to say nothing of the many signs or gestures – applause, the hearty handshake, boos and gestures of contempt, the light in the eye and the nod of approval. We may not agree with the sentiment conveyed but we are in no doubt about the meaning of the communication. If we could not rightly interpret these messages we would be regarded as completely lacking in comprehension.

When we begin to consider the term 'good' within ethics, we find that difficulties and complexities begin to arise. What do we mean when we say Brian is a very good man or has done a good deed? Do we mean he is considerate, helpful and that he can be trusted? Do we mean he is not daunted by danger, that he shows courage and is willing to sacrifice himself for others? Is this what we mean by the use of the word 'good'? Are we not merely listing the qualities which entitle a person to be called 'good'? It is because of these factors that a person is deemed to be good. We imply that considerate action and regard for others are things to which goodness belongs and by which its attribution is earned. What is this goodness which considerate action and dauntlessness seem to have? Is there anything to which we can point, beyond the characteristic of conduct or character by which we describe these terms? When we have said that the action was considerate, and the like, what more is there that the word 'good' conveys? Do we strictly need such a word?

How can we dispense with a word in such common use? It is hardly sufficient justification for its use to say that it helpfully holds together such qualities as already described. Why should we want to hold these words together unless the term 'good' indicates something which characterizes them all? What sort of thing can we ascribe to an action which is not part of the description of the action?

A way of dealing with this situation has been to think of goodness not as a quality strictly belonging to actions or persons but as interpretable in terms of the reactions of people to them. Yet we all tend to think of goodness as belonging expressly to the good deed or person, irrespective of our recognizing it or applauding it.

The foregoing remarks set the scene for the lengthy, complex and obtuse discussions of modern moral philosophers on the understanding of the term 'good'. Moral philosophers have presumed that they could find out more about moral goodness if they could be more definite about what 'good' means when used as a moral term.

G.E. Moore, the prominent writer on the matter, claims that it is impossible to define 'good' since it is the name of a simple unanalysable characteristic of things. He does not mean that we cannot recognize things that possess this unanalysable characteristic. He is sure that we can, if we think about it hard enough, recognize intrinsically good things. It is a matter simply of recognition. No evidence can be adduced to show that something is intrinsically good; it is just a matter of seeing that it is so.

Moore thought that there were three possible meanings for the term 'good' in its ethical sense. It denotes

(1)   something simple and indefinable, standing for some simple property or characteristic that things or actions may have;
(2)   something complex; or
(3)   no property either simple or complex, so that it means nothing at all and there is no such subject as ethics.

He rejected possibilities (1) and (2) and argued that this indefinable something must be a non-natural quality.

Moore thought that those who tried to define 'good' and give it a descriptive meaning confused the question of what sort of things are good with the question of what goodness itself is: the former can no doubt be answered in descriptive, natural, terms; but only an answer to the latter would constitute a definition or analysis of 'good'. Secondly, he relied on what has been called the 'open question' argument. Take some proposed analysis of 'good', say 'conducive to pleasure'; we can surely understand the view of someone who says 'I admit that such-and-such is conducive to pleasure but is it good?' The same holds true if we substitute for 'conducive to pleasure' any other proposed definition, for example 'more evolved', 'socially approved', 'in tune with the universe' or 'in acordance with God's will'. It is still an open question whether what is so described is good; or at least we can understand the view of someone who holds that it is still open. If the proposed definition had been a correct account of 'good', this question could not still be open.

An action may be good because it is generous, but its goodness is not identical with its generosity; this is different from a figure being square because it has four straight sides equal in length and each of its angles a right angle, where we can hardly distinguish the squareness from the features that together make the figure square. We may talk in a condemnatory tone of an act that is generous as being too generous, impling that it is not good. We could not in the same way call into question the squareness of a figure with four equal sides and every angle a right angle.

Moore gave no ground on his strong opinion on the indefinability of the term 'good':

> 'If I am asked "What is good?" my answer is that good is good and that is the end of the matter. Or if I am asked "How is good to be defined?" my answer is that it cannot be defined, and that is all I have to say about it.'
>
> (Moore 1903)

Moore goes on to use an analogy between 'good' and 'yellow' to establish two further points. The first point is that though it is as impossible to define colour words as it is to define the taste of chocolate, it is possible to state the physical concomitants of the colours. We may state that light vibrations must strike the normal eye in order that the colour may be perceived. Moore says, these light vibrations are not what we mean when we talk about the colour. The colour word is the name of a property perceptible to the normal eye, not the name of something which it needs scientific measurement to discover. He argues that with 'good' it may be possible to state what else besides being good, all good things are; for instance, it might turn out that if ever anything was good it was also pleasant, or the object of approval. This would not, however, imply that when we talked of a thing being good, we meant that it was pleasant or the object of approval. To identify the light waves with the colour or the pleasantness with the goodness is to commit the fallacy (naturalistic?) of trying to define what is simple and indefinable. This fallacy rests entirely on the assumption that 'good' is the name of a discernible property of things.

The second point, which the analogy with colour is used to make, is this: nobody thinks that because 'yellow' is indefinable it is impossible to say what things have the property of being yellow. Nobody thinks that there can be only one thing which is yellow, nor that all the other properties which the yellow thing has are identical with the property of yellowness.

Moore's reasoning was mainly aimed at the naturalistic fallacy – the failure to distinguish clearly that unique and indefinable quality which we mean by good. The naturalistic fallacy he associated with hedonism – the identification of the 'good' with the 'pleasurable' – but the particular form of hedonism he attacked the most was the utilitarianism of John Stuart Mill. Moore suggests that Mill tries to prove that pleasure (in a very broad sense) is the only thing desirable as an end, by appeal to the fact that people do actually desire it and it alone as an end. This attempted proof is, Moore says, a glaring example of the naturalistic fallacy.

Mill's proof consists in arguing that 'desirable' is like 'visible'; and just as you could establish what things are visible by finding out what things people actually see, so you could find out what things were desirable by discovering what people actually desired. What they do desire, Mill says, is pleasure and therefore pleasure is desirable and therefore is good. Since pleasure is all that people desire, it can be said not only to be 'good', but to be 'the good'.

R.M. Hare suggests a catch-all definition of the term 'good' 'such as to satisfy requirements (etc.) of the kind in question'. Hare stresses the evaluative nature of the term 'good'. The proposition 'This is good chocolate' is evaluative. It is legitimate to infer from this phrase: 'Take it.' If this is inferring too much, a more complicated imperative might be substituted: 'If there is any question of taking chocolate, other things being equal, take this one.'

Mackie sums up this convoluted, and for some sterile, dispute concerning the term 'good'. It is true that the general meaning of the term 'good' leaves it open that the word may be used in moral contexts with reference to supposed intrinsic requirements; but it equally leaves it open that the term 'good' in moral contexts may be used for egocentric commendation. The general meaning of the term is neutral as between these rival views. Further, if the main ethical use does refer to supposed intrinsic requirements, this does not necessarily require that there are objective values (Mackie 1990a).

The term 'ought'

Like the term 'good', the term 'ought' has been a source of much disputation amongst moral philosophers. The classic tradition of moral philosophy has always held that the idea of 'ought' is not primary and irreducible, and that judgements containing it can be derived from more ultimate judgements concerning what is 'good'; while it has also commonly been held that these in turn can be reduced to propositions about the nature of humankind and the world, together with the expressions of or propositions about human desires and purposes. What I ought to do depends on what it would be best that I should do. That in turn depends on what I am and what other things and people are, and what we all most constantly desire.

Sidgwick holds that the fundamental notions represented by the terms 'ought' or 'right', which moral judgements contain expressly or by implication, are essentially different from all notions representing facts of physical or psychical experience. He refers such judgements to the 'reason', understood as a faculty of cognition. By this he implies:

> 'that what ought to be is a possible object of knowledge, that is, that what I judge ought to be, must, unless I am in error, be similarly judged by all rational beings who judge truly of the matter'.
>
> (Sidgwick 1874)

Hume remarked that writers on morality often move imperceptibly from statements joined by 'is' to ones joined by 'ought' and 'ought not'. These, he protested, express some new relation, make some new sort of claim, which needs to be explained:

'A reason should be given, for what seems altogether inconceivable, how this new relation can be a deduction fom others which are entirely different from it.'

This protest has since hardened into a dictum called Hume's Law – that one cannot derive an 'ought' from an 'is'.

'Ought' and 'must' and 'shall' and 'should' are constantly used in non-moral as well as moral contexts, and as with 'good' it is not likely that their moral uses are completely cut off from other uses. The meanings of these words can easily be perceived as varying, according to the context, from an absolute imperative to less commanding modes such as when they are used to describe the rules of a game, for example chess.

Some attempt has been made to outflank Hume's Law by arguing from this milder application of such words as 'ought' and developing quite logically, the notion of 'ought', etc. being used within agreed sets of circumstances such as an obligation to fulfil promises. John Searle (b. 1932) presents this line of argument, claiming that 'ought can take its force from its accepted meaning' within what he calls an 'institution'. It may be argued that in this way 'is' can become 'acceptable' and without undue stretching of reasoning 'acceptable' can become 'ought'.

An 'institution' in the ethical sense

Any institution is constituted by many people behaving in fairly regular ways, with relations between them which transmit, encourage and perhaps enforce those ways of behaving. An institution will have rules or principles of action, or both, which the participants in the institution will formulate fairly explicitly, allow to guide their own actions, and infringements of which they will discourage and condemn. They will use concepts closely associated with these rules which cannot be fully explained without references to these rules and principles. The rules and principles in turn will usually be formulated partly in terms of those concepts. An institution can be described in an abstract and formal way simply by stating and explaining the rules and principles and concepts – the game of chess, for example, could be fully described in this way.

To speak within an institution is to use its characteristic concepts, to assert or appeal to, or implicitly invoke its rules and principles, in fact to speak in those distinctive ways of speaking and thinking with which the participants help to constitute the institution.

An institution, in this ethical sense, does not need to be instituted. It need not be such an artificial creation as the game of chess. 'Promising' may well be a universal human practice, to be found in all societies; it is certainly one that could grow very naturally out of the ordinary conditions of human life. That does not alter the logical status of conclusions that can be established only within and by invoking that institution. A promise, and the apparent obligation to keep a promise, are created not merely by a speaker's statement of intention in conjunction with the desire of the person to whom the promise is made that it should be fulfilled, or even by these together with the hearer's reliance on the statement. What creates the ethical 'institution' of promising is all these factors being embedded in and reinforced by general social expectations, disapprovals and demands. Promising, in contrast to merely stating an intention, entails a complex of all these attitudes.

The term 'right'

W.D. Ross (1877–1971) in *The Right and the Good* examines a number of attempts to define 'right'. He approached the term 'right' in a similar fashion to the way Moore dealt with the term 'good'. Ross concluded that rightness was indefinable. If it can be put into some more general category such as 'suitability' its 'differentia' cannot be clearly stated. To quote Ross:

> 'Just as red is a species of colour, what distinguishes it from other clours can be indicated only by saying that it is the colour that is red.'

As to what things have this indefinable characteristic of rightness, Ross allows that a number of things may be said to possess it but, properly speaking, only actions can be said to be 'right'. He is cautious about saying that a whole overt action can be right, since he thinks that the whole complete action contains some elements for which one is not responsible and are independent of our action. Ross acknowledged that his views derived from H.A. Pritchard's article 'Does moral philosophy rest on a mistake?' (Pritchard 1912). The term 'right' used here must not be confused with 'a right', dealt with at length later.

The inadequacy of ethics

The ethical material already presented is hardly the sort that is noised abroad constantly in an animal unit, nor does it strike one as relevant to the acceptability of a rabbit biopsy for purposes of research. It might even be disappointing to students keen to study ethics, as it appears to be so remote from practical problems. Indeed, where practical problems are referred to, they tend to be inserted merely to illustrate some theoretical point.

A sparsity of positive statements

One might have imagined, naïvely, that ethics could be of some use in deciding what we ought to do. A.J. Ayers, a leading modern philosopher, dismisses such a fantasy in a pre-emptory manner:

> 'It is silly, as well as presumptuous, for any one type of philosopher to pose as the champion of virtue. And it is also one reason why many people find moral

philosophy an unsatisfactory subject. For they mistakenly look to the moral philosopher for guidance.'

(Ayers 1959)

C.D. Broad gives reasons for the lack of answers in ethics:

'It is not part of the professional business of moral philosophers to tell people what they ought or ought not to do. Moral philosophers, as such, have no special information not available to the general public about what is right and what is wrong; nor have they any call to undertake those hortatory functions which are so adequately performed by clergymen, politicians or leader-writers.'

(Broad 1952)

B. Williams sums up the negative approach of modern ethics:

'I have tried to say why ethical thought has no chance of being everything it seems. Even if ethical thought had a foundation in determinate conceptions of well-being, the consequences of that could lie only in justifying a disposition to accept certain ethical statements rather than in showing, directly, the truth of those statements.'

(Williams 1985)

The obtuseness of the subject matter

Mackie, like other modern writers on ethics, stresses the absence of firm conclusions and at the same time perfectly illustrates the recondite nature of the subject. He defends valiantly the sceptical approach of moral philosophers in modern times. For him this scepticism is a form of an error theory – admitting that a belief in objective values is built into ordinary moral thought and language – but holding that this ingrained belief is false. There is, therefore, a need for strong arguments in support of ethical scepticism against common sense. According to Mackie, those arguments exist. The bases of arguments against the popular acceptance of objective values in ethical matters, according to Mackie, are:

(1) The relativity or variability of some important starting points of moral thinking and their apparent dependence on actual ways of life.
(2) The metaphysical peculiarity of the supposed objective values, in that they would have to be action-guiding and motivating.
(3) The problem of how such values could be consequential or supervenient upon natural features.
(4) The corresponding epistemological difficulty of accounting for our knowledge of value entities or features and of their links with the features on which they would be consequential.
(5) The possibility of explaining, in terms of several different patterns of objectification, traces of which remain in modern language and moral

concepts, how even if there were no such objective values, people not only might have come to suppose that there are, but also might persist firmly in that belief.

(Mackie 1990b: p. 49)

The complexity of ethical studies

Moral principles, of their nature, are various and complex. Any attempt to explain the moral life in terms of one or two principles of high generality, or to resolve a particular moral issue in that way, will fail to do justice to the demands of concrete situations. The clash of various ethical theories also confuses moral issues. Furthermore, the lack of agreement on clear universally accepted definitions of ethical terms obviates the presentation of a solid-based morality.

A similar situation where there is a lack of clarity in defining concepts occurs in aesthetics where a simple universally accepted explanation of the crucial term 'taste' proves wholly elusive. The resulting vagueness does not call into question the existence of an acknowledged beautiful object, however much opinions may differ about its worth. 'Beauty may be in the eye of the beholder'; a phrase that really smacks of subjectivism but this phrase does not negate real beauty.

Some redeeming features of ethics

For good moral order to be maintained in the real world, even the most commendable ethical principles need legal backing of the coercive type. Universal observance depends on sanctions. After Plato wrote his seminal work on ethics, *The Republic*, he wrote *The Laws*, no doubt when he was older and wiser. The benefit is not, however, completely one-sided. Within a free society the formation of a moral consensus is essential to the general acceptance of law.

There are occasions in life when a person encounters moral dilemmas and a choice of modes of behaviour about which they are unsure. In the absence of any awareness of any inner faculty, of the nature of a categorical imperative, or a demanding or even nagging conscience, or a rigidly formed conscience from a religious education, they may find a rational discussion of ethics of some worth. Even when someone has ignored or consigned to the subconscious some concern or even worry about the justification of their way of life or the means whereby they earn their living, they might find that if there does not seem to be any other reasonably accessible means of gaining peace of mind when the buried thoughts surface, perhaps, due to a challenge or confrontation or an encounter with uncomfortable facts, an investigation of ethical attitudes on the matter may help them to untangle the moral quandary in which they find themselves. It may be that all that is needed is to think the challenge through rationally by the use of ethics in order to arrive at a satisfactory solution.

In the ever-present bustle of life, the niceties of moral rectitude cannot always be given considered attention. Rule-of-thumb moral axioms may be easily accepted and aptly quoted when appropriate. They tend then not only to express the moral stance of the person but also to form it and certainly to reinforce it. This moral stance more and more becomes the fixed attitude of the person, needing no defending until challenged from an outside source. It will be found that however deeply held these moral views are, the mere repetition of them with greater and greater emphasis, is inadequate in proving their value to others, unless they agree with you. Indeed such method of argument is insufficient even to justify rationally your own adherence to such tenets. It might prove merely to be a whistling in the dark. A study of ethics may sometimes prove disturbing ('There are few who have the courage to think what they know', Nietzsche), calling for the sacrifice of sacred cows. Ethics, for the thinking person, can indicate the direction in which to look for rational arguments to justify an opinion. In this way ethics may be able to provide the comfort of mental satisfaction with one's outlook on the morality of one's own actions.

There must be hardly an area of morality that is not a potential arena for ethical controversy. All too often the approach of the contenders is in line with the valuable marginal note to a sermon, 'argument weak, shout loud' or Truman's (Harry S) Law: 'If you can't convince them, confuse them'.

Ethics, perhaps, can provide a more effective approach and certainly a more rational one. Accepted modes of argument can be hammered out and independent appraisal of opinions can be constructed. Within ethics and, perhaps, *only* within ethics, can be found clear definitions of the popular terms associated with morality. These form the necessary equipment to achieve any advance in polemics between opposing moralists. Without any agreed definitions and some agreed basic principles, any dialectic is futile, mere shadow-boxing. Only ethics can provide principles broad enough to be accepted by moralists of widely divergent schools and to enjoy popular acceptance in a plural society such as ours.

Unfortunately, in some prominent debates of great importance to every-day existence there occurs a dialogue of the deaf. All there is on either side is the eye that sees not and the echoing ear. No form of persuasion is going to get to first base. Not only are the protagonists coming from opposite directions but they seem to be determined to remain on parallel lines so they can never meet. Furthermore, both sides may be sincere and therein lies a further danger – fanaticism. In such cases, even the prayer of Oliver Cromwell (himself no wimp), 'I beseech you in the bowels of Christ, think it possible you may be mistaken' (Cromwell 1650), would be a useless plea. The crucial difficulty is that they base their arguments on completely different premises, each of the premises wholly unacceptable to the opponent. For example, according to Aristotle and many who followed in his wake, animals existed for the use of humans; on the other hand many animal pressure groups use terms such as 'fascism' even when referring to painless research. One might add a similar sentiment; animals are entitled to empowerment.

While opposing opinions at the extreme ends of the spectrum may be irre-concilable, the influence of such extreme views may be counteracted by providing a bridge between the moderate exponents of contrary views. This can be done by finding, through ethics, moderate premises which may be, albeit grudgingly, accepted by both sides. One side might be persuaded to accept that animals have a standing in nature independent of man and on the other side it may be possible to convince some of them that there can be productive reaction between humans and animals to the benefit of both. By such a rational approach it may be possible to establish a tentative common ethical ground for the discussion of animal–human relations.

The present pattern of dialectics on this topic is reminiscent of the anecdote about the two ladies of Oxford. Two ladies (the term is used with some hesitation) were indulging in acrimonious verbal abuse of one another. They were hurling their somewhat profane oral missives at one another from opposite balconies across an Oxford thoroughfare. A passing haughty don observed superciliously to his learned colleague: 'They will never reach agreement, they are arguing from opposite premises.'

One practical aspect of ethics

Ethical studies may be of some use to members of ethics committees in respect to the use of animals in research. The topic of an ethical review process will be discussed in detail in Chapter 14. Often such bodies will be in-house scrutinizing committees looking at the application of the three Rs (replacement, reduction and refinement of animal use) or cost–benefit assessment. The acceptability of the use of animals in research in principle will have already been presumed. The application of secondary principles affecting decisions to use particular animals in specific ways could be a useful function of such committees. To operate efficiently and in an acceptable manner to researchers, it is paramount that the decisions should be consistent, to a certain extent predictable and delivered without due delay. These desirable qualities can best be found where there exists within such a committee a consensus opinion on the ethical aspects of animal use. This consensus should also be present for the proper interpretation of the ethical justification of the use of animals in the variety of cir-cumstances which can occur in scientific research.

Such a consensus as regards first-order ethics – the reasons why particular pro-cedures are acceptable or unacceptable – is best formed by the members of such a committee having a sufficiently broad knowledge of ethics and a skill in using the relevant ethical arguments. In this context it is only first-order ethics we need consider.

There are, of course, a variety of other types of ethics committees besides those concerned with the scientific use of animals. Each such committee deals in its own way with the moral nature of some human activity, for example the acceptability of specific forms of medical treatment (Elster & Herpin 1994).

The prevalence of such committees in a variety of professions indicates, if not a need, at least a use for such bodies. As was indicated as regards ethics committees on research using animals, so in other cases a knowledge of ethics, and an ability to apply the principles of ethics in practice, are essential to the proper functioning of such committees. It could be that a demand for the study of ethics is on the increase (Whitehorn 1995).

To summarize this introduction we may venture to suggest that ethics is a rational attempt to prove Terence wrong in his suggestion that each man has his own individual morals (see page 1). Ethics is perhaps a valiant effort to find some common intellectual basis for a morality acceptable, if not to all, at least to many.

References

Ayers, A.J. (1936) This appears in Ayers' influential book *Language, Truth and Logic.*

Ayers, A.J. (1959) In *Philosophical Essays*, p. 246, London, Ayers forcefully indicates the deficiency of ethics.

BBC (1994a) This distinction was aired on the religious radio programme on Sunday mornings, BBC Radio 4 *Sunday* 17 July.

BBC2 (1994b) This strange juxtaposition of terms was uttered on *Newsnight*, 12 July.

BBC1 (1995) The programme in which this expression occurred was on BBC1, 7.30 PM 24 April. It was a useful exposition of welfare and the lack of it in respect to poultry.

Broad C.D. (1952) The same message, as for Ayers (1959), is given in *Ethics and the History of Philosophy*, p. 244, London.

Cromwell, O. (1650) This uncharacteristic plea for scepticism occurred in his Letter to the Church of Scotland, 4 August.

Dalrymple (1994) This is a summary of one of Dr Dalrymple's superb weekly articles which appeared in the *Spectator* 2 April. It is merely one example of his wise reflections on moral matters and modern attitudes to morality. Their realism comes from the fact that as a doctor dealing with patients in prison, he has more experience of the real issues of good and evil than a speculative moral philosopher.

Dostoyevsky, F.M. (1880) This is the challenge uttered by the Nietzschian atheistic brother in *The Brothers Karamazov*.

Elster, J. & Herpin, N. (1994) Human medical ethics is dealt with at length in *Ethics of Medical Choice* (eds J. Elster & N. Herpin), Pinter Publishers, London, in a series of publications on social change in Western Europe.

Fontana (1977) *The Fontana Dictionary of Modern Thought*, (eds Bullock & Stallybrass), p. 214. Fontana/Collins, London.

Freud, S. (1913) His book *Totem and Taboo* 1913 was a ground-breaking work in psychoanalysis. It presented insights into human morality.

Hare, R.M. (1952) In his best-known work, *The Language of Morals*, Oxford, 1952, this most influential moral philosopher of his generation dealt in depth with the terms current in modern ethics.

Hefner, H. (1994) This cavalier remark appeared in Life, the *Observer*, 6 November.

Kuhn, T.S. (1997) The high standing of Kuhn as a worthy successor of Popper in the undefined area where philosophy encounters science, and speculation entangles with deduction, is acknowledged by Paul Strathern in *Aristotle in 90 Minutes*, Constable, London, 1997.

Lewis, C.S. (1963) *Mere Christianity.*

Linzey, A. (1994) *Animal Theology*, p. 118. SCM. This book is based on a series of Oxford lectures *The Theology of Animal Rights* 1993. Andrew Linzey is a leader in the field of theology on animals and an ardent apologist for animal rights.

Mackie, J.L. (1990a) Here is the most comprehensive exposition of an explanation in ethical terms of the term 'good'. *Ethics (Inventing Right and Wrong)*, pp. 50–63, Penguin.

Mackie, J.L. (1990b) He defends moral scepticism in his *Ethics*, pp. 48–49, Penguin.

Moore, G.E. (1903) *Principia, Ethica* (as illustrated by the Myth of the Cave in *The Republic*.

Nietzsche, F.W. (1885) This declaration occurs in his *Also Sprach Zarathustra*.

Oppenheimer, J.R. (1995) This striking admission is quoted in the *Spectator* 18 July, p. 12.

Popper, K. (1959), (1972) The great philosopher of science in the twentieth century expounded his strict demands for constant testing of scientific hypotheses in such works as *The Logic of Scientific Discovery*, London 1959 and *Objective Knowledge*, Oxford 1972.

Rawls J. (1971) His theory is fully expounded in his book *A Theory of Justice*.

Sidgwick, H. (1874) A later but leading Utilitarian, Sidgwick expounded his own ideas of moral philosophy in *Methods of Ethics*.

Terence (*c.* 166) This variously translated quotation is from his work *Phormio*, verse 454.

Ward, B. (*c.* 1940) *The Good Pagan's Failure*.

Warnock M. (1963) *Ethics since 1900*. Oxford University Press, Oxford.

Whitehorne, K. (1995) Katherine Whitehorn stresses a growing interest in ethics in business and other walks of life in her article in the *Observer* 23 July. She valiantly makes the case of 'Obedience to the unenforceable', an astute reflection on the nature of ethics. These words she attributes to Lord Moulton.

Williams, B. (1985) The same opinion as expressed by Ayers (1959) and Broad (1952) is reiterated by Williams in *Ethics and the Limits of Philosophy*, p. 199, Harvard University Press, Cambridge, Massachusetts.

Chapter 2

Ethical Theories

'Myself when young did eagerly frequent
Doctor and Saint and heard great argument
About it and about; but evermore
Came out by the same door as in I went.'

The Ruba'iyat of Omar Khayyám, edn. 1, xxvii

Introduction

The Socratic Question was among the first of the numerous ethical problems propounded by moral philosophers down the ages. Some of the proposed theories in answer to these problems have been referred to in Chapter 1, for example Stoicism and the less restrained outpourings of Nietzsche. There is a need to consider other attempts, of perhaps a more sophisticated nature, to elucidate ethical thought.

In spite of the proliferation of ethical theories, especially in modern times, Williams still claims that the Socratic Question is crucial to all later development of ethical opinions.

'How should one live?' is not about what I should do now, or next (should I test this substance on that rat?). It is about a manner of life. The Greeks themselves were much impressed by the idea that such a question must, consequently, be about a whole life and that a good way of living had to issue in what, at its end, would be seen to have been a good life. Impressed by the power of fortune to wreck what looked like the best-shaped life, some of them, Socrates one of the first, sought a rational design of life which would reduce the power of fortune and would be to the greatest possible extent luck-free. This has been, in different forms, an aim of later thought as well. The idea that one must think, at this very general level, about a whole life may seem less compelling to some of us than it did to Socrates. His question presses the demand for reflection on one's life as a whole, from every aspect and all the way down, even if we do not place as much weight as the Greeks did on how it may end.

The only serious enterprise is living and we have to live after the reflection; moreover (though the distinction of theory and practice encourages us to forget it), we have to live during it as well (even carry on with testing that substance on that rat).

Williams, in the very beginning of his work, accepts the sceptical approach to ethics:

'The aims of moral philosophy and any hopes it may have of being worth serious attention, are bound up with the fate of Socrates' question, even if it is not true that philosophy, itself, can reasonably hope to answer it.'

(Williams 1985a)

Socrates just talked with his friends in a plain way, and the writers he referred to (at least with any respect) were the poets. Within one generation Plato had linked the study of moral philosophy to difficult mathematical disciplines, and after two generations there were treatise on the subject – in particular, Aristotle's *Ethics*, still one of the most illuminating.

It is obvious that Williams' speculations are of a most general character. His main concern is with second-order ethical questions of a fundamental and obtuse type. Before embarking on consideration of these higher notions, it may be a consolation to know that there are some works on ethics of a more practical nature, for example *Applied Ethics* by Peter Singer (Singer 1992).

Absolutism

Certainly absolutism is the most comfortable form of ethics, particularly for those for whom it hurts to think. Clear directives and dogmatic stances deliver certainty; unfortunately, certainty is not the same as truth. The opposite to certainty is doubt, which is uncomfortable for many. The opposite of truth is falsity. Falsity is a quality necessarily adhering to at least one contradictory premise of which both contenders in a dispute are so certain that their premise is true. Both premises can be false but both cannot be true if they are logically contradictory: 'Between contradictories there can be no middle ground'.

Absolutism has been a difficulty endemic to many moral systems in the past. There were immutable moral principles bearing little tolerance of varying circumstances or individual cases, epitomized in the harsh righteous dictum: 'Hard cases make bad laws'. Peter Abelard (1079–1144) was a lone and heavily censured voice amongst Christian moralists. He boldly speculated on the acceptability of a relative approach to right and wrong conduct. He accepted solid moral principles but stressed the importance of considering specific circumstances in assessing the morality of an action. Even someone as identified with the Christian establishment as Lord Tennyson, in a time noted for its conformity, indicated the danger of moral absolutes.

'The old order changeth, yielding place to new,
And God fulfills himself in many ways,
Lest one good custom should corrupt the world.'

Idylls of the King, Merlin and Vivien

The absolute moralist denies that circumstances alter cases and that consequences need be considered. He is driven to the extravagance of saying, with Newman, that it would be better for everyone in the world to perish than for a man to save the world by telling a lie. The absolutist must hold that since there is a moral law, all men can discover it – that there is a wide measure of agreement about what is right and what is wrong. Unfortunately, it is difficult to find such widespread agreement on such issues as nuclear development, genetic manipulation, birth control, etc.

According to those who hold by absolutism the morality of actions is perceived by the intellect, just as are number, diversity, causation and proportion. Morality is eternal and immutable. Right and wrong, immutably and necessarily belong to those actions of which they are truly affirmed. Right and wrong, as having a real existence outside the mind, can only be discerned by the understanding. This discernment is accompanied with an emotion. Impressions of pleasure or pain, satisfaction or disgust, generally attend our perceptions of virtue and vice. These are merely their effects and concomitants, not the perceptions themselves.

Objections to absolutism

There are occasions on which a mother's love for her own children or a man's love for his own country have to be suppressed or they will lead to unfairness towards other people's children or countries. Objectors to absolutism deny the existence of good and bad impulses. They point out that a piano has two kinds of notes – right and wrong ones – but every single note is right at one time and wrong at another. The moral law does not reside in any one instinct or one set of instincts. It is something which makes a kind of tune of goodness or right conduct by directing often very diverse instincts.

The most dangerous thing you can do morally is to take any one impulse of your own nature and set it up as the thing you ought to follow at all costs. There is not one instinct that will not make us into devils if we set it up as an absolute guide. Even love of humanity in general may become questionable. If justice is left out, agreements may be broken and evidence faked 'for the sake of humanity'. True statements may be withheld because of political correctness. Some who have intended to set up a Heavenly Kingdom based on unquestionable divine commands have finished up with Hell on Earth.

Intuitionists who are ready to produce answers with no shadow of doubt, to any possible dilemma or trilemma, often show by their response that they have lost contact with the actual world with which their intuitions were designed to cope. Relativists, like utilitarians, realize that they need to look at what is going on in the real world so as to assess the usefulness of moral intuitions.

Defences of absolutism

The failure to find a rational way of harmonizing incompatible moral principles does not, *per se*, prove that no rational solution exists. It simply proves we have not yet found the rational solution. Absolutists have presented various attempts to deal with this difficulty of moral demands apparently contrary one to the other.

Here is an example of an attempt to deal with the ethical difficulties of an absolutist. Consider the maxim: 'People should always be frugal with their money.' Suppose you are a fund-raiser for families left destitute by a flood and suppose a rich lady turns down your appeal because she stands by the frugality maxim and claims to be an ethical absolutist. One tactic for dealing with the rich lady is to say that the frugality maxim may be true for her but that, as far as the flooded families are concerned, it is false. Using that tactic backs you into moral incompatibility, which leaves you with an apparent relativism. The frugality maxim is as false for one person as it is true for another. A better tactic is to avoid an incompatibility confrontation; you can point out that frugality is indeed a virtue but that the short frugality maxim states only a half-truth. A fuller truth is captured by the longer frugality maxim: 'Poor people should be frugal with their money.' There is a longer frugality maxim that fits the rich lady's case: 'Rich people should not be frugal with their money if it can be used to benefit some other person.' In making the frugality maxim longer, you are adding further conditions to which the virtue of frugality is relevant. This has the logical effect of avoiding incompatibility because the frugality maxim about poor people is perfectly compatible with the one about rich people.

Adding conditions does not concede to relativism (?). The rich lady cannot refuse you on absolutist principles alone because you are no longer caught in the relativism she opposes on ethical theory grounds. By using the longer maxim tactic, you force her to consider the moral issues rather than ethical theory issues. She is forced to choose between rational moral options or arbitrary refusal.

In a hypothetical case, often presented in the past when obstetrics was not so advanced, if a doctor could save the life of an unborn child only at the cost of the mother's life and could save the life of the mother only at the cost of the child's life, then if we did not invoke the principle of the double effect we should have to say that whatever the doctor did, even if he did nothing, he may be regarded by some as morally responsible for the death of one presumably innocent person. If we use the principle of the double effect we can retain absolute moral rules. We can say that the doctor can save one of the two persons at the cost of the death of the other, provided that this death is a second effect and not a means.

Even under duress, on this principle one could refuse to kill an innocent person even though many others will die as a result of this refusal because consequent deaths would be a second effect. In this way, absolute prohibitions can be maintained about directly intended actions, chosen ends and means. It would be difficult to sustain the observance of such absolute commands if their scope were extended to include obliquely intended actions, side-effects and further consequences. In this absolute attitude to moral tenets there is the need to distinguish between positive acts and omissions. Moral commands would only apply to positive acts so that conflicting cases would not arise since in any conceivable set of circumstances all prohibitions of positive acts could be obeyed by complete inaction. An example of such an attitude is: 'Don't kill but you can let die.' Likewise, 'It is forbidden to take life but there is no obligation to strive unduly to save life.'

It is argued in favour of absolutism that a non-absolutist could be blackmailed, for example, into killing one innocent person in order to avert the worse evil of the blackmailer killing a larger number. An absolutist could not accept this proposition and a potential blackmailer, knowing this, would not be tempted to try such a heinous form of persuasion.

Relativism

Relativism allows for the existence of incompatible moral maxims which vary between cultures and regards moral concepts as emotional and therefore falling outside the category of truth.

Relativism avoids the strait-jacket of absolutism. Many, however, regard the necessarily general maxims of relativism as lacking moral bite and as destructive of moral fibre. They point to the obvious weakness of relative morality as being 'wet'. Various metaphors are used to illustrate the dangers of relativism, e.g. the slippery slope, snowballing, the salami effect and the rat nibbling at the bag of sugar.

Relativism, unlike more traditional forms of ethical thinking, does not become enmeshed in speculative principles. Westermark makes the case for relativism:

> 'Far from being a danger, ethical subjectivism seems more likely to be an acquisition for moral practice. Could it be brought home to people that there is no absolute standard in morality, they would be perhaps more tolerant in their judgements and more apt to listen to the voice of reason. If "right" has an objective existence, moral consciousness has certainly been playing at blind-man's bluff ever since it was born. Who will admit this? The popular mind is always inclined to believe that it possesses the knowledge of what is right and what is wrong and regards public opinion (a most variable commodity) as the reliable guide to good conduct.'
>
> (Westermark 1932)

To quote Williams:

> 'Relativism is not peculiar to ethics; it can be found even in the philosophy of science. Relativism aims to take views, outlooks or beliefs that apparently conflict and treat them in such a way that they do not conflict. Each of them turns out to be acceptable in its own place.
>
> The simplest method and the one that is in the most precise sense relativistic, is to interpret the original claims as each introducing a relation to a different item. Protagoras, probably the first relativist, started from conflicting sensory appearances; as when I find the wind cold and you find it warm. He claimed that there was no answer to the question whether the wind was really in itself warm or cold. According to Protagoras, the fact of the matter is simply that it is cold for me and warm for you.'
>
> (Williams 1985b)

Protagoras, thousands of years ago, easily produced his example of the relativity of experience, even in the physical world. It is even easier to think of numerous illustrations of how moral norms vary from culture to culture. Attitudes to animal welfare are salient examples of differences of mores in this matter from different countries. Variations in morality in different cultures are obvious to any traveller and in the past formed a cultural shock to devout wayfarers. Often it was the practical expression only of moral principles that varied. The underlying motivation of actions, when fully understood, could go some way to make strange practices understandable. Perhaps the celibate missionary may not have always immediately appreciated that the compelling generosity of the Eskimo husband with his wife's favours (that is, of course, the Eskimo's wife), was an unconscious eagerness to enrich the gene pool of the tribe. The moral perception of cannibalism may be amended when seen from within the social structures or having regards to needs in exceptional circumstances. These illustrations may mitigate somewhat the tendency to extreme relativism and an inclination to deny any generally acceptable standards of human behaviour across disparate cultures.

In spite of the obvious variation in the acceptability of types of conduct in different races, it may be possible to posit some common moral principles, of which these types of conduct are peripheral expressions. An example of such a basic principle might be loyalty to one's kin even though, in some cases, that might be expressed in a distinctively savage manner of dealing with outsiders, unacceptable in other civilizations.

This topic, because of its crucial nature in ethics, will be referred to later. Important aspects of ethical studies, for example the notions of the mores of a community and the 'social contract', are relevant to relativity in ethics.

The deontological and teleological approaches in ethics

There is an even more marked divide in modern ethical literature than that between absolutism and relativism. Ethical systems are considered as deontological or teleological (see pages 46–47 for definitions). These two attitudes to right and wrong may overlap. The deontological–teleological divide of ethics supposes that the ethicist either stresses the moral attitude of the agent, for instance his respect for duty, or looks to the consequences of a proposed act in order to decide on its righteousness, for instance a cost–benefit assessment is brought into operation. The issue between deontology and teleology is often raised by asking: 'Are there some actions that must be done and/or others that must not be done whatever the consequences?' or 'Should we always act so as to bring out the best possible results on the whole?'

Various philosophers from the past are often trotted out as examples of deontologists and teleologists. Kant heads the list of deontologists and is accompanied by such as Spinoza (1632–1677) and Newman. The prime candidate among the teleologists is naturally Machiavelli (1469–1527) but Bentham (1748–1832) and John Stuart Mill follow closely. In real life it may not matter so much whether we classify such philosophers as Aquinas among the deontologists or Marx as a teleologist. What really matters is how each one of us individually addresses morality in this respect.

Having been heavily involved in ethical discussion in the last few years, I have noticed again and again how individuals separate out along this divide. It becomes obvious quite quickly in discussion that some delegates are deontological and some are teleological. Perhaps as in the Gilbert and Sullivan opera, like little Conservatives and Liberals, we are born that way.

There are others who have become aware of this philosophical phenomenon lurking in each one of us. According to various reports in the press, a professor at New York University, Dr Louis Marinoff, was successfully ousting Prozac as a treatment for emotional dilemmas by bringing philosophy off the campus and on to the street. In some cases of distress, for example of a matrimonial nature where continuation in the relationship was desired, he would tune into the deontological inclination of the client. He talked in terms of Kantian deontology with its stress on loyalty to a higher power. In other situations, he said he was quite prepared to talk in terms of consequences. He and other colleagues were readily harnassing both deontology and teleology as practical tools in therapy. His main consideration in this form of treatment was the philosophical insight most helpful to the client (*The Times* 1998).

Deontology and teleology are by no means exclusive one of the other. In fact a moral decision of a teleological nature, because it is made with a view to the consequences of the action, may have a crucial deontological element. The perception of the goodness of the consequences may be purely intuitive and so be deontological in nature.

This close association of the two approaches is most marked in the practical application by an individual of ethical principles. We may find that although we tend to be usually deontological in our judgements – quite definite that right is right and wrong is wrong – occasionally we may be swayed by circumstances. On the other hand, we may regard ourselves as tolerant, flexible and practical, not hidebound by rules. We make our decisions in the light of consequences like true teleologists. However, on some occasions we think enough is enough, sometimes a line must be drawn in the sand.

An illustration of this intermingling of the deontological and teleological approaches is the following Reuter's report:

> ' "Really, it's a question of respect for the deceased and their relatives", said Baptist Pastor Lennart Nilsson, protesting about plans by a Swedish crematorium to burn corpses for use as fuel. "I know that the crematorium in Boras has been providing heat for local restaurants for the past six months, but we here in Helsinborg think differently. After all, on a cold November day, recently bereaved relatives might have felt awkward about Aunt Astrid being used to heat up their houses. It may be environmentally sound but it isn't polite".'
>
> (*Private Eye* 1997)

Ecological correctness is certainly teleologically acceptable but deontology surfaces with a vengeance at the name of Aunt Astrid.

Deontology

The word 'deontology' comes from the Greek word *deon* meaning duty. Deontology includes such ethical systems as intuitionism which looks for an intellectual support for ethical opinions and emotivism which, to put it in a homely fashion, is associated more with a 'gut reaction'. Deontology is the form of moral philosophy that supports the notion of duty and principle, the supremacy of conscience and is expressed in Kant's concept of the categorical imperative.

Deontological principles essentially involve the agent and the special relationships between him, what he does and other people affected by his attitudes and actions. It allows for self-reverential altruism and expresses many of the natural tendencies in human nature. Because of the personal feature of deontology there is provision for that special preference in choice of actions as regards those who are near and dear to us. Special relationships are of significance and so the cold calculating process which may be associated with teleological consequentialism is obviated. One may censure such selectivity in moral attitudes but they mirror real life. Few researchers would be ready to use their pet cat as an animal model. The special one among the rest of the rabbits is not unknown in an animal house.

Deontology caters for duties arising from promises and contracts. Such altruistic pursuits as generosity fit easily into a deontological life style. True remorse and justifiable revenge, natural reactions to one's own crime or that of another, are provided for in deontology. There need be no concern about the need for beneficial consequences (deterrents) to justify punishment. Of course there may be a teleological justification for such actions as fulfil one or other of these duties but the case would need to be made out in each instance and may be obviated by other teleological arguments. Where deontology scores, is that it can make actions described in terms of such special relations to the agent obligatory or wrong as such. Deontology delivers that welcome security of certainty.

There are, in practice, great advantages in acting on principle – that is, deontologically – and in having predetermined principles on which to act.

The intuitionist, with his deontological approach, reports what the moral consciousness of most people in the society say on those moral questions on which a moral judgement has been reached. Deontological ethics can tell us what the moral judgement of our contemporaries says we ought to do. If, however, we ourselves have reached a certain level of critical awareness, it has no means of convincing us that we ought to do it.

Teleology

Teleology, derived from the Greek word *telos* (genitive case *teleos*) meaning, 'end' or 'purpose', is used in ethics in association with such theories as consequentialism and utilitarianism. These two expressions of the teleological approach in ethics will be dealt with in some detail. The exposition of these two forms of teleology should sufficiently elucidate the nature of the teleological aspect of ethical thought.

The consideration of the motives and the consequences of a proposed action as indicative of its moral rectitude moderates the influence of dogmatic principles which may not be relevant to the situation or may even prove to be counter-productive in practice; for example, pacifist appeasement leading to bloodshed. Some negative arguments illustrate the worth of a teleological approach in ethics. The casuistic contortions of men of principle, like the Pharisees, trying to save the truth by the use of the half-truth, is hardly edifying. Even the most exalted principles seem occasionally to cause embarassing difficulties to their apologists.

Some deontologists, while standing by their principles, tend to have a new principle for each occasion. In such cases, undue deference is frequently shown to what is immediately vivid or pressing. It is, however, a primary function of a principle to counteract such subjective preference. In a controversy (October 1994) about the use of rubella vaccine, developed from human fetuses, Ampleforth College rejected the practice. Their spokesman, on television, compassionately regarded its use as justified, however, in the case of pregnant women. Not so much a change of principle, perhaps, as an example of movement from deontology into teleology.

Skipping from an awkward principle to a more acceptable one, by an honest man of principle, (the plain blunt man) occurs occasionally in politics. It was asked, concerning one shady politician on a certain issue: 'Would he stand firm or act on his principles?' Immutable principles impair desirable activities of even the best. It was said of the truly heroic figure, Bonhoeffer – the pacifist involved in the plot to kill Hitler – 'that he did not make a God of his principles'.

Rightly did Socrates quote the poets, and only the poets, as authorities on ethics. Like Kipling in his poem *If*, they often better encapsulate moral truths than philosophers.

Consequentialism

Consequentialism regards the results of an action as a definitive factor of its moral worth. If this means that any end which could be seen in itself as good would justify the use of any means, however bad, then the consequentialist would have to explain how ends differed from means and why this difference was of such moral significance that only an end matters, and means count for nothing. Not even Machiavelli held this view. The consequentialist's view is rather that there is no morally relevant distinction between means and ends. Any badness in the proposed means has to be balanced fairly against the expected goodness of the end, with no special weighing for either (akin to the cost–benefit balancing procedure). It may be possible even for a means which is in itself very bad to be outweighed and therefore 'justified' by a sufficiently good end. Consequentialism requires that everything known to be involved in a course of action should be taken equally into account. It is thus no easy option for it demands, perhaps even on a case-by-case basis, the serious consideration in an ethical light of the chosen end, the means adopted to achieve it, possible side-effects and further consequences of the result. Moderate consequentialists may concede that there are cases in which some aspect of an action may determine its moral quality absolutely. Such an action would be thereby judged either obligatory or wrong without further ado, no matter what else is involved.

It was not only Machiavelli who held that:

> 'A prince, especially a new prince, cannot observe all those things which are considered good in men, being often obliged, in order to maintain the State, to act against faith, against humanity and against religion. A prudent ruler ought not to keep faith when the reasons which made him bind himself no longer exist.'

Hume confirms this view.

> 'There is a maxim very current in the world, which few politicians are willing to avow, but which has been authorized by the practice of all ages, that there is a system of morals calculated for princes, much more free than that which ought to govern private persons.'

Hume argues that treaties of princes are less binding and may be lawfully transgressed for a more trivial motive. The reason he gives is that:

> 'Though the intercourse of States be advantageous and even some times necessary, yet it is not so necessary nor advantageous as among individuals.'

With growth of world trade and multinationals, this is not so true in modern times.

Even within Machiavellism and in international politics, honesty may still be the best policy. If France promises Bosnia that if the Bosnian Serbs attack Sarajevo they will go to war against the Bosnian Serbs, should the promise be kept? In some circumstances this may be hard to decide. Indeed it is difficult to say when it is right to give such assurances. Perhaps it is better to turn from particular cases to regular patterns of conduct. The giving of shaky assurances of this sort, promises which may or may not be fulfilled, is likely to be worse than either giving no such assurances or giving only ones which will be fulfilled, and of which it is known that they will be fulfilled, if the occasion arises. Where there are shaky assurances, the opposing parties are likely each to interpret them optimistically from their own point of view. The Bosnian Serbs are likely to believe that the French will not actually go to war against them if they attack Sarajevo while the Bosnians are likely to believe that the French will go to war against the Bosnian Serbs. The Bosnians are then likely to take greater risks than they otherwise would in their dealings with the Bosnian Serbs. History abounds with examples of unreliable promises being more dangerous than either reliable promises or no promise at all. Remember Munich.

Utilitarianism

For Jeremy Bentham and John Stuart Mill the maximization of happiness was to be the determinant in any situation which appeared to raise moral issues. They devised the 'felicific calculus' for determining the moral worth of any specific action. Bentham incorporated the essential basis of moral equality into his utilitarian system of ethics in the formula: 'each to count for one and none for more than one'. The interests of every being (even the smallest animal?) affected by an action are to be taken into account and given the same weight as the like interests of any other being. Bentham maintained that words like 'ought', 'right' and 'wrong' have no meaning unless interpreted in accordance with the principle of utility. James Mill was of the opinion that the very morality of an action lies, not in the sentiments aroused in the one who perceives or contemplates it, but in the consequences of the action and the fact that the agent intends those consequences. He adds that a rational assertor to the principle of utility approves an action because it is good and calls it good because it conduces to happiness.

A later utilitarianist, Henry Sidgwick, states:

'The good of any one individual isof no more importance, from the point of view of the Universe, than the good of any other.'

Bentham, in his attack on natural law, claims that there is nothing in *a priori* principles which cannot be better stated as an induction from experience and that there is no means of distinguishing true principles from irrational prejudices except by applying this test. Utilitarianism makes the point that principles, whether *a priori* or empirically grounded, are general and abstract but the reality to which they refer and for whose sake they are formulated is the lives of human beings, their satisfactions and their frustrations. That is why utilitarianism became the great bulwark of advances in social reform. Its protagonists pressed constantly for enlightened legislation, particularly in the area of the Poor Law. Restrictions of liberty and support for outmoded moral attitudes were challenged by the Utilitarians. To them, people mattered more than rigid principles or venerable institutions.

The principle of utility

The popularized form of the principle of utility in its most general sense was simply expressed as a desire to produce the greatest happiness of the greatest number. Primarily, the principle was of concern to the individual making decisions of a moral nature. It was the principle which approves or disapproves of actions according to the tendency it appears to have, to augment or diminish the happiness of the person making the decision. Utility is the property of an object or action to produce benefit, advantage, pleasure, good or happiness or to prevent evil, mischief, pain or unhappiness. These desirable or undesirable consequences are initially associated with an individual but also apply to communities since communities are made up of individuals. The interests of the community are the sum total of the interests of the individuals who make up a particular community. It is in the community that the full expression of utilitarianism is to be found. The taking of a poll within a group may be seen as an effort to ascertain what action or conduct is regarded as most conducive to the greatest happiness within that group. Such soliciting of individual opinions may be seen as a way of calculating the 'felicific calculus' associated with utilitarianism.

Formal utilitarianism stated the need for universalization of moral prescriptions. Substantial utilitarianism was the practical expression of this ethical theory. It provided factual beliefs about the interests of people in the real world and what would be the effects of such beliefs.

Act utilitarianism

Where an agent has a choice between courses of action or of inaction, the right decision is the one that produces the most happiness not only for himself but also for those affected by the results of the decision. The greatest resulting happiness was usually interpreted hedonistically – that is, a balance of pleasure over pain. It is in the working-out of this balance that utilitarianism, particularly act utilitarianism, runs into daunting difficulties. There is a far from realistic suggestion that for each alternative course of action it is possible in theory to measure all the amounts of pleasure it produces for different people in different situations. These estimations would be added up. Similarly, all forms of predictable distress from the course of action would be assessed. The sum total of the resulting pleasure and the sum total of the resulting displeasure, both of these terms being used in the broadest sense, would be weighed one against the other. If such an equation could possibly be established, the recommended morally correct decision would be the one choosing the action that would produce the greatest positive or the least negative balance of pleasure over pain.

It seems natural to seek pleasure and to avoid pain and distress and it seems sensible to balance these against each other, even to put up with a certain amount of pain in order to achieve a quantity of pleasure that outweighs it. In taking the general happiness as the standard of right actions, this proposal seems to satisfy at once the presumptions that moral actions should be unselfish and that moral principles should be fair. This seems to provide a coherent system of conduct. All decisions about what is right or wrong would flow directly from a single source, whereas in other proposed first-order moral systems we find a multiplicity of independent rules and principles, even perhaps in certain circumstances conflicting with one another. Indeed many common-sense or intuitive rules can be justified by their tendency to promote general happiness but where two common-sense rules come into conflict we need to appeal to utility to decide what to do.

Rule utilitarianism

Rule utilitarianism differs from act utilitarianism in that it makes the general happiness – not directly but only indirectly, by way of a two-stage procedure – the criterion of right action. It is summed up in Austin's (1911–1960) dictum: 'Our rules should be fashioned on utility; our conduct on our rules.' Austin continues 'To find out whether an individual action is right or not, we must discover its "tendency".' The 'tendency' of an action is the probable effect upon general happiness, if acts of the class to which this one belongs were generally done rather than generally omitted. Even act utilitarians regularly admit the use of rules of thumb, since it would be either impossible or absurdly laborious to calculate in detail the utility of each action. What is distinctive of rule utilitarianism is the suggestion that the two-stage procedure, and the rules which in it intervene between utility and the individual choice, have some substantial merit besides the economy of quick decision.

It has been suggested that rule utilitarianism can escape some of the more violent conflicts that break out between act utilitarianism and common moral beliefs or 'intuitions'. There may be cases where an act utilitarian would have to say that it is right to kill an innocent person (perhaps to save others), to invade rights, to torture suspects, to break solemn agreements or to cheat. The rule utilitarian, however, can say that each individual act is wrong because the general performance of acts of each of these classes would plainly have a very bad effect on the general happiness. Rules as well as actions may be justified by their own type of utility.

Numerous objections against utilitarianism

Who are included in the 'happiness of the greatest number': all human beings or all sentient beings? A theory that equates good with pleasure and evil with pain can hardly exclude any creatures capable of feeling either pleasure or pain. Does this concern embrace only those who are now alive or also future generations (enter ecology), and if so, only those who will exist or also those that might exist? We may have to compare alternative courses of action, one of which would lead to there being a large population each of whose members was only moderately happy and another course of action which would lead to a smaller population in which each person was very happy. In the first case there may be more total utility or happiness; in the second case higher average uitility or happiness. Which of the two, then, is it whose maximization is to be the criterion of right action? Is it really possible to measure quantities of pleasure and pain of various qualities even for the same person in different sorts of experience? Is pleasure sufficiently of the same type of experience as pain to be measurable on the same scale and so to allow a quantity of one to balance a quantity of the other? Interpersonal (and what about inter-species?) measurement presents greater difficulties.

Is the proposed criterion simply the greatest happiness or average happiness? Does it matter how happiness is distributed? Is a state of affairs in which one person is supremely happy and nine are miserable (equivalent situations have existed in many cultures and were accepted and perpetuated), better than one in which all ten are equally happy, provided only that the total balance of happiness is greater?

Utilitarians might try to deal with interpersonal distribution by the familiar rule that happiness should be proportionate to merit. This rule may act as an incentive device for increasing the aggregate of happiness, if merit is measured by a person's contribution to the happiness of others.

Bernard Williams has argued against utilitarianism. He suggests that in becoming capable of acting out of universal concern, people would have to be stripped of the motives on which most of what is of value in human life is based, for example close affection, private pursuits and many kinds of competition and struggle. He thinks that the utilitarian trimming-down of morality to fit present human capacity might bring morality into contempt. He is dissatisfied with the prosaic presentation of a morality bereft of ideals.

Utilitarianism lacks the more forceful sanctions which readily attach themselves to other systems of morals. Conscientious feelings and guilt can be firmly associated with breaking specific rules such as those of justice; for example:

- the rules against invading what are recognized, in a particular society, as some-one's rights
- respect for agreements.

The making of moral decisions on calculation alone seems to lack the emotional warmth associated with human actions. It would seem that, for many, because of the influence of feelings on behaviour, accepted established rules rather than general utilitarian principles form the core of common morality.

In some cases the stress on the absolute role of utility in deciding the morality of an action may lead to ludicrous results. A benign enslavement could indicate the acceptability of slavery. An extreme Utilitarian could condemn capital punishment of fanatical terrorists, regarding it as an inadequate deterrent. On the other hand he could argue for its use against those who wrongly park their cars. Such carelessness reduces excessively communal happiness and could be the occasion of much suffering by delaying unduly the emergency services, even costing lives. He would have no doubt that in such cases it would act as an efficient deterrent against slovenly drivers. Road hogs are not the stuff of which martyrs are made.

Beneficence – an endowing with benefits – may be a suitable basis for a relationship with associates in a common enterprise but is inadequate as a basis of a relationship with friends. It fails to characterize the close relationship we experience in a fellowship. A relationship within a fellowship is a kind of being-for-others and appears to be superior in moral tone to hedonistic utilitarianism.

The final objection in this list has a similar tone to some of the previous complaints against utilitarianism. It is based on the difficulty of defining essential details for the application of a utilitarian ethic. No intellectual enlightenment, no scrutiny of facts, can decide how far the interests of the lower animals should be regarded when conflicting with those of men (Bentham claimed his pleasure of eating meat outweighed the pain involved in the slaughter of the animal) (Bentham 1789). Similarly, what enlightenment or scrutiny could decide how far a person is bound, or allowed, to promote the welfare of his own nation, or his own welfare, at the cost of other nations or other individuals? Not only would Sidgwick's moral axiom, 'I ought not to prefer my own lesser good to the greater good of another', not appear in any way self-evident in many cultures in the past but would even be regarded as absurd in some cultures in modern times. Who is that 'another' to whose greater good I ought not to prefer my own lesser good? A fellow-countryman, a criminal, another mammal, a fish – all without distinction?

Finally, an evil propensity in society is the 'I'm all right Jack' syndrome. Each is concerned with his own interest. The utilitarian stress on the interest of all counters that.

Scepticism

Scepticism, in this context, embraces all those ethical theories which cast doubt on the possibility of arriving at an objective and universally acceptable basis for moral rectitude. Early among such sceptical moral philosophers were some of the Sophists of ancient Greece but scepticism in ethics has come to the forefront in more recent times. The main outlines of this approach to ethics have already been explored in the sections on such topics as the term 'good' and the term 'ought' (see Chapter 1).

It is sufficient here to point out that the leading figure in ethical scepticism, as in scepticism as such, was David Hume. Hume's Law, the denial of any rational justification to pass from 'is' to 'ought', was a watershed in the history of Western morals. Later moral sceptics followed in his wake and those seeking certitude in ethics were often obsessed with the need to refute Hume's challenge.

Hume (1711–1776) was not typical of moral philosophers of that era. In the previous century, Spinoza (1632–1677) had produced his mystical work *Ethics Mathematically Demonstrated* and Bishop Butler (1692–1752) had expounded intuitionism in his sermons. A little earlier, Thomas Hobbes (1588–1679) and John Locke (1632–1704) had considered ethics within a political and legal frame. It was from their learned works that Rousseau (1712–1778) developed his theory in his *Social Contract*.

Hobbes had argued that the concept of a primitive social contract created mutual obligations which did not exist prior to the constituted State. Locke, however, argued that moral principles and obligations existed before the creation of the State, so that men could change the State if it failed to uphold these principles. The idea is of ancient origin and is referred to by both Plato and Lucretius (first century BCE). Although in the main a neglected theory without having a factual base in history, it is not completely rejected. John Rawls (b. 1921), a modern ethicist, in his work *The Cry of Justice*, presented his idea on a theoretical level (Rawls 1971). This attitude to ethics did attempt to provide some perceptible basis for social morality but was sceptical of the existence of any universal criterion of righteousness, either within a person themselves or from authority or objectively, except within the scope of a supposed agreement. There seems to be a similar pattern of thought in this approach to that found in the modern ethical concept of an 'institution'.

Immanuel Kant (1724–1804)

The complex and comprehensive philosophy of Kant, one of the greatest of thinkers, was a direct reaction to the scepticism of Hume. Kant reinstated the sense of duty as a standard of right conduct. He presented it as subjective rather than objective, as personal rather than as imposed from outside. Kant called this commanding sense of righteousness, the 'categorical imperative'. He explained this concept in his *Critique of Practical Reason* as a personal inner dictate defining and ordering right conduct irrespective of intention or consequence. He attempted to graft objectivity on to this subjective moral force by claiming that we should only feel compelled to act upon a maxim which we would wish to see accepted as a universal law. Kant thought we should act as we would wish others to act; a sort of 'do as you would be done by'. By urging this form of universalization, Kant did not imply that everyone would agree with a proposed regulation but that an acceptable lifestyle would be maintained if everyone abided by it. His suggestion could provide both the assurance of internal conviction and the objectivity of general acceptance. The notion of the categorical imperative fitted in well with authoritarian culture to which Kant belonged, in which 'befehl ist befehl' (an order is an order) became the shibboleth of the good Prussian citizen. The thoughts of Kant, a dominant philosopher of the modern period (*c.* AD 1500 to the present day), deeply influenced later views on ethics, particularly the theories of intuitionists.

The Kantian ethic, with its emphasis on equality and no exceptions before the law, seems to be an excellent analysis of the distinctive nature of associate morality, concerned with relations within the community. Unfortunately, rigoristic theories of this type go wrong, not in their analysis or associate morality, but by presenting it as the *only* morality.

Intuitionism

An early exponent of intuitionism was Joseph Butler (1692–1752). He taught the existence of a moral faculty which apprehended one's duty in specific circumstances. Adam Smith (1723–1740) referred to these moral faculties as the: 'viceregents of God within us', who:

> 'never fail to punish the violation of them by the torments of inward shame and self-condemnation; and, on the contrary always reward obedience with tranquility of mind, with contentment, and self-satisfaction'.

It may be worth noting that these are the words of a famous economist, not of a hell-fire preacher. They come from a time when such unfortunate words as guilt, shame and punishment were considered politically correct terms. Even Hutcheson (1694–1746), who raises the question why the moral sense should not vary in different men as the palate does, considers it 'to be naturally destined to command all the other powers'.

Later intuitionists like Rashdall (1858–1924) developed and refined this moral faculty akin to the conscience in Christianity and the categorical imperative of Kant. Intuitionists accept that we have a capacity to discern *a priori* truths which some regard as self-evident like mathematical axioms. Moral truths are perceived in the form of general principles, for example one should tell the truth.

A major difficulty with intuitionism is that there are mortals who seem to be merrily unaware of these fundamental moral principles, categorical though they are for intuitionists.

Conscience

This an old-fashioned word with a religious flavour yet a concept which even in the vicissitudes of total war has been given credence by hard-headed politicians, in the recognition of the reality of conscientious objection. Perhaps, because of its devout connotations, the term 'conscience' is not now so prevalent in the Groves of Academe. Less positive and more scholastically acceptable terms have come to the fore. Where once people spoke of a lack of conscience, a wider term tends to be used – 'amoral'; or in more defined cases of ignoring the directives of a conscience – 'judgemental withdrawal'. In spite of such niceties in the area of moral awareness, many ordinary people in the outside world talk in terms of conscience, of having a conscience, of not 'being allowed to do' something by their conscience, of the duty to respect somebody's conscience and condemnation of those who have no conscience. Granted, such people do naïvely talk of evil people rather than of those 'who are morally challenged'. Conscience belongs more to the area of moral awareness than to the field of ethical speculation. Perhaps that is why it is the most commonly used term in popular parlance on moral decisions. Conscience is considered to be at the sharp end (occasions when each one must deal with moral questions for herself or himself) of the assessment of right or wrong conduct.

Conscience is a tangible practical expression of the ethical theory of the intuitionists. Obviously, descriptions of the common term 'conscience' vary tremendously. For some it is never more realistically described than in the form of the mythical cricket on Pinocchio's shoulder or as the alleged enlarging of the puppet's sensitive nose in the absence of truth. Conscience has been described in many ways which were in much more learned form than the fairy-tale portrayal. Among the most ponderous is the definition from Scholasticism:

> 'It is the proximate subjective criterion of a moral act or a practical judgement indicating that some determined act must be done because it is good or must not be done because it is bad.'

The term 'conscience' may refer to our rational judgement of the situation before us, based on apprehension of the factors involved in that situation, and the values and principles of conduct which we have accepted as being normative. In this sense, the dictates of our conscience are in fact the final conclusions of our understanding of the matters at issue.

So far as we are aware of conscience in ourselves and in others, it may appear, because of its immediacy, to be a kind of 'simple divination'. In fact, its conclusions are the products of a 'multiform and intricate process' of unconscious reasoning by which we take into account the cumulative significance of a range of probabilities which are independent of each other and too fine to avail separately, too subtle and circuitous to be convertible into syllogisms, and too numerous and various for such conversion, even were they convertible. This process of reasoning in any particular case is impossible to express in the cumbersome apparatus of verbal reasoning. Its conclusions, nevertheless, are the product of reasoning and, furthermore, they are very much our own conclusions because they are in great measure made by ourselves and belong to our personal character and apply our own principles.

By 'conscience' we refer to our awareness of the conclusions of an unconscious process of reasoning, so it is not only legitimate but also necessary for us to regard them as authoritative for us. They declare what we fundamentally assess to be our duty. To go against them is to go against our best judgement. At the same time, we must not forget that these conclusions – and so the deliverances of conscience as understood – are only as sound as the reasoning which produces them. Because that reasoning may be partly based on mistaken principles and values, because it may have misapprehended the situation, and because its connection of items may be faulty, its conclusions in any particular case may be in error even though we suppose it to be binding upon us. The moral danger of using the conscience as an absolute guide of conduct is that it may be wholly subjective, blissfully ignoring the realities of the outside world.

The downside of conscience

The unquestioning acceptance of the dictates of conscience can produce the most unfortunate results. This is not surprising when we consider how a conscience might be formed. A conscience may be the product of childhood programming or may be formed within the dogmatism of a narrow cult. Frequently, the rejection of religiously instilled strict rules of conduct in youth can evolve in later life into a contempt for accepted morality (Joyce 1914). Even taking the most optimistic view of conscience and presuming that it had been moulded by evolutionary forces, the best we could suppose is that the conscience might lay down principles which may prove useful (Mackie 1990).

Because of the dangers of non-conformity associated with conscience, moral theologians insisted that the individual has a moral duty to form her or his conscience in keeping with authoritarian teachings. In this context it was presumed that a right conscience was based on divine revelation as interpreted officially in ecclesiastical circles. Conscience in this setting was by no means seen as a purely human phenomenon, evolved by evolutionary forces.

Emotivism

Emotivism, as an ethical theory, stems from the presumption that to name an act as good or bad, ultimately implies that it is apt to give rise to an emotion of approval or disapproval in the person who pronounces the judgement. Moral concepts, for the emotivist, are essentially generalizations of tendencies in certain phenomena to give rise to emotions which inspire praise or condemnation.

Moral judgements as value judgements are expressions of the speaker's emotions about the action, person or situation to which they refer and not, as they grammatically appear to be, statements of fact, true or false. Emotivists emphasize the distinction between utterances that express feelings, such as ejaculations or expletives, for example 'Dear dear me!', and utterances that state that a certain feeling is being experienced. It is to the former that they assimilate judgements of value; the latter are regarded as descriptions of the emotional state of the speaker.

Emotivism was set out as an explicit theory by A.J. Ayer (1910–1989) and was developed by C.L. Stevenson (1908–1979). This ethical theory grew out of the speculation on the apparent irresolubility of disagreement about morality. For many emotivists the distinctive feature of value judgements was that their acceptance by someone committed that person to acting in a certain way, whereas the acceptance of a statement of fact committed him only to the adoption of the corresponding belief. If this is correct, value judgements are more like imperatives than merely expressive utterances. As a result, emotivism, notably in the influential works of R.M. Hare, has largely given way to imperativism or prescriptivism (Hare 1972).

Although rooted in the emotional side of our nature, our moral opinions are in a large measure amenable to reason. In every society the traditional notions as to what is good or bad, obligatory or indifferent, are commonly accepted by the majority of people without further reflection. By tracing them to their source it will be found that not a few of these notions have their origin in sentimental likings and antipathies, to which a scrutinizing and enlightened judge can attach little importance; whilst on the other hand, he must account blameable many an act and omission which public opinion, out of thoughtlessness, treats with indifference. It will, moreover, appear that a moral estimate often survives the cause from which it sprang.

Whilst the import of the predicate of a moral judgement may be traced back to an emotion in the one who pronounces the judgement, it is generally assumed to possess the character of universality or objectivity as well. The statement that an act is good or bad does not merely refer to an individual emotion; it has reference to an emotion of a more public character. Very often it even implies some vague assumption that the act must be recognized as good or bad by everybody who possesses a sufficient knowledge of the case and of all attendant circumstances and who has a 'sufficiently developed' moral consciousness. We are not willing to admit that our moral convictions are a mere matter of taste and we are inclined to regard convictions differing from our own as errors. This characteristic of our moral judgements has been adduced as an argument against the emotionalist theory of moral origins and has led to the belief that moral concepts represent qualities which are discerned by reason.

Our tendency to objectivize moral judgements is not sufficient ground for referring them to the province of reason. If there is a difference between moral judgements and others that are rooted in the subjective sphere of experience, it is, largely, a difference of degree rather than in kind. The aesthetic judgements which have an emotional origin also lay claim to a certain amount of 'objectivity'. By saying that a piece of music is beautiful, we do not merely mean that it gives ourselves aesthetic enjoyment, but we make a latent assumption that it must have a similar effect upon everybody who is sufficiently musical to appreciate it. This objectivity ascribed to judgements which have a merely subjective origin springs in the first place from the similarity of the mental constitution of human beings, and, generally speaking, the tendency to regard them as objective increases proportionally with the consensus of opinion. If 'there is no disputing tastes' that is because taste is so extremely variable. Yet even in this instance we recognize a certain 'objective' standard by speaking of 'bad' and 'good' taste.

Some modern moral philosophers

G.E. Moore (1873–1958)

The *Principia Ethica* of Moore (Moore 1903) epitomizes the highly general, speculative and sceptical approach to the study of ethics. Moore laid great emphasis on the fallaciousness of any attempt to define 'good' in any way. He particularly condemned any attempt to define 'good' in terms of a natural object. The whole thrust of Moore's speculation was analytical and any positive indications within his writings were towards intuitionism.

His theory of conduct is extremely simple. There is no such thing as a moral obligation which is not an obligation to produce the greatest amount of good. 'Our, "duty", therefore, can only be defined as that action which will cause more good to exist in the universe than any possible alternative.' What we ought to do is always to be determined by a calculation of the consequences of our acts, and the assessment of the goodness or badness of these. Thus, on the question of conduct, Moore is in far closer agreement with the utilitarians than with any other moral philosophers. Moore talks about consequences recognized intuitively as good, not consequences which can be proved to be useful empirically. Utility is not his criterion for 'good'; that is utilitarianism. An empirical assessment of 'good' would involve the naturalistic fallacy so forcefully rejected by Moore.

Like all forms of intuitionism Moore's moral philosophy depended on a surrounding philosophical environment hospitable to metaphysics. That means an intellectual atmosphere in which there is an acceptance that there are real properties and states of affairs that are distinct from the properties and states we can experience and which the natural sciences study. Furthermore, if intuitionism is to have credibility there must be some hope of eventual agreement on ethical insights. If ethical disagreements are sufficiently deep and unresolvable and if neither one side nor the other can make a creditable claim to better insight, then it will be doubted that there is an objective truth to be known. These requisites of any acceptable form of intuitionism increasingly failed to hold in the first half of the twentieth century. This was partly because of the initial analytic impetus of Russell (1872–1970) and even, in fact, of Moore himself, who had rather weakened his own cause by his sceptical approach. On a wider canvas, Anglo-American philosophy became more naturalist and empiricist, and the metaphysical underpinnings of both con-sequentialism and deontological intuitionism began to seem less plausible. An equally important cause of the rejection of intuitionism was the increasing erosion of ethical consensus.

Eventually, the negative emphasis of Moore's teaching came to the fore. Moore had said that while intrinsic goodness is a property, it is not an intrinsic property. He said that intrinsic properties seem to describe the intrinsic nature of what possesses them, in a sense in which predicates of value never do. Part of what was distinctive about ethical terms for Moore, then, was that they do not describe things in the ordinary way. To say of aesthetic enjoyment that it is intrinsically good is not further to describe what it is. To accept Moore's view of the property of intrinsic value, one had to be willing to believe that reality contains properties that are neither part of anything's (describable) nature nor capable of any sort of empirical confirmation. In a climate of increasing empiricism, such statements tended to be understood as implying that the characteristic of ethical terms is that they are not used to refer to any aspect of reality at all.

The negative aspect of Moore's ethics was further confirmed, for many, by his claim that the fundamental propositions of ethics do not admit of proof. He did not see this as problematic as long as there could be agreement on ethical matters: 'What we seek in ethics is agreement, rather than proof.'

Moore had set the pattern for ethics in the twentieth century. He had begun his *Principia Ethica* with the charge that philosophical dispute in ethics was largely due 'to the attempt to answer questions, without first discovering precisely what question it is which you desire to answer'. Stevenson, and other moral philosophers who fol-lowed him, could not have agreed more. They appreciated his questions but they did not accept his suggestions of the directions from which answers might come.

Charles Stevenson (1908–1979)

The intuitionism of Moore was considered by the non-cognitivists such as Charles Stevenson. For the non-cognitivists ethics is an ongoing human activity of moral debate that is complete within itself and not responsible for objective ethical facts. Indeed, for them there are no ethical facts. Stevenson further argued that what makes the meaning of ethical terms irreducible, as he believed Moore had shown, is that they have an emotive meaning that non-ethical terms do not. Ethical terms are used both to express and excite emotion. (There are shades here of the lin-guistic philosophy of L. Wittgenstein (1889–1951) and J.L. Austin (1911–1960).) They are instruments used in the complicated interplay and readjustment of human interests. Ethical terms are not intended to express propositions that are lit-erally true or false. That is not what ethical language is for. It is used not to say something about the world, but to express an attitude towards it, and to encour-age others to do the same. Moore had indeed said 'What we need in ethics is agreement rather than proof' but he had said it from a metaphyscial background very diverse from the reality envisaged by the non-cognitivists (Stevenson 1937 and 1944).

W.D. Ross (1877–1971)

This deontological intuitionist defended common sense morality (a non-starter in philosophy). Unfortunately his ordinary man's approach suffered, as had Moore's intuitionism, because of the collapse of a consensus of opinion on ethical matters in modern times.

Ross, like Moore, believed that fundamental ethical propositions could be directly known through what he called intuition. Both were fundamentalists in moral epistemology; they believed that ethical convictions are justified if, and only if, they are self-evident or deducible from others that are justified. Ross likened ethical insight to the sort of insight a mathematician might have into the truth of mathematical axioms. He was careful to insist that only propositions about *prima facie* duty can be evident in this way and not propositions about what it is right to do, all things considered. Ross, however, vehemently attacked Moore's deontological consequentialism associated with the awareness of the goodness of a state of affairs intuitively perceived. Ross thought that Moore's consequentialism oversimplified the complexity that reflection on common moral convictions reveals.

The centrepiece of Ross's ethics was a plurality of *prima facie* duties that includes:

(1)   duties of fidelity to promise and contract
(2)   duties of reparation
(3)   duties of gratitude
(4)   duties of justice
(5)   duties of beneficence
(6)   duties of self-improvement
(7)   duties of non-maleficence.

While rough generalizations can be made about the relative incumbency of *prima facie* duties, for example that it is more incumbent not to harm than to benefit, there are no hard-and-fast rules. While we can know what our *prima facie* duties are in a particular instance, we generally cannot know with certainty which is most incumbent, what would be right on balance. Ethics cannot provide any certain standards here. That is beyond its competency.

Ross claimed he had the support of common conviction for his list but it could still be argued that his theory gave no deeper explanation for his selection of those particular ethical duties (Ross 1930).

Naturalism (the naturalistic fallacy)

Naturalism, in an ethical setting, is a general term usually applied to various forms of consequentialism, except, of course, to the deontological consequentialism of Moore. According to naturalists the criterion of right action is some empirical feature of the natural world such as the happiness of sentient beings, following in the tradition of hedonistic utilitarians; or the self-preservation of an individual or the group, as in the case of Marxism. For naturalists, moral statements are genuine propositions, the truth or falsity of which can be tested. Naturalists maintain that the facts that verify moral statements are of an ordinary empirical kind. They are not of a supernatural character as supposed in moral theology; nor constituents of an autonomous realm of moral values, accessible only to a special moral faculty as proposed by the intuitionists.

It was the ethical theory of naturalism that Moore first branded as the naturalistic fallacy. He described this fallacy as the mistake of defining 'good' in terms of ordinary empirical expressions such as 'pleasant' or 'desired'; or indeed of giving any analysis of 'good', that is to say any definition intended to elucidate its meaning.

Pragmatism

The early pragmatists, such as William James, held that all possible kinds of value judgements were judgements of means to ends. To say that anything is good is to say that it is fitted for some special purpose and that it was conducive to the general end of the action, namely the good (James 1898).

This form of empiricism was developed in the USA by C.S. Peirce (1839–1914) and John Dewey (1859–1952). They interpreted the meaning and justification of their beliefs in terms of their 'practical' effects or content.

Dewey's influence on American philosophy has been considerable. Several of his writings were concerned with ethics, and in particular with the problem of how to distinguish ethical from non-ethical terms. His theory on value judgements was extended to cover not only value judgements ordinarily so called, but all judgements. 'True' and 'real' were also viewed as part of 'the good'; they were each a particular kind of satisfaction of desire. Therefore any fact whatsoever would be judged by the same standard. If I state that something is red, or if I state that it is good, what I say will be allowed to be true if regarding it as red or regarding it as good are conducive to the satisfaction of desires of different kinds. Thus the distinction between judgements of value and judgements of fact has been obliterated. Let us look at Dewey's own words:

> 'A judgement about what is to be desired and enjoyed is . . . a claim on future action; it possesses a *de jure* and not merely a *de facto* quality. It is in effect a judgement that the thing "will do". It involves a prediction; it contemplates a future in which the thing will continue to serve; it will do. It asserts a consequence that the thing will actively institute; it will do.'

Situation ethics

Situation ethics is the most obvious expression of relativism. Its relativity avoids the most crippling effect of absolutism in ethics. In the past, absolute moral stances have changed but slowly and often after centuries of circuitous arguments as in the case of usury. Occasionally, the rules of right conduct were bent in practice, for example as regards monogamy or when strict concern for righteous observance deteriorated into ludicrous forms of casuistry, such as the observance of the Sabbath.

It is true that these controversies were more often argued out in moral theology, the more dominant force in the ages of faith, than in moral philosophy. The existence of the controversies, however, and the changing attitudes illustrate the need for flexibility in ethics, at least as regards first-order ethical judgements, particularly those of a lesser degree of generality.

This more flexible and modern approach to morality insists against the legalism of traditional morality, that the right solution to any moral problem depends much more on the situation itself than on any general external code. This flexibility goes beyond the ordinary acceptance of established exceptions to mandatory rules or the presumed agreed priority of moral obligations. Even in the past, few disputed the suspension of the serious commandment 'Thou shalt not kill', in cases of self-defence. It may be a caricature of situation ethics to say that it implies that the exception does not prove the rule but that the exception becomes the rule, but this phrase indicates where the emphasis lies.

This ethical system avoids such heart-searching as is seen in the first book of Plato's *Republic*. The essence of that dispute was whether the supposed absolute moral dictum 'to each his due', binds one to return the weapon of a roaring drunk or raving maniac to its rightful owner. If morality is perceived after the manner of the laws of the Medes and Persians, then with absolute unchangeable rules hard cases proliferate and intractable self-righteous stances abound. It was J. Fletcher who expounded this modern and understanding approach to morality. He drew attention to the importance of circumstances and motives which are the realities of moral acts rather than cold facts and rigid laws. It is not difficult to perceive a distinction between a wrong action done for the right reason (the ubiquitous white lie) and a good deed done for an evil motive (officiously, for purposes of inheritance or insurance, reviving a person who has attempted suicide.)

Where there is a clash of principles, Fletcher claimed that the decisive factor was love. (He was probably thinking more along the lines of the Greek term *agape* (fellowship, friendship) than the other forms of love expressed by the Greek terms *philos* (liking, affection) or *eros* (fondness and sexual love).) This moral outlook is reminiscent of the great moral maxim 'Love your neighbour as yourself'. The old question must automatically follow this directive: 'Who is my neighbour; the laboratory rat?'

Situation ethics is no mere passing expression of permissiveness. Perhaps, because of the relative stability of modes of behaviour in a single generation we may deceive ourselves into believing that these principles or generalizations are stable for all time. Yet the ethical precepts which governed attitudes and practice a century ago with regard to child labour, colonization and women's rights, would hardly be acceptable today. Situation ethics may deteriorate, no doubt, into mere expediency or at worst be an expression of personal preference. (Unfortunately such preference may be contingent upon the digestion of the chief technician, the hormonal imbalance of the director or the pet aversion of the inspector.) The inherent weakness of situation ethics was exposed in *Tom Brown's Schooldays*, long before the expression was in vogue. 'He never wants anything but what's right and fair; only when you come to settle what's right and fair, it's everything he wants and nothing that you want.'

Usually, however, those who hold by situation ethics are realists. They do not regard society as some ideal structure which can be governed by abstract and absolute rules. They deal with the problem in hand and provide an ethical framework for discussion.

Utilitarians, on the whole, held that established moral rules, such as the rule not to commit murder, must be regarded as universally binding for two reasons: first because the wisdom of past generations had discovered that the consequences of murder are in fact conducive to misery rather than happiness; second, because even in the case of an apparent exception, where the murder might seem certain to have good consequences (e.g. the assassination of a tyrant), the rule should still be kept, because in general it is right, and one breach of it has, among other things, the consequence of weakening the authority of the rule which we wish to see generally observed. But John Stuart Mill does not deny the possibility that sometimes these general moral principles may conflict with each other, or may seem inadequate to the complexities of the situation, and in this case a direct consideration of the particular contemplated action, without reference to general principles, may be necessary, and an attempt must be made to assess the consequences of this individual act. In general, Moore is in complete agreement with this view. He states more clearly than any utilitarian that there can be no certainty attaching to moral rules. Since moral rules lay down duties, and since duties are determined by consequences, they can never be more than probably right, since certainty about the consequences of actions is impossible. In the case of fairly broad types of action, such as lying, stealing or murder, the probability that the consequences will be harmful are fairly high, and Moore would subscribe to the two reasons given, particularly by the rule utilitarians, for not breaking these general, well-worn moral rules.

Moore, like act utilitarians, is far more explicit than John Stuart Mill in allowing that there may be a great number of cases in which the only moral rule which would apply would be a new or revolutionary rule, or where, owing to the complexity and particularity of the circumstances, no rule can be formulated at all. Sometimes where there is no stock rule to help us, we have to make our own predictions and assessments. For example, views on cannibalism in extreme circumstances may vary. Each case must be decided on its own facts. In short, situation ethics.

Situation ethics may provide a practical solution when other ethical theories may be found wanting. It allows for the difference between those cases where the possession of a principle, the avoidance of breaking a rule, is the paramount consideration; for instance, where we feel we must keep a a promise because there is a principle against breaking promises. In other cases we may feel it would be immoral to be bound by any ready-made principle, since none would be adequate to the situation. The classic case discussed at length by moral theologians was King Herod's evil pledge to the dancing Salome which cost John the Baptist his head.

It should be realized that it is in second-order ethics that scepticism predominates rather than in first-order ethics. It is first-order ethics which are the grass roots of accepted morality, in so far as we can say that any particular form of morality is generally accepted. Morality, in turn, may be regarded in modern terms as applied ethics.

The reader may rightly ask: 'Is all this speculative material leading anywhere?' Some conclusions may be drawn even if only of a negative nature. It may be suggested that though simplistic theories in this complex matter are inadequate, the more sophisticated theories are not credible enough to be obviously true, albeit acceptable to some.

That is hardly a satisfactory result of two-and-a-half millennia of philosophical speculation. It does, however, provide a salutary warning against naïve acceptance of plausible falsehoods presented as axioms. The inability to find a solution does not *per se* prove a solution does not exist. Absence of evidence is not evidence of absence although it is a good hint on which to base a doubt. There is always the possibility that one is looking in the wrong direction.

It is reasonable for a newcomer to ethics to be a little bewildered by the diversity of ethical theories. Rightly they may feel a certain empathy with the phrase: 'the triviality of the debate over "is"/"ought".'

Once again, Omar Khayyám injects a little common sense into ethereal speculations:

> 'The grape that can with logic absolute
> The two-and-seventy jarring sects confute.'

I am aware that some of my students have been more vociferous on moral philosophy in the local hostelry than in the lecture hall.

References

Bentham, J. (1789) This telling admission by Jeremy Bentham occurs in Chapter XVII on Penal Law in his *An Introduction to the Principles of Morals and Legislation*. His more famous opinion, 'The question is not; "Can they reason?" nor "Can they talk?" but "Can they suffer?"', was a reflection on Descartes's dismissive comment: 'Animals cannot talk, therefore they cannot think, therefore they cannot feel'. This expression of Bentham's concern for animals will be referred to later in the text. It is fitting here to quote more fully his opinion on the eating, or in his case the enjoyment, of meat:

> 'There is a very good reason why we should be suffered to eat such of them as we like to eat: we are better for it, and they are never the worse. They have none of those long-protracted anticipations of future misery which we have. The death they suffer in our hands commonly is, and always may be, a speedier, and by that means a less painful one, than that which would await them in the inevitable course of nature.'

Fletcher, J. (1966) *Situation Ethics*.
Hare, R.M. (1972) Emotivism, as an ethical theory formulated primarily by Hare, appears in his book *Applications of Moral Philosophy*, London.
James, W. (1898) An early expression of the pragmatic approach to ethics occurs in William James' book *Philosophical Conceptions and Practical Results*.
Joyce, J. (1914) Joyce strikes painful chords in the memories of those who have experienced programming or even brain-washing in their early years, done for one's own good and

with the best of intentions by devoted educationalists. The theme has never been better expounded than in his *Portrait of the Artist as a Young Man.*

Mackie, J.L. (1990) Mackie clearly delineates the limited role that can be realistically played by conscience in the formation of a morality. *Ethics*, p. 124, Penguin.

Moore, G.E. (1903) *Principia Ethica.*

Private Eye (1997) Reuter's report, 29 July.

Rawls, J. (1971) *The Cry of Justice.* Harvard Press.

Ross, W.D. (1930) Ross's theory introducing the idea of a popularly accepted form of morality appears in *The Right and the Good.*

Singer, P. (ed.) (1992) *Applied Ethics.* Oxford University Press, Oxford.

Stevenson, C.L. (1937), (1944) Stevenson appears to have distanced ethical thought from the real world and from facts, more so than is even implicit in the writings of Moore. Stevenson's speculations on ethics are certainly at the far end of the spectrum from the so-called naturalistic fallacy which had been attributed by his predecessors to earlier moral philosophers such as the down-to-earth Utilitarians. Stevenson's extreme view of ethical terms as purely emotive is presented in his works *The Emotive Meaning of Ethical Terms* (1937) and *Ethics and Language* (1944).

The Times (1998) A full report of the services provided by this enterprising philosopher, Dr Louis Marinoff, was published in *The Times*, 8 March.

Westermark, E. (1932) Westermark aggressively argued the case for relativisim in ethics in his work *Ethical Relativity*, London, 1932.

Williams, B. (1985a) The exposition of the 'Socratic Question' is the theme of the whole of *Ethics and the Limits of Philosophy*, Harvard Press, 1985.

Williams, B. (1985b) Williams comments on the earliest form of relativism in moral philosophy in *Ethics and the Limits of Philosophy*, p. 81, Harvard University Press, Cambridge, Massachusetts.

Chapter 3

Seeking a Norm of Morality

Introduction

The concept of a norm of morality, a criterion of right and wrong conduct, belongs more to the practical application of morality in everyday life, than to philosophical discussion. An acceptable and effective norm of morality would enable us to assess readily the righteousness of an action or a mode of conduct.

Even in ordinary social behaviour there is a continual application of standards to conduct. Standards that are immediately perceived and easily understood. To return to a topic alluded to earlier (perhaps a subject which may be of little consequence to many but to a committed client of public transport is of more than passing interest), there is nothing more practical than the prosaic morality of the queue. Most experienced passengers readily acknowledge the wisdom of this procedure. One who contravenes this accepted custom is immediately identified as acting unjustly. Such conduct is quickly and unequivocally condemned. There is no doubt in the minds of the affronted, patiently awaiting their turn, that an objective and recognizable standard of conduct, a norm of morality, granted of a low order, has been breached. If reaction to 'jumping the queue' is forceful, the defaulter may offer an excuse based on an urgency of a personal nature.

An excuse may be accepted but it will have been duly considered by the interested parties. It will have been measured against a standard, a norm of morality. Even the unmitigated bully will not be unaware of the standard against which his misbehaviour is being assessed. He would probably not deny that the notion of the ordered queue was a desirable principle of behaviour. This homely illustration of the awareness of the man in the street, of the existence and usefulness of objective standards of conduct, may be dismissed by a high-flying ethicist. It may be regarded as merely a display of local mores of little significance in moral philosphy. There is, however, in this scenario a hint of a readiness to accept and abide by an objective norm in certain circumstances, trite though they may be.

It is the lack of a universally agreed norm of morality, an absolute standard for distinguishing good from bad behaviour, which is one of the endemic disagreements in ethical studies. Among the scholastic philosophers of the Middle Ages it was held that there was a universal natural law written in the heart of man, whereby evil could be distinguished from good. The real existence of this reflection of divine law was readily accepted by Christian teachers over the centuries. It would follow from this notion of a universal natural law that all men in all ages would be readily aware of what was right or wrong. Each would have an inbuilt, God-given norm of morality as an ever-present personal guide – a correctly formed conscience. Unfortunately, there has been little success in ascertaining what this supreme moral law lays down in detail. In fact it has proved impossible to establish the universal acceptance of even generalities of a natural law. Full proof of the existence of it is not available and indeed the identity of the Lawgiver is usually regarded as a matter of faith rather than of experience. Such a natural law, if it exists and is echoed in the human conscience, would seem to be flexible in the extreme. What has appeared as grossly immoral to one generation has perhaps appeared harmless to a later one and vice versa. If a universal norm of morality exists it has certainly not been perceived as applying to everyone in the same way. Apparently, different modes of conduct have been acceptable to Asians, Europeans and Polynesians

It was in response to Hume's blatant scepticism in matters ethical that Kant sought assiduously for some fundamental and universally acceptable basis for discerning right from wrong conduct. Like other intuitionists, he presented a deontological solution. For him the norm of morality was *a priori*, based on analytical thought and he presented it as the categorical imperative – a sort of all-compelling, immediately perceived, sense of duty.

It would seem that the certainty and amount of pleasure foreseen as the consequence of an action or line of conduct could be regarded as a guide to right behaviour as a practical and indeed universal norm of morality. There was, however, the tendency within utilitarianism to regard secondary principles, framed in terms of kinds of action that are or are not to be performed, as the immediate guides to right conduct – practical norms of morality. This replacement within utilitarianism of principles rather than consequences as such, as standards of behaviour, was forced by reality. Any calculation of the consequences of an action beyond the most immediate and obvious ones, even if it were possible, would be absurdly wasteful of time and effort. Even after the event, and even if all the events were known, there would be seriously theoretical problems about what to assign as consequences for my having done this rather than that, particularly when this act is overlain by many others, and what has happened can be traced causally not only to my choice but also to many independent choices of other agents. In practice then even apparently practical utilitarianism has neither an obvious nor simply discernible norm of morality. (Think of the complexities of the cost–benefit balance.)

The various forms of naturalism, like utilitarianism, looked outside the individual's own moral attitude for a basis of right and wrong, such as self-preservation. John Rawls appears to despair of any accepted norm of morality: 'In a just society the rights secured by justice are not subject to political bargaining' (as supposed in the notion of the social contract) 'or to the calculus of social interests' (the direction in which utilitarians might look). Existing societies seldom adhere to this principle; for what is just or unjust is usually in dispute. In a utilitarian tone even the sceptical Hume admits to the benefit of a solidly based morality, difficult though it might be to find a standard by which it could be consistently assessed. 'A man is more useful to himself and others, the greater degree of probity and honour he is endowed with.'

Perhaps for most of human history, religion of one form or another, readily supplied, if not imposed, an absolute and fundamental norm of morality. Assuring as this has been for millions in providing comforting and secure certainty, there have been difficulties as the inadequacies of such norms of morality have come more to the fore in modern pluralistic societies. It is one of the undisputed truths of history that religions differ in moral teachings. Even within the same religion, disputes occur concerning the application of fixed rules to a changing reality. Not all religious teachers have been in full accord on such crucial and pertintent moral issues as the indissolubility of marriage, birth control, nuclear warfare, etc.

Sam Shuster (Professor of Dermatology at Newcastle), summed up the modern rejection of the traditional in morals:

> 'Modern knowledge and technology are too complex to be powered by an outdated ethic, a blinkered understanding and a wet sentimentality.'

Whether this extreme comment is true, or not, the demise of religious morality based on a norm of morality stemming from revelation is an observable fact. It is this diminishing influence of religion on how people live that has given not only space for, but in fact a need for, a greater awareness of ethics. Increasingly, professional people look to ethics to provide a practical simple norm of morality.

Other forms of human awareness of morality, akin to religion, have supplied the need for a norm of morality. In the dim past there was the savage and crystal clear imperative of the taboo. It may have lingered on as a mere shadow of its former self as an indication of the in-thing within a closed group. Some might still consider the taboo as important, as a form of social cement protecting and reinforcing the bonds of a community by norms, without its previous strict sanctions. Culture also provides, within its own setting, a guide to right conduct. Indeed, such social attitudes as for example social mores, are often the after-taste of a state dominated by a specific religion which has lost its authority or its drive. The Protestant work ethic of America may be a case in point.

In this general area of religious morality there has been no lack of definite norms of morality. Unfortunately, no particular one has met with universal acclaim, in spite sometimes of very vigorous legal and violent support.

The law as a norm of morality

For many, perhaps, law is a sufficient criterion of acceptable behaviour: 'Does it matter if it's honest as long as it is legal?' This may sound cynical but for many it expresses their way of life. (For example, showing greater concern about the details of a project licence for experimentation than attention to ethical justification.) Acceptance of the law of the land as a norm of morality is an efficient way to escape from endless ethical controversy. The practice has a long heritage and strong pedigree from the time of Thrasymarchus the Sophist (*c.* 380 BCE). After all, the law can bite.

When we look at the history of law we find that there have been bad laws since the time of the horrific legal system of Draco, the Athenian tyrant, and probably from before that. The acceptance of the existence of bad laws, in the moral sense, implies that there is a standard beyond law by which the morality of a law may be assessed or even condemned. History is strewn with discarded laws which did not have moral support and consequently fell into disrepute (eg. the poll tax). Morality is a foundation for law rather than law being a producer of morality.

Ethics, being philosophical, tends usually to be argued in conformity with reasoning. Any close alignment of law and reason is sometimes merely coincidental. It is axiomatic that 'the law is an ass'. This would hardly suggest that law as such would be fully acceptable as a universal norm of morality.

Some minor laws, for instance as regards traffic or trade, are from their very nature concerned with detail far removed from morality. In such cases, even one with the most tender conscience would feel no shame after a breach of such trivial regulations. This implies a real distinction between law and morals, each, therefore, having its own standards. This in no way diminishes the paramount influence of law in human affairs. Plato, the great moral philospher, when he was older and perhaps wiser, followed his seminal work on ethics, *The Republic*, by his much larger work, *The Laws*.

In the past, scholastic moral theologians used the term 'penal laws' in reference to state laws to which no moral connotation was attached. Here the use of the word 'penal' is to be distinguished from its use as applied to laws which persecuted religions unacceptable within a state. In the former sense 'penal' referred to the penalty imposed and regarded by these moralists as sufficient for the maintaining of good order within the State. These moral theologians taught that the moral force of such 'penal' laws was merely the obligation to pay the appropriate penalty for the breach when imposed. An example of this type of legislation not carrying a direct moral implication was customs duties. Hardly theological but indicative of ecclesiastical understanding in such illegal pursuits may be:

> 'Brandy for the parson,
> Baccy for the Clerk.'
>
> *A Smuggler's Song* Rudyard Kipling

On a more serious level refer to Davis (1945).

Reference

Davis, H. (1945) This moral latitude (for some surprising) is to be found among past moral theologians. It is clearly expounded upon by Henry Davis S.J. in his monumental work on moral theology *Moral and Pastoral Theology*, Vol. 1, pp. 142–148), Sheed and Ward, London.

Chapter 4

The Nature of Freedom

'It is he that saith not "Kismet";
It is he who knows not fate;'

Lepanto, G.K. Chesterton

Introduction

We freely talk of 'will', particularly of her will, of his will and, with special emphasis, our own will but probably give little thought to the true nature of this concept. The will, but especially the freedom of the will, is essential to any value that ethics may have. Whether 'good', 'right' or 'wrong' have any real meaning is of little importance unless one is free to choose between a right or wrong action. Praise or blame, always in the background of moral judgements, are of no significance, unless when an agent is praised for doing a certain action, it is presumed they did not do it under compulsion. Likewise when one is condemned for committing a wrong action, such condemnation would be completely misplaced if the wrongdoer had not been free to avoid the offence. This all seems as obvious as stating that celibacy is not inherited but the freedom of the will has been called into question in many disciplines: theology; philosophy; and science, particularly in psychology. Things are not what they seem and determinism is rampant. What does a will weigh? What does it look like?

What then is the will we so readily talk about yet rarely seriously consider. In the schools of the Middle Ages it was defined as: 'Voluntas est facultas immaterialis seu spiritualis qua ens intelligens tendit in bonum intellectu cognitum.' Which means that they regarded the will as an immaterial faculty by which an intelligent being recognizes what is good and has a tendency towards it (that is, if it is a good will). It is difficult to find a better definition for a gift which we probably think we have but which some philosophers might even deny exists. If we suppose this will is free, in what does that freedom consist? It would seem that such freedom, if it is real, is the power to act or not to act in respect to a particular end or object. It may be physical in the sense of being free from coercion, restraint or the compulsion of physical forces or it may be psychological immunity from natural necessity.

Free will

The common-sense acceptance of the freedom of the will reflects the facts of life. Our normal reaction to an accidental injury, as in a car crash, and to an assault, are based on the fact that in the latter case the assault need not have taken place if the aggressor had so willed. The distinction, between obeying the laws of nature, such as gravity when one falls, and observing a moral law, such as respecting an other's property, is beyond question. In the former instance one has no option, in the latter case there is apparently no such compelling force and one feels free to act as one wills.

The idea and reality of moral obligation is essentially bound up with the idea and reality of freedom. There can be no meaning to the sense of shame on account of having done or omitted to do this or that; there can be no meaning in ascribing to a person responsibility for any particular occurrence, except on the assumption of contingency – that he need not have done what he did do – that its occurrence under the circumstances was not inevitable. If all occurrences are in truth equally and absolutely determined in the physical sequence of events, it cannot be denied that the whole language about responsibility and guilt is the language of illusion. If a man were genuinely convinced that his every action was absolutely predetermined, so that he was no more justly to be blamed for anything he might do, than a vegetable or an animal, and were to allow this conviction to dominate his life, he would cease to be a fit member of society. Bishop Butler (1692–1752) (in *Opinion of Necessity*) calls the determinist theory absurd. He claims that no man can act as if this theory is true without becoming less than human and being treated as such.

No doubt the latent forces of heredity, the strength of habit, etc., limit the freedom of an individual. It may be that, as acts form habits and habits form character and character forms stereotypes, it is possible for an individual actually to cease to be free to a certain extent and in some areas not to have any longer the alternative of choosing good or bad. In general, however, these are pathological conditions or may be induced by intensive programming such as brainwashing.

We ourselves, if we reflect, find that we can be conscious of making choices, and can become aware of the working of our free will. Various motives, which are to be relatively judged good or bad – pleasure, acquisitiveness, ambition, pride – present themselves to our consciousness at crucial moments, and are estimated at their relative value by us. We, by a deliberate act of choice, so attach ourselves to one or the other, so that our resultant action becomes decisively this or that, the other motives being ignored. It may even happen that the consciousness of the strong pressure of some motive contrary to that which we choose only seems to increase the vigour we put into that which we have chosen. If freedom of choice in this sense is denied to be possible for all normal human beings, it appears that such a denial is simply a refusal to face the facts, as revealed directly in human consciousness.

What takes place when an act of the will occurs is something special but unmistakable in quality. It is totally different from what takes place when distinct and opposing physical forces are acting simultaneously upon a physical body. The motion of the body is then the mixed resultant of the different forces. In the case of a variety of motives acting upon the will, the will acts on account of one and ignores the others. They are neutralized. As previously noted, often the very intensity that the rejected motives had, far from diminishing the force of the accepted motive, may even add to the vigour with which the successful motive is embraced. Truly, one does the right thing all the more forcefully or the wrong thing all the more impulsively because of the strong pressure experienced against the choice eventually made. (This may, perhaps, be due to just sheer cussedness, for which we may be programmed by our genes, leaving us little leeway in the matter – some are born contrary.)

As the physical sciences are coming to recognize the abstractness of their subject matter and since the dominance of mechanical materialism has been relaxed, within scientific circles there is more tolerance of the idea that real freedom is a quality of intelligent beings.

Professor Eddington, the physicist (1882–1944), writes:

> 'Meanwhile we may note that science thereby withdraws its opposition to free will. Those who maintain a deterministic theory of mental activity must do so as the outcome of the study of the mind itself, and not with the idea that they are thereby making it more conformable with an experimental knowledge of the laws of organic nature.'
>
> (Eddington 1933)

Professor Eddington finds indeterminism in nature at its very basis (Eddington 1933). He thought in terms of the quantum theory but since then has come quarks and the unpredictable dance of the 'selfish gene'. The concept of human freedom does not require that the will acting freely should produce any augmentation or reduction of the physical energy which passes into the human body and passes out of it in action (akin to the crass proposal that thoughts are the secretion of the brain as insulin is of the pancreas). All that is required from the ethical point of view is a certain restricted control over its direction, as in this or that kind of activity.

Determinism

Theological determinism is the trickiest of all. The religion of the ancient Greeks encouraged a type of fatalism. Greek tragedy is overshadowed by the concept of a mysterious Fate, to which even the Olympian gods were subject. The Pharisees developed a fatalistic aspect of Judaism, while early Christianity distinguished itself by its enthusiastic insistence on the reality of free will and moral responsibility. Under the influence of Augustine (396–430), however, in his extreme antagonism to Pelagius (*c.* 354–420) (the first Briton to win fame as a writer and a thinker), Western Christianity adopted the teaching of predestination. The logical (perhaps not the practical) implication of this, cut at the roots of any real sense of moral responsibility. Christianity never quite recovered from this Augustinian determinism. Popular Christianity tended to accept and favour the notion of free will. Indeed in the conflict with Islam it was the Christian knight of whom it was said:

> 'It is he that saith not "Kismet";
> It is he who knows not fate.'
>
> *Lepanto* by G.K. Chesterton

Thomas Aquinas and the other scholastic philosophers tried to save free will for Christianity. Skilful intellectual acrobatics were indulged in. The Thomists talked in terms of the grace moving the will by physical premotion. This moving of the will was said to be in accord with human nature and, as man was free, his will must be moved freely. This was a valiant attempt to square the circle. The Jesuit, Molina (d. 1600), was the scholastic theologian who moved the farthest from determinism. He taught that there was a distinction between sufficient and efficacious grace. Efficacious grace worked. Sufficient grace did not. The crucial difference between the two was the acceptance or rejection of the proffered grace by the human will. Such a solution aroused the fury of the puritanical Jansenists associated with Blaise Pascal (1623–1662) at Port Royale in Paris. With fervour they prayed to be delivered from mere sufficient grace: 'A gratia sufficiente, libera nos domine.' Augustine's determinism lived on. It had been strongly reinforced by Calvin (1509–1564) and John Knox (1514–1572). Predestination with its implied determinism still thrives and is well and living in Scotland among the Wee Frees.

'There go I but for the grace of God', was a thinly disguised statement that the only difference between the saint and the sinner, is the grace of God, not human free will. One Protestant who dealt effectively with this dilemma of the impotence of man and the omnipotence of God, but on a practical not a theological level, was Cromwell. Before the Battle of Naseby, he told his troops: 'Put your trust in God but keep your powder dry.'

Determinism in philosophy has a long history and the theory has been widespread among philosophers. In ancient Greece the religious idea of Fate was secularized by Leucippus and Democritus, as abstract necessity. Everything that happened was attributed to the movement of material atoms and consequently everything was determined. The Stoics identified the immutable order of nature with divine providence which excluded freedom of the will. Stoical determinism was expressed in the Hymn of Cleanthes and confirmed in the *Meditations* of Marcus Aurelius.

The philosophical aspect of determinism, particularly in regard to the motives influencing decisions, was a popular topic of dispute in the Middle Ages. The classic analogy used was Buridan's ass, starving equidistant between two equal piles of hay. Friar Buridan suggested that as the stimulation of either bale of hay was identical, the attraction of each would cancel out the other. If the donkey was completely at the mercy of outside forces alone, without free will, it was doomed. I have been unable to trace an account of the outcome of such a predicament. I have no doubt the beast would have sorted the matter out pretty quickly.

Spinoza (1632–1677) was adamant on the matter of determinism:

> 'There is in the mind no absolute or free will; but the mind is determined in willing this or that by a cause, and this by another, and so on to infinity. Men think themselves free because they are conscious of their volitions and desires, but are ignorant of the cause by which they are led to wish and desire.'
>
> (Spinoza 1982)

Schopenhauer (1788–1860) agreed with and confirmed the rejection of free will by Spinoza. Diderot (1713–1784) presented the same teaching:

'Since I act in this way, anyone who can act otherwise is no longer myself; and to declare that, at the moment I do or say a thing, I could do or say another is to declare that I am myself and someone else'.

(Diderot 1754)

(Do we act out of necessity from our own individuality?)

Surprisingly even the great utilitarian, John Stuart Mill, accepted determinism:

'That, given the motives which are present to an individual's mind and given likewise the character and disposition of the individual, the manner in which he will act might be unerringly inferred; that if we knew the person thoroughly, and knew all the inducements which are acting upon him, we could foretell his conduct with as much certainty as we can predict any physical event. This proposition I take to be a mere interpretation of universal experience, a statement in words of what everyone is internally convinced of.'

Aristotle taught that man had the power to choose between good and bad actions. He pointed to the universal practice of rewarding the good and punishing the wicked as indication of the validity of his teaching.

The bluntest defence of free will, based on intuition, is that of Dr Johnson: 'Sir, I know the will is free and there's an end on't.'

Kant defended the freedom of the will on the basis of moral necessity. He argues from the fact of moral obligation (his own categorical imperative). If it can be truly said that it is a duty to perform (or to avoid) an act, it must have been possible for the agent to perform it and possible for him not to perform it.

One modern philosopher who was deeply committed to the doctrine of free will was Bergson (1859–1941). He approached the problem from an intuitionist and anti-scientific attitude. He taught that we do not discover the truth by the intellect; on the contrary, the intellect falsifies our experiences. The intellect constructs an abstract scheme (the world of theory as opposed to the practical?), according to which one state of consciousness succeeds another, instant by instant (discrete states not a flux of awareness); and this sort of scheme must land us in complete determinism. He argues, the flow of consciousness cannot be thus divided up into instants of time; true knowledge of it can be obtained only by direct insight, or intuition. Hence the paradox that we are convinced that we are really free, though intellectual arguments show that we are determined. Our freedom consists in our ability to create the future and that would be impossible if we were slaves of the past. (Does this necessarily follow?)

If there must be some causal explanation possible for everything that a man does, it looks as if it cannot be true that when he does one thing he really at that time has the power to do something else, things being as they are. A genuine causal explanation cannot, of its very nature, leave this possibility open. If I explain that your tyre is flat because I stuck a tack into it, although obviously I can allow that had things been different the tyre would not have been flat, I cannot allow that, with things as they are, the tyre being capable of puncture by a tack and having had a tack stuck into it, the tyre could be other than flat. If I had allowed for the tyre not being flat after the puncture, I would have failed to give a causal explanation of an event that demanded an explanation. It must be possible to justify a properly causal explanation by saying: 'Whenever this happens, that happens.' This is precisely what would not be possible if it were really open to a person, in a given set of circumstances, to do either of two things.

It must be pointed out that the concept of 'cause' belongs more to philosophy than to science but the terms 'cause' and 'effect' are used in the everyday language of science and the demand for a defined cause of a phenomenon is relevant in science. It is not surprising then that not only in psychology, and particularly among the behaviourists, but throughout science, determinism was acceptable and accepted.

Ernst Haeckel (1834–1919) is definite on the matter:

> 'We know that each act of the will is as fatally determined by the organization of the individual, and as dependent on the momentary condition of his environment as every other psychic activity. The character of the inclinations was determined long ago by heredity from parents and ancestors. The determination of each particular act is an instance of adaptation to the circumstances of the moment wherein the strongest motive prevails according to the laws which govern the statics of emotion.'

Haeckel, with a philosophical pseudo-scientific flourish, sums up the situation:

> 'Ontogeny teaches us to understand the evolution of the will in the individual child. Phylogeny reveals to us the historical development of the will within the ranks of our vertebrate ancestors.'

This is by no means an isolated scientific attitude to determinism (Richardson 1997).

A leader in the English scientific field, Thomas Henry Huxley (1825–1895), puts the matter more soberly and perhaps a little more enigmatically:

> 'We are conscious automata endowed with free will in the only intelligble sense of that much abused term – inasmuch as in many respects we are able to do as we like (is this "liberty"?) – but none the less are parts of the great series of causes and effects which, in unbroken continuity, compose that which is, and has been and shall be – the sum of existence.'

Einstein (1879–1955) accepted determinism: 'Everybody acts not only under external compulsion but also in accordance with inner necessity' in *The World as I See It*.

Sir William Bragg (1890–1971) though approaching the problem from a scientific angle, defends free will, using the argument from experience. This seems to be the strongest argument in favour of free will. It has a more scientific flavour than, for example, the arguments of Kant from moral necessity and of Bergson from intuition or of Scholasticism from logical arguments based on Aristotelian principles. Bragg's argument is worthy of consideration. He uses the analogy of two laboratories: one being strictly scientific and deterministic; the other being real life where there exists a vivid awareness of free will in the sphere of human relationships. In this latter laboratory we feel that we have some control over what we do and may act selfishly or unselfishly. He points out that even if the lessons of the two laboratories seem to contradict each other, the clash is not even so definite as that which in the world of physics may set the wave theory and the particle theory in apparent contradiction, if we confuse the uses to which the two theories may be put.

Is this problem of free will more verbal than real? Is it a pseudo-problem – a mere matter of semantics? This latter cliché is a popular gambit for avoiding an embarassing checkmate in involved polemics. Could the perplexities of the dilemma be removed by reformulation of the question? Should we edge towards the mind-set of the 'sprachspiel' (philosophy as a word game) of Wittgenstein?

There can be no doubt that, when we scrutinize some of the forms in which the free will controversy is stated, the issue is extremely confused. It appears that some writers are really talking about the relation of mind to body; others are discussing the status of a law of universal causation and others are concerned with the mathematical theory of probability. Yet another fundamental question which arises is whether or not we can trust our intuitions.

Obviously Moore had some profound thoughts on this topic. For him free choice implied the choosing of an act which a man was not compelled in any recognized way to perform. It is worth reiterating that the opposite of 'free' is not 'caused' but 'compelled' or some similar word. Thus the supposed inconsistency between freedom of choice and universal causation is shown to be non-existent since 'freely chosen' and 'caused' do not rule one another out. Hume had offered a solution to the problem on these lines and still earlier, so did Hobbes (Warnock 1963).

Is the real distinction that the act which is done is caused but the choice is not caused, but could be decided by compulsion, in which case it would not be free?

It has been suggested that a great deal of argument about free will is due to differences about locating the causes of an action. If the person who acts can be treated as the cause, and not some external or environmental agency, some think that we may retain the law of causality without losing the essence of freedom.

Does 'determined' simply mean that which is 'predictable'? This is an attractive suggestion but how can any human action be truly predictable? How can any outsider become aware of all the motives influencing another person's decision? For some of the things which the other person would have to know in order to predict your choice, would be what features in the situation would appeal to you as reasons. You could not discover this for yourself without weighing them up as reasons. As soon as you started to do this instead of trying to predict your own choice you would actually be choosing. For an important part of choice is deciding what is a reason worth taking into account and what is not. Thus it seems unlikely that the concepts of decision and choice would conceivably be eliminated, whatever the theoretical possibilities of prediction might be. But it is conceivable that the language which we use of our own choices and that which we use of other people's might tend to become rather different.

In the past, punishment was probably a more common and accepted part of life. Generally, the notion of punishment implied blame and blame implied responsibility which is, I am sure now quite obvious, associated in the minds of many with the freedom not to have done the offending act. However mischievous Mr Punch has been throughout the performance, the operator who then belaboured the puppet after the show for his misdemeanours would hardly be regarded as rational. The same would be thought of one who similarly belaboured an animal for a past delinquency. The material that appears in *The Criminal Prosecution and Capital Punishment of Animals* by E.P. Evans (Evans 1988) is surely evidence of an aberration of a legal system. In 1978 the World Wildlife Fund saw fit to protest about the public execution in an Italian village square of a stray dog, sentenced to death by poisoning for killing chickens.

Most people would agree that punishment, in such a case, is out of place because of a lack of free will but would accept the justice of some punishment in the case of erring humans in similar circumstances. That is not to call into question some minor forms of correction of pets, where the immediacy of the correction acts as a deterrent. It is only in the role of a deterrent that many would now accept punishment as having any moral worth. A deterrent is of no use unless it deters and it can only do that if the person contemplating a crime fears and anticipates possible punishment. The extreme determinist might argue that the threat of punishment is a factor so influencing the decision that it determines it.

An unfortunate fact about deterrents is that to be effective they need to be impressive. The criminal might scoff at a petty avoidable sanction but be in fear of an inevitable and severe penalty. Even severe penalties are not always effective because of lack of responsibility, implying in such cases a loss of freedom on account of an inability to make wise decisions.

> 'And the burnt fools bandaged finger
> goes wabbling back to the fire.'
>
> *The Gods of the Copybook Headings* R. Kipling

The same pattern of ethical thinking was the basis of the M'Naghten rules which allowed for the plea of insanity.

Plato, long ago, had considered the part played by punishment as a determining factor in behaviour. In *The Republic* he uses the fable of Gyges' Ring which was reputed to endow its wearer with invisibility. He makes the point that the best of us will get up to mischief if our peccadillos will remain undetected and therefore unpunished, even if only by shame.

The very strong argument in favour of the existence of free will from the popular acceptance of the practice of punishment does not prove the freedom of the will. It does prove that there is popular belief in the existence of free will. (Can 100 000 lemmings be wrong?)

Existentialism (the farthest reaches of freedom)

Sartre (1905–1980) claimed that existentialism asserts the radical freedom and responsibility of human beings. This concept he expressed in the slogan 'existence precedes essence'. This is only possible if there are no rules prior to human existence, which determine what a human being is and what a human being must do. Belief in the reality of God, however, is held to entail the reality of rules. Sartre takes up Dostoyevsky's remark that 'If God did not exist, everything would be permitted' and then goes on to assert that it is because God does not exist that everything is permitted and a human being is radically free. Each individual is responsible for the values and conduct of his or her own life. We choose for ourselves what we shall be and what we shall value. Sartre explains this approach.

> 'When I confront a real situation . . . I am obliged to choose my attitude to it. I cannot avoid choosing nor can I avoid bearing responsibility for the choice. Since God is excluded, we must be seen as those who invent "values". To assert this, means that there is no sense in life *a priori* . . . but it is yours to make sense of, and the values of it is nothing else but the sense that you choose.'
>
> (Sartre 1943)

Although Sartre vaunts human freedom, he holds that human beings are not free not to choose. They are under a demand to choose and are responsible for their choices. It would seem that there is in fact some essence before existence in the sense that the essential freedom of the human being precedes his existence. Only a reading in depth of the writings of Sartre could elucidate the previous sentence. It seems to have all the clarity of a mind-trap of Zen.

Liberty

Liberty is an easier concept to comprehend than the more abstract, internal and in some respects subjective notion of freedom. Liberty is more concerned with the lack of perceivable compulsion or restraint and is closely associated with law and politics.

For many 'liberty' is sacrosanct; any process which in any way endangers it, such as censorship, is anathema. Yet all must agree that ultimate unrestrained liberty leads to anarchy. Most people agree that the liberty of others inevitably demands control of any one individual's liberty. Crudely put: my liberty to swing my fists is limited by another's liberty to retain an intact nose.

The utilitarians were very involved in this area of ethics because of their deep involvement in both social and political affairs. John Stuart Mill wrote copiously on the matter and dealt seriously with the concept of power – a notion directly involved in both the restriction and the protection of liberty. Mill proposed the principle that the only purpose for which power can be rightfully exercised over any member of a civilized society against his will is to prevent harm to others. Further, the only part of the conduct of any one for which he is answerable to society is that which concerns others. In the part which merely concerns himself, his independence is of absolute right. A person's own good, either physical or moral, is not sufficient warrant for any interference with his liberty. Mill excluded the moral coercion of public opinion as well as legal penalties. Mill excused paternalism if it maximized what is ordinarily called happiness. Historically, various benign industrial enterprises were material expressions of this attitude.

Freedom of speech

Although many readily agree that any part of one's conduct that only concerns one's self should enjoy complete liberty, there is very little of one's conduct that does not have some influence on others, particularly for example in the matter of thought and discussion. Mill therefore defends freedom of speech, not on the grounds that it is only of concern to the speaker but on the grounds that freedom of speech is liable, overall, to be more beneficial than harmful.

This will not always be true. People can be persuaded to destroy not only the freedoms of others but also their own, including the freedom of discussion, even by persuaders exploiting that very freedom. Yet it would seem that restraint on freedom of discussion is unlikely, in the long term, to be in the interest of freedom of speech; it could prove to be counter-productive. The solution to this dilemma seems not to lie in a supposedly self-evident principle of non-interference but in principles of legitimate interference, rules which distinguish acceptable from unacceptable ways of affecting other people (especially children), perhaps quite radically; where the acceptable ways are those that in the concrete situation harmonize with the general form of conditions for the good life.

Liberties conflict with one another, and almost any policy whatever can be represented as a defence, direct or indirect, of some sort of liberty. What is needed is not a general and spectacular defence of liberty but a more prosaic adjudication between particular rival claims to freedom; not a single-issue politics but viable compromises.

Education is an ideal opportunity for affecting the freedom of thought. Parents commonly claim the right to bring up their children as they think fit and to hand on to them their own beliefs and their own moral outlook. Rousseau was very outspoken on this subject, holding that parents and teachers alike should refrain from any pre-rational indoctrination, leaving all these subjects to be discussed rationally after the children are old enough to take part critically and intelligently in such discussions. It seems unrealistic to demand the postponement of all consideration of morals and religion in a world where from their earliest years children are confronted with all sorts of information, influences and opinions. Perhaps there should be a caution against subjecting children to one-sided teaching coupled with the view that it would be wicked even to consider any contrary opinion.

Liberty and the commons

This agro–economic concept, with a historic basis and of great practical significance, illustrates well the impossibility of tolerating absolute liberties and the need to weigh carefully the worth of conflicting liberties.

Commons were pastures open to all; each local citizen could have the inalienable right to graze as many of his cattle as he wished on this community land. It is to be expected that each herdsman will try to keep as many cattle as possible on the commons. This beneficial arrangement may work reasonably well for centuries because wars and disease keep the numbers of both man and animal well below the carrying capacity of the land. Finally, however, comes the day of reckoning; that is, the day when the long-desired goal of social stability becomes a reality. At this point, the inherent logic of the commons remorselessly generates tragedy.

As a rational being, each herdsman seeks to maximize his gain. Explicitly or implicitly, more or less consciously, he asks: 'What is the utility to me of adding one more animal to my herd?' This utility has one negative and one positive component:

(1) The positive component is a function of the increment of one animal. Since the herdsman receives all the proceeds from the sale of the additional animal, the positive utility is nearly +1.
(2) The negative component is a function of the additional overgrazing created by one more animal. Since, however, the effects of overgrazing are shared by all the herdsmen, the negative utility for any particular decision-making herdsman is only a fraction of −1.

Adding together the component partial utilities, the rational herdsman concludes that the only sensible course for him to pursue is to add another animal to his herd and another and another. This conclusion is reached by each and every rational herdsman sharing a commons. Therein is the tragedy. Each man is locked into a system that compels him to increase his herd without limit, in a world that is limited. Ruin is the destination to which all men rush, each pursuing his own best interest in a society that believes in the freedom of the commons. Freedom in a commons brings ruin to all.

Ethics and pollution

In a reverse way, the tragedy of the commons reappears in problems of pollution. Here it is not a question of taking something out of the commons, but of putting something in – sewage, chemical and radioactive waste and dangerous fumes into the air. The rational man finds that his share of the cost of the wastes he discharges into the commons is less than the cost of purifying his wastes before releasing them. We are locked into a system of 'fouling our own nest' so long as we behave only as independent, rational free-enterprisers. The pollution problem is a consequence of population. It did not matter so much how a lonely American frontiersman disposed of his waste. As population becomes denser the natural chemical and biological recycling processes become overloaded, calling for a redefinition of property rights.

Analysis of the pollution problem as a function of population density uncovers a not generally recognized principle of morality, namely: the morality of an act is a function of the state of the system at the time it is performed. Using the commons as a cesspool does not harm the commons under frontier conditions because there is no public. The same behaviour in a metropolis is unbearable. One hundred and fifty years ago a plainsman could kill an American bison, taking only the tongue for his dinner and discarding the rest of the animal. It would not be condemned as being wasteful. Today with only a few thousand left, we would be appalled at such behaviour.

The fact that morality is system-sensitive escaped the attention of most codifiers of ethics in the past. 'Thou shalt not ...' is the form of traditional ethical directives which makes no allowance for particular circumstances. The laws of our society follow the pattern of ancient ethics. Therefore they are poorly suited to governing a complex, crowded and changeable world. Our solution is to augment administrative law. It is practically impossible to spell out all the conditions under which it is safe to burn trash in the back yard or to run an automobile without smog-control but we try frantically to devise more detailed regulations. Ancient liberties must be curtailed. The Englishman's home can no longer be regarded as his inviolable or impregnable castle.

Population and the commons

The tragedy of the commons is relevant to the population problem facing the modern world. In a society run on a dog-eat-dog basis, parents who bred too exuberantly would leave fewer descendants, not more, because they would not be able to adequately provide for their numerous offspring. Although rabbits seem to do quite well, the negative feedback associated with the aforesaid principle appears to control the fecundity of birds. Humans, however, are not birds and have in no way acted like them for millennia (Lack 1954).

Although there is a certain amount of self-righteous and adverse propaganda from the chattering classes against the callousness of modern humanity, support systems and caring for the needy exist after a fashion. The piety of past ages did not so readily throw up an Oxfam, or its like, on a scale which now operates. Within cultures such as a welfare state where most people have access to the commons in various forms of community support, how can the tragedy of the commons be prevented? Is there a way? Is it ever justifiable to curtail the family, the class, the religion, the race or any distinguishable and cohesive group, that adopts overbreeding as a policy to secure its own aggrandizement? To associate the concept of the freedom to breed with the belief that everyone has an equal right to the commons is to lock the world into a tragic course of action. Does humanity speak with one voice on this ominous prospect? Opinions on the matter have been expressed by the great and the good. For example, The Universal Definition of Human Rights describes the family as the fundamental unit of society. It follows that any choice and decision with regard to the size of the family must irrevocably rest with the family itself and cannot be made by anyone else (U Thant 1968).

It would be a mistake to think that we can control the breeding of mankind in the long run by an appeal to conscience. People vary and some will respond to such a plea but others for various reasons will not. Those who have more children (in a world where the benefits of the commons exist) will produce a larger fraction of the next generation than those with more susceptible consciences. The difference will be accentuated, generation by generation. Could it be supposed that in hundreds of generations, a progenitive instinct would possibly eventually develop? Would Homo contracipiens be completely replaced by Homo progenitivus? (Darwin 1960.)

Liberty and rights

A liberty and a claim-right are two important forms of rights. Any claim for either of these must be within some legal or moral system. (This is implied only if we talk solely in terms of value judgements and ignore objective values within ethics because then there can be no place for self-subsistent rights.) To say that someone has a certain liberty is to say that the system in question does not forbid him to act in the way he intends or (speaking within the system) he is permitted so to act. To say that someone has a certain claim-right, may be to say that if he claims whatever it is that he has this right to, the system will support his obtaining what he claims; or (speaking within the system) to say that he has the right to be given support, by the imposing on one or many the duty of fulfilling the claim if it is made. A liberty and a related claim-right may go together. Often the liberty to do something is associated with the claim-right not to be impeded by others from doing it. Such systems of right, for example as regards ownership of property, secure for people areas of freedom of action. As an indivdual's pursuit of his own happiness is a large and central part of the good life; he needs a secure area in which to make choices that contribute to that pursuit.

Such considerations support the view that some rights exist but they hardly determine which rights should be recognized. Jefferson's formulation of a right to the pursuit of happiness is too vague. It does not specify any definite content of the right. It could be maintained that specific rights cannot be determined *a priori* on general grounds and that whatever rights are recognized should not be absolute. This follows from the fact that in practice rights have to be determined (unless we admit the objective existence of *a priori* rights on a deontological basis) by a politico-legal process, typically by partial modification of an existing system through conflict and compromise between rival ideals.

Unfortunately, reconciliation of a variety of rival claims can call forth a plethora of detailed regulations. This may perhaps be beneficial but is often destructive. A promising remedy for, say, migraine may be sunk beyond trace by demands for conformity to irrelevant safety regulations by overzealous bureaucrats. The outcome of conflicts between such rival claims may depend purely on the mind-set of the dominant contender. The mind-sets of the disputants on rival claims in political and social debates usually fall into one of four modes:

(1) *Egalitarian.* All for the underdog or the crated calf. Everyone must have their say, however uninformed or irrelevant it might be. Often they are 'nimbys' and 'notes' ('Not in my back yard' and 'Not over there either'). The realm of single-issue politics, direct action and the universal put-down: 'You don't know all the side-effects.'
(2) *Hierarchic.* 'Auntie knows best.' 'You can leave it to government' (rarely heard nowadays). 'She is a leading scientist, she must be right.'
> 'Do cling tightly on to nurse,
> Lest perhaps there's someone worse.'
(3) *Individual.* 'Laissez faire, laissez passer.' Allow market forces to reign. Let people make up their own minds. '*Caveat emptor*' (let the buyer beware).
(4) *Fatalistic.* People of this mind-set rarely enter into discussion on important controversial topics. They accept the opinions of their betters. 'Que sera sera' and 'Let it be, let it be.'

Is the right to liberty absolute?

A world founded on the four essential freedoms is a most desirable ideal – The dream of slaves and serfs down the ages (Roosevelt 1941). Unfortunately, the uncritical worship of liberty can be political suicide. It can result in social chaos. In the past, subversive elements have sheltered under the banner of freedom until they were powerful enough to contemptuously trample upon it. Liberty is indeed precious but the preservation of liberty is essential.

While in no way a latter-day Torquemada, I can talk with some expertise on one of these four freedoms – i.e. freedom of speech and censorship – having in the past penned my signature, with authority, under the official phrase *Imprimi potest* (It can be printed). Freedom of speech may be regarded by many as sacrosanct. There must, however, be limits. Nobody should be able to feel free to yell fire in a crowded theatre.

Slavery

Who would not agree that slavery is wrong? Yet there are logical difficulties in taking for granted that something is wrong. We might assume that it is absolutely wrong and consequently presume that it is also obvious why it is wrong. This mode of thought can lead to the development of weak arguments based on a supposed absolute value of human freedom. If we can think more clearly about *what* is valuable about freedom and *why* it is valuable we might avoid the rhetoric of the exponents of rightism – the modern peril. Rightists, the moment anything happens that is dis-advantageous or distasteful to them in their opinion, start complaining or threatening to sue, about some supposed infringement of their liberty. Claiming the absolute value of liberty, they see no need to produce reasons why it is wrong that they should be prevented from doing whatever they wish to do.

Those who were involved in the negotiations which led to the formulation of the Convention for the Protection of Animals used for Experimental and other Scientific Purposes (March 1986), will recall that they were delayed for some years. A source of contention in the discussions which caused the blockage was the concept of the 'humane endpoint'. This is now an essential factor in the implementation of our Animals (Scientific Procedures) Act 1986 and an important feature in the refinement of research projects. It prevents undue suffering of laboratory animals. In each project licence granted under this Act, a limit is set on the level of the severity of animal suffering permitted in that piece of research. There were those who contended that such a restriction imposed on the use of experimental animals would infringe the liberty of the scientist, a liberty which they thought should be paramount in research. Fortunately, consideration for the suffering of the animal triumphed over the respect for the liberty of the scientist. This was a recognition that even in the pursuit of knowledge there is a principle of a 'hurt too far' which annuls a claim to absolute liberty in animal experimentation. Excessive suffering of an animal, at least in law, outweighs any absolute rights of a researcher. This digression is not completely irrelevant. Some might say that the state of the captive animal is akin in ways to slavery.

Curtailment of rights may be wrong but until we have some way of judging when it is and when it is not, we shall be at the mercy of every kind of demagogy. In any consideration of contending claims, even in regards to human liberty, it is essential to be clear on the factors involved. In the controversy on slavery – and there was controversy even among theologians, at least in modern times – the clash of rights was between the right to liberty and the right to property. Clarification is also needed on what is meant by the term 'slavery'.

What is slavery?

Even ignoring broad uses of the term such as 'wage-slave' in the writings of Marxists for example, it is clear that the word 'slave' and its near-equivalents such as 'servus' and 'doulos' have had slightly differing meanings in different cultures. Slavery is primarily a legal status or rather the lack of a legal status. It is defined by the disabilities or the liabilities which are imposed by law on those called slaves. These legal restraints may vary from one jurisdiction to another. Slavery involves a status in society and a relation to a master. Firstly, a person is called a slave because he occupies a certain position in society, and because he lacks certain rights secured by law to others and is subject to certain liabilities from which others are free. Secondly, the person is the slave of another person, or even of a corporate body such as the State itself. So it cannot be said that members of a low caste are slaves, because although they lack certain legal rights (as often women did in the past), they do not belong to someone. The status of slaves was defined by the Greeks in terms of four freedoms which a slave lacked. These were: a legally recognized position in the community, conferring a right of access to the courts; protection from illegal seizure and detention and other personal violence; the privilege of going where he wants to go; and that of working as he pleases. The Institutes of Justinian (AD 532) legislated in detail on slavery.

Similar to slavery was indenture, military service and imprisonment, but they differed from slavery even though in fact the personal suffering involved may have been even more severe. Indenture took place only by contract, as in the case of apprenticeship and was for a fixed period like a football-player's agreement. Military service, again, was a fixed period as was, usually, imprisonment. It is difficult to distinguish serfdom from slavery, especially in the case of a villein in gross (tied to the feudal lord), rather than a villein regardant (tied to the land).

Utilitarianism and slavery

Opponents of utilitarianism challenged the utilitarian principle on the grounds that although Utilitarians were opposed to slavery, the greatest happiness of the greatest number could on occasions justify slavery. The argument took the form of a fantasy. It was supposed that two isolated Caribbean islands, having become independent, had adopted two opposite types of social organization. One, Juba, retained slavery of a very enlightened and benign form. The other island, Camaica, rightly abolished slavery and each slave seized what land he could. There was a population explosion. In the ensuing economic chaos, starvation and misery prevailed. Camaica lacked what Juba had, a government with the will and the instrument, in the shape of the institution of slavery, to control the economy and the population. Its prosperous but slave society became the envy of its neighbours. Large numbers of slave coastguards had to be employed to repel floods of people trying to enter from Camaica (Hare 1979).

Faced with these facts, if he cannot deny them, the liberal Utilitarian finds himself forced into admitting that within the terms of utilitarianism, slavery may be justified – a horrifying thought. Has the Utilitarian any way out of this ethical difficulty?

One answer may be that the principle of liberty which forbids slavery is a *prima facie* principle admitting of exceptions. This imaginary case could be one of these exceptions.

No doubt the Utilitarian could drive home the defence of his position by stressing the fantastic nature of the example and insisting on the inevitability of abuses in the practice of slavery. Principles, he could claim, are framed to deal with slavery as it actually occurs. Further, it may be argued that some would find it difficult to accept any exception in the case of slavery because having been imbued with current thinking on the topic, the man in the street would hardly be inclined to consider the special case on its merits.

Utilitarians could justify abandoning their principle, of the greatest happiness of the greatest number, in this special case. The world being as it is, we should be morally worse if we abandoned the principle against slavery because then slavery may be condoned if it could, by propaganda, be presented as beneficial. In fact, the abuses within slavery have been so terrible that the Utilitarian could argue that the just man could hold only those moral convictions which condemn slavery without qualification.

The Utilitarians' main defence of their benign but paradoxical stand against 'benevolent' slavery turns on the wholly unreal nature of the example of benign slavery proposed. Is the fable of the two islands so preposterous?

I recall from Kipling:

> 'Why brought you us from bondage,
> Our loved Egyptian night?'

The White Man's Burden, Kipling

The above quotation may seem fanciful but it echoes Holy Writ: 'So the people ... murmured against Moses, saying: "Why didst thou make us go forth out of Egypt?" ' (Exodus 17:3). The Hebrews harked back with a certain ambiguous nostalgia to their enslavement in the House of Pharaoh.

This is not a solitary instance of an abnormal assessing of the benefits of freedom. There was great rejoicing, fully justified, in Western Europe at the triumph of Solidarity and the freeing of the suppressed peoples of Eastern Europe in the 1980s. The Poles, after having thrown off the yoke of Communism, eventually elected Communists once again to rule them in the 1990s.

Does it really matter what judgements people reach about imaginary or extraordinary cases as long as this does not have an adverse effect upon their decisions in real cases?

The ethical consideration of the slavery controversy is not a dead historical topic. Slavery still exists and the trade in human organs has given it a new poignancy and urgency. Slavery with its overtones of racism can be relevant to the discussion of speciesism in regard to animal use. The controversy on the abolition of slavery illustrates well the varying mores in different periods of history and the insensitive moral views of respected leaders in apparent civilized societies (Dallas 1968).

The real wickedness of slavery

There is a fundamental difference between the ownership of a human being from ownership of any other form of property. Men are different from other animals in that they can look a long way ahead and therefore can become an object of deterrent punishment. Other animals, we may suppose, can only be the object of Skinnerian reinforcement and Pavlovian conditioning. These methods may be cruel but they fall short of the peculiar cruelty of human slavery. A piece of human property, unlike a piece of inanimate property or even a brute animal in a man's possession, can be subjected to a sort of abuse from which other kinds of property are immune; and human owners being what they are, many will inevitably take advantage of this fact. That is the reason for the atrocious punishments that have been inflicted on slaves. There would have been no point in inflicting them on animals. A slave is the only being that is both able to be held responsible for actions and yet has no escape from or even redress against the threat from another person who has the power to oppress him. If the slave were a free citizen, he would have rights which would restrain the exercise of the threat. If he were a horse or a dog the threat would be valueless because it would not be understood.

References

Dallas, R.C. (1968) The real evils of slavery are apparent in a tract based on personal accounts from the times of the slave trade in his book *The History of the Maroons*, Frank Cass.

Diderot (1754) *Peusées sur l'interprétation de la nature.*

Eddington, A.S. (1933) Professor Eddington was moving away from the acceptance of determinism by many scientists when he expressed his views on the subject in his book *The Expanding Universe.*

Evans, E.P. (1988) *The Criminal Prosecution and Capital Punishment of Animals.* Faber and Faber, London.

Evolution after Darwin (1960) Possible direction of future evolution was speculated on in the review, *Evolution after Darwin*, **2**, 461, S. Tax University, Chicago Press.

Hare, (1979) This allegorical presentation of the difficulties inherent in a utilitarian opinion on slavery appears along with other relevant and telling arguments on the whole subject of slavery in: What is wrong with slavery? *Philosophy and Public Affairs*, Winter, **8**, No. 2.

Lack, D. (1954) The research and speculation by Lack has relevance to the subject of overpopulation. David Lack deals with the problem dispassionately in *The Natural Regulation of Animal Number*, Oxford Clarendon Press.

Richardson, M. (1997) The basic theory on ontogeny presented by the famous biologist of the nineteenth century, Ernst Haeckel, is claimed by Dr Richardson to be deeply flawed. Dr Richardson, in the August (1997) issue of *Anatomy and Embryology*, calls into question the authenticity of Haeckel's series of portrayals of human embryos alongside those of other creatures such as the fish, salamander and pig. So fundamental is this feature of Haeckel's work to his central claim that 'ontogeny recapitulates phylogeny' that any use of false evidence in making his case calls into question Haeckel's credibility. Haeckel's views on the evolution of the will, it must be pointed out, do not in any way suggest that such an evolved will is free.

Roosevelt, F.D. (1941) Roosevelt proclaimed his view of the essential freedoms in his speech on 6 January.

Sartre, J.-P. (1943) Existentialism, a modern, virulent but abstruce philosophy, is presented in Sartre's own work *L'Être et le Néant* (Being and Nothingness).

Spinoza, B. (1982) *The Ethics and Selected Letters to Samuel Shirley* (Indianapolis).

U Thant (1968) This proclamation of U Thant appeared in *International Planned Parenthood News*, Feb., No. 168, 3.

Warnock, M. (1963) These comments, and similar ones on this topic which follow, are more fully dealt with in her book *Ethics since 1900* pp. 90–100, Oxford University Press, Oxford.

Chapter 5

Personal Morality

'... The sin they do by two and two they must pay for one by one.'

Tomlinson, Rudyard Kipling

Introduction

When Socrates asked 'What should I do?', he sought the answer in the context of the actions of an individual. This emphasis on the importance of personal morality was heightened by the Stoics. This strong sense of personal obligation taught by the Stoics may have contributed as much to the moral sense of the past two millennia as did the New Testament. Deontologists have invariably given prominence to the personal aspect of morality, using such terms as the 'dictates of conscience'.

While morality may appear to some to be purely personal, it would hardly be justified to argue that each one should or could have their own morality. What is profitable to one man in helping him to persevere in the way of life he has decided upon may well be profitable to another man who is trying to follow a similar way of life. To pass on information that might prove useful would surely be morally acceptable. Although egotism may form a part of any viable moral system (love of self can be a measure of your love of your neighbour even in the best moral circles), it is in the interest of everyone that there should be a stable and accepted system of morality. Even if a prevailing moral system is found unsuitable by an individual, it is more desirable that it should be modified rather than destroyed.

Unfortunately, in real life there is often a challenge between what I want to do and the demands of a moral system which I agree is essential to the smooth-running of the society of which I am a beneficiary. I may ask the question, why should I not at the same time profit from the moral system but evade it? Why should I not encourage others to be moral and take advantage of the fact that they are, but myself avoid fulfilling moral requirements, if I can? There will certainly be some occasions when I could do so with impunity and without detection. Often the point of morality is that it is necessary for the well-being of people in general that I should act to some extent in ways that are not egotistically prudential. Indeed, morality may have the function of checking what would be the natural result of egotistical prudence alone.

Plato, in *The Republic*, presents a solution to this personal quandary, as follows. The just man is happy because his soul is harmoniously ordered; because he has an integrated personality. The unjust man's personality is disintegrated and the man who represents the extreme of injustice is psychotic. His soul is a chaos of internal strife. This is a forceful argument against extreme injustice. Is it of any avail against injustice in moderation? Perhaps it could be argued that one who, in the pursuit of self-interest, evades on occasions a morality which he not only professes and encourages but allows ordinarily to control his conduct will probably be incurring costs in the form of psychological discomfort. In old-fashioned, perhaps in politically incorrect terms, he would feel guilty, suffer from remorse or have a bad conscience. In spite of a pervasive cynicism in some quarters, regret for moral lapses, on a purely humanist level, is not unknown. As Plato, agreeing with Socrates, pointed out, the poet seems to be best able to reflect with greater clarity the reality of moral feelings.

> 'If we fall in the race though we win,
> The hoof slide is marked on the course.
> Though Allah and Earth pardon sin,
> Remaineth for ever remorse.'
>
> *Certain Maxims of Hafiz*, Rudyard Kipling

Are these vague immaterial considerations enough to keep us on the straight and narrow path? May they only be effective in the case of idealists or people of a nervous and sensitive disposition? It appears that most of us have moral feelings. We tend to think in set moral ways, thus it is natural for each of us to conform to such accepted morals even if on occasions it causes us difficulties.

There are general motives that operate on both a conscious and unconscious level as driving forces for the observance, even in difficult circumstances, of a popularly approved morality. The reasons for such observance may be summarized accordingly:

- Because it increases our satisfaction with our own behaviour.
- Because it enhances our personal relationships.
- Because caring is supportive.
- Because well-earned respect increases our appreciation of others.
- Good actions produce a good inter-personal environment.

Coercion

In *The Republic*, the seminal work of ethics, it is difficult to decide how much is the teaching of Socrates and how much has been contributed by Plato. When older and wiser, Plato wrote his own complete and longer work, *The Laws*. Even in the ethical codes of learned professions, effective sanctions to ensure their observance are contained within the document. In practice it seems that however philosophically valid an ethical theory may be, its observance as a form of morality demands the underpinning of law.

The social arrangements that produce responsibility are arrangements that create coercion, of some sort. Consider bank-robbing (speculatively as a topic in ethics not as a career, of course). The man who takes money from a bank acts as if the bank were a 'commons' (see Chapter 4 'Liberty and the Commons'). How do we prevent such action? Certainly not by trying to control his behaviour solely by a verbal appeal to his sense of responsibility. Rather than rely on propaganda we insist that a bank is not a commons. We seek definite social arrangements that will prevent it from becoming a commons. We neither deny nor regret that such arrangements will infringe on the freedom of the would-be bank-robbers. The majority readily accept prohibitions with appropriate sanctions on bank-robbing. The reasons for such procedure are easily understood and no one expects exceptions to be made. Other less serious contraventions of established morals can be inhibited by appropriate penalties. Even for the encouragement of virtues, such as consideration for others, coercion (or some may prefer to call it persuasion, a nicer word), may prove to be appropriate. Taxing can be a good coercive devise. Parking meters can limit the obstruction caused by selfish prolonged parking. Fines can dissuade more persistent road-hogs. By making obstructive prolonged parking increasingly expensive, carefully biased options are offered in the place of prohibition.

To many liberals, coercion is a 'dirty word'. When it is fully understood, it need not be. Coercion is not necessarily arbitrary decisions of distant and irresponsible bureaucrats. Mutual coercion can be agreed upon by the majority of the people affected. To say that we mutually agree to coercion is not to say that we are required to enjoy it. Who likes taxes? We accept compulsory taxation because we realize that voluntary taxation would favour the less conscientious. We introduce various coercive devices to escape the horror of the 'commons' referred to previously; to obviate the hazards of the 'free-for-all approach' – the unacceptable face of capitalism.

'If I don't do it, someone else will'

I may fully admit that the consequences of an action which I intend to carry out are most certainly bad and it would be better if it were not performed at all. I assuage my concern by persuading myself that there is really no significant, if any, difference in the end result if it is I or someone else who performs the act in question.

Roger, an expert in many fields, takes on a job developing means of chemical and biological warfare. He admits that it would be better if such research did not take place but says correctly: 'If I don't do it, someone else will.' The same could be said about selling arms to a rogue tyrant. If we accept Roger's excuse as justification, it is hard to see what acts, however wicked, could not be defended in the same way – a gas operative in Belsen? Does it make any real difference to the total resulting suffering, who accepts the job? Is the refusal by one specific person to do such tasks of any real import?

One approach to this moral predicament springing from the argument 'If I don't do it, someone else will' is to consider the various effects, if the argument is accepted, and the alternatives. The very fact that Roger takes the job means that, because of who he is, there are bound to be various side-effects that may not be associated with another candidate accepting the position. Roger, because of his multifactorial skills, could be a valuable asset lost to more socially worthwhile endeavours if he takes the proffered position in ammunition work. Others taking the job may not have been of such great benefit to industries of use to the community.

There is also the question of the influence Roger, because of his standing, may have on others. If he takes a job connected with biological warfare it may have a small effect on others in his circle to the extent that it makes such work appear respectable. The matter at issue here is not the rightness or wrongness of involvement in research as regards biological warfare. It may be justified for the purposes of national defence. It is merely being used here as an example of the type of work frowned upon by some, as a model for the moral quandary being discussed. If Roger refuses the job on moral grounds he may make a good, if small, impact on the moral climate of science and it could leave him free to campaign against others doing such work.

Suppose Roger takes the job, even though he thinks it would be better if such research were not done, but persuades himself that by inefficient work he can ensure that it is less productive. He may have underestimated the effects of bad faith and find it difficult to prevent the bad faith contaminating other relationships. Consequentialism can condone the use of untruths but strong arguments are needed to sustain constant deception because of the psychological difficulty of keeping one part of one's mind sufficiently cordoned-off from other parts. Emotional responses are not always governed by beliefs. Roger may occasionally feel disgust at working on chemical warfare and be unable to dispel this self-loathing even by rehearsing to himself his complex reasoning which he thinks justified his taking the job. Such tension could damage his self-esteem which is necessary if he is to persevere in being moral.

> 'I waive the quantum o' the sin,
> The hazard of concealing;
> But oh, it hardens a' within,
> And petrifies the feelings.'
>
> *Epistle to a Young Friend*, R. Burns

A purely deontological approach to this moral poser is much more simple and clear. An action which is perceived as morally unacceptable is rejected outright. A subtle discussion of possible consequences do not enter into the decision-making process (Smart & Williams 1973). A striking example of this deontological approach to moral challenges is the Solzhenitsyn Principle as presented in his book *The First Circle*:

> 'And the simple step of a simple courageous man is not to take part in the lie, not to support deceit. Let the lie come into the world, even dominate the world but not through me.'

This is a rallying cry for opponents of utilitarianism and a rejection of purely consequentialist morality. Solzhenitsyn's attitude was far from utilitarian but generated a display of independence and bravery which achieved good in Russia that we cannot calculate. In consequential terms it was well worth the risk taken. Even in Western society, acts of moral independence may have helped to create a climate where prejudice and malign social pressures have decreased (Williams 1985).

Doing good by stealth

To return to Roger who as a committed Utilitarian has justified his actions to himself by complicated, personal and esoteric reasoning which he would need to keep to himself because the uninitiated might not understand the logic of his position. Sidgwick, a latter-day but leading Utilitarian, writes knowingly on this aspect of utilitarianism.

> 'Thus the utilitarian conclusion, carefully stated, would seem to be this; that the opinion that secrecy may render an action right which would not other-wise be so should be kept comparatively secret; and similarly it seems expedient that the doctrine that esoteric morality is expedient should itself be kept esoteric.'
>
> (Sidgwick 1874)

There seems to be a hint here of ethical snobbery, a sort of 'not in front of the children'. The watchword seems to be expediency which has been defined as the saving of the truth by the half-truth. Is such truth worth saving? Perhaps it is; reality itself is untidy. Jonathan Glover has dealt masterfully with the whole of this theme (Glover 1975).

To return to the 2 by 2 and 1 by 1. The quotation at the beginning of this chapter is not completely irrelevant. If we follow the popular coverage of news in some parts of the media (at least in this August of 1998) we may get the impression that sensuality is the prime subject of ethics and even of politics (even the politics of the most powerful nation). Likewise if we have hearkened to religious moralists in the past we would have been convinced of the wickedness of sexual lapses. Both these sources of influence on public opinion seem to be obsessed with that particular area of wrong-doing. The activities of humankind are far more varied than merely physical pursuits, however pleasurable they may be. Any human action with consequences either good or bad affecting others, including animals, and the state of the world we live in, are of moral import. The moral dimension of human activity has an impact on every facet of life. The moral implication of all our actions, especially those outside the scope of narrow partisan religious conformity, was indicated by the quaint old adage:

> 'Mr. Jones went to Church
> He never missed a Sunday;
> But Mr. Jones went down to Hell
> For what he did on Monday.'

References

Glover, J. (1975) The comprehensive arguments put forward on this important moral topic by Jonathan Glover appear in *Proceedings of the Aristotelian Society*, Vol. XLIX, pp. 171–190.

Smart, T.J. & Williams, B. (1973) Discussion on the value of utilitarianism is well presented in their book *Utilitarianism: For or Against*, Cambridge.

Sidgwick, H. (1874) This peculiar notion of 'doing good by stealth' is discussed in his book *The Methods of Ethics* p. 490.

Williams, B. (1985) Bernard Williams contributes much to this theme of the worth of a deontological approach in his *Ethics and the Limits of Philosophy*, Harvard University Press, Cambridge, Massachusetts.

Chapter 6

Society and Ethics

'Some people . . . may be Rooshans and others may be Prooshans; they are born so, and will please themselves. Them which is of other natures thinks different.'

Mrs. Gamp in *Martin Chuzzlewit* by Charles Dickens

Introduction

Fundamental to Aristotle's ethics is that man is a political animal. Essentially he belongs to the *polis* (the community). His social and moral attiudes reflect the opinions of those around him even if his moral stance is instigated by an ingrained antipathy to the prevailing mores. Even in religious inclinations, atheism does not occur in a vacuum. The atheist rejects the God of his own group – like it or not, he is a Jewish or a Christian atheist, etc. Human life, except in the rare anchoritic form, is gregarious.

'No man is an island, entire of itself;
Every man is a piece of the continent,
A part of the main.
. . . . . .
Any man's death diminishes me,
Because I am involved in Mankind;
And therefore never send to know
For whom the bell tolls;
It tolls for thee.'

Devotions, J. Donne

The universality of the popular remark defining what is perceived as wrong conduct, 'It can't be wrong because it doesn't do anyone else any harm,' testifies to the general acceptability of the view that morality is a social affair. Morality is seen as serving society.

Even on a more idealistic level, this close association of morality and the community prevails. Morality has been perceived as serving society. The right thing to do is not what suits oneself but what is good for the group. In the long run what is good for everyone is good for each one. In keeping with this line of thought, acceptable conduct does not mean what suits each particular person at a particular time but what suits the human race as a whole. People realize that they cannot have real safety or happiness except in a society where everyone plays fair. It is because of such considerations that people try to behave properly according to accepted standards.

The early form of ethics found in the Bible, a primordial source of Western morality, is communal in the extreme. Even sanctions for transgressions were imposed on the group. The destruction of Sodom and Gomorrah is of a whole community as such (Genesis 18:33). In Joshua, Chapter 7, when Achan is executed for stealing some valuables which had been seized in battle but which had been dedicated to God, his entire family is executed with him. Such attitudes may horrify us but we will see that even in supposed advanced cultures like those of ancient Greece, the heinous crime of infanticide was considered acceptable for the good of the community in some situations.

A salient force within primitive groups has been the taboo. It was much more real in the past than an internal construct producing guilt feelings in keeping with the teaching of Freud. It was a real factor within the community. The neglect of the taboo was seen as a threat to the well-being of the tribe. If, as some would claim, morality grew out of this primitive notion of right and wrong conduct, then certainly morality is solidly grounded in society as such. The observance of the taboo was seen as essential to the preservation of the integrity of the group. If we accept that moral motivations work in our pattern of conduct, they work because we are capable of feeling guilt. The consciousness of guilt is the counterpart of taboo (in a broad sense) whereas the fear of punishment is related to the force of law (since the passing of the primitive preternatural sanctions of the taboo). The two kinds of motivation and the two kinds of inhibition must not be confused; they differ in psychological as well as in anthropological terms. That is why there are grounds to expect that in a society where all taboos (in the sense of indications of acceptable behaviour within the group) have been done away with, and consequently the consciousness of guilt has evaporated (both can obviously continue to operate for a time, by the inertial force of tradition), only legal coercion would remain to keep the entire fabric of communal life from falling apart and all non-coercive human bonds from dissolving. Are we in fact, approaching such a chaotic state in inner cities in some parts of the world?

Whatever is the actual content of the taboo in a given society, and whatever its origin, it is irreducible to, and inexpressible in terms of, any other form of human communication; it is *sui generis* (out on its own), both in the perception of those who feel its presence and in reality. No matter how frequently violated, taboos (in this broad sense) are alive as long as their violation produces the phenomenon of guilt. Guilt, and its outward expression shame, is all mankind has, except sheer physical compulsion, to impose rules of conduct on its members; and that also is all it has to give those rules the form of moral commandments. Obviously, the group needs the taboo and the taboo is integral to the group in which it occurs. It has been said that culture is a set of taboos; for example, dietary taboos feature prominently in many cultures.

The leading political philosophies of this century were deeply committed to the domination of the individual by society – Communism, Falangism and the other forms of Fascism. In Marxism, ethics was purely a communal affair. There has been a solitary political voice, Margaret Thatcher, that had the temerity to deny the existence of 'society'.

The social contract

Hobbes was the leading early exponent of what had been a form of ancient speculation on the origin of law and morality. It had been suggested that acceptable conduct within society had sprung from agreements of mutual benefit within primitive communities. There are traces of this theory in Plato's *The Republic*.

Hobbes expounded in depth on this vague notion of a primordial social contract. The main import of his argument is that there was of necessity a slow movement towards peace out of conflict. Fear of death and the desire to preserve themselves, and, by industry, to acquire the means to a decent life and to be secure in their possession of them, give men a reason to seek peace. What is needed for peace is an agreement to limit competitive claims. Even if such an agreement is made, no one has a sufficient incentive to abide by it unless he has some assurance that the other parties to it will do so too. The only kind of agreement that will achieve this purpose of establishing peace, and so making life more secure and more comfortable, is one which sets up a mechanism for enforcing that agreement itself. This, Hobbes thought, must be a political sovereign, a man (or body of men) that is not, as such, a party to the agreement but whom (or which) all the parties agree with one another that they will obey. The moral principles that Hobbes offers as the necessary solution to the problem of natural competition and distrust are stated as a series of 'laws of nature'. These 'laws' were intended to:

- seek peace if there is a hope of attaining it;
- accept mutual limitation of competitive claims;
- keep agreements;
- show gratitude in return for benefits;
- accommodate oneself to others;
- pardon past offences of those who repent and give assurance of not repeating their offences;
- refrain from harking back to the past (the mutual annihilation of the vendetta, and Ulster 'whataboutary' – the spontaneous reference to a past atrocity in defence of a tit-for-tat terrorist action);
- accept the introduction of retributive punishment.

Hobbes readily admitted that even these 'laws', alone, were not sufficient. The essential device was a form of agreement which provided for its own enforcement. Each of the parties would have a motive for supporting the authority which would itself have the job of punishing breaches of the agreement, and would itself have a motive for doing so. Consequently, each party would have a double reason for fulfilling his side of the bargain: the fear of punishment for breaking it, and the expectation of benefits from keeping it.

Hobbes speaks, without historical justification, of men in a state of nature coming together, setting up a civil society and a sovereign power. It could be maintained, however, that such a pattern of contract is implicit in human societies in order to prevent that decay of the relations and motivations to which Hobbes draws attention.

Such decay would be liable to lead to unrestrained conflicts and radical insecurity of life.

Hume is in this tradition which leads eventually to the developed and crystallized form of the theory as expounded by Rousseau in his work *The Social Contract*. Hume says that it is only from the selfishness and confined generosity of man, along with the scanty provision nature has made for his wants (he did live in Scotland) that justice derives its origin. Justice (by which he means particularly respect for property and for rules governing its possession and transfer, honesty and the keeping of promises) is an artifical virtue. It is not something of which we would have any natural, instinctive tendency to approve, but a device which is beneficial because of certain contingent features of the human condition. If men had been overwhelmingly benevolent, if each had aimed only at the happiness of all, and everyone had loved his neighbour as himself, there would have been no need for the rules that constitute justice. There would have been no need for them if nature had supplied abundantly and without any effort on our part, all that we could want, if food and warmth had been as inexhaustibly available as air and water seemed to be. The making and keeping of promises and bargains is a device that makes possible mutually beneficial co-operation between people whose motives are mainly selfish. Hume insists that a single act of justice, considered on its own, may do more harm than good: 'It is only the concurrence of mankind, in a general scheme or system of action, which is advantageous.' The essential connection between morality and society could not be more clearly stated (Mackie 1990).

Social conventions

The suggestion that morals are merely more serious forms of social conventions hardly warrants consideration. No doubt some social conventions, for example those concerned with fundamental hygiene, ought to be observed and have survival value and are far more important than points of etiquette concerned merely with modes of dress, but few have difficulty distinguishing between bad manners and morally reprehensible behaviour.

It is granted that mores vary from country to country but polite behaviour can differ tremendously within the same nation, particularly in matters of speech. Accepted conduct within a society is essentially based on conformity whereas moral codes tend to originate from moral reformers who were non-conformists within their own society; frequently, 'they marched to another drum'.

Society and mores

It would appear that society is a ubiquitous, essential and natural expression of human endeavour. We have already referred to a lone voice in politics relegating society to limbo (i.e. Margaret Thatcher). In philosophy, Nietzsche stands out from his peers in divorcing morality from society:

'It is the duty of the free man to live for his own sake, and not for others. Exploitation does not belong to a depraved or an imperfect and primitive state of society; it is a consequence of the intrinsic Will to Power, which is just the Will to Live.'

This attitude is against the flow of the tide in both ethics and sociology. The consensus is that mores are indigenous to a particular society and some would posit that they have been produced by that society. In short they are the moral mind-sets of that society. The size of an ethical unitary society may vary considerably from intercontinental to a single primitive village community; similar, in a way, to the great variability in language-spreads.

The concept of society is common enough to be easily understood; the meaning of 'mores' calls, perhaps, for a little elucidation. Mores may be defined as customs enforced by social pressures. They are established patterns of action to which the individual is expected to conform and from which he deviates only at the risk of disapproval and punishment. Mores vary from society to society and the mores of a society produce and are the product of its culture. A web of customs reinforced by multiple sanctions, varying from hardly noticeable subtle influences to public outrage at an unacceptable form of conduct, may be regarded as constituting the ethical matrix of a society.

Society is the school in which men learn to distinguish between right and wrong. Custom is the teacher and the lessons are the same for all. Public opinion issues the pronouncements on moral judgements. Public approval and public indignation are the prototypes of moral emotions. In early societies there seems to have been little difference of opinion. Consequently, a character of universality or objectivity was, from the beginning, attached to moral judgements.

The effect of custom, in preventing any misgiving respecting the rules of conduct which are imposed on each individual, is all the more complete because the subject is one on which it is not generally considered necessary that reasons should be given, either by one person to others or by each to himself. People are accustomed to believe that their feelings, on matters of this nature, are better than reasons and render reasons unnecessary. The practical principle which guides them to their opinions on the regulation of human conduct, is the feeling in each person's mind that everybody should be required to act as he, and those with whom he sympathizes, would like them to act. No one acknowledges to himself that his standard of judgement is to his own liking; but an opinion on a point of conduct, not supported by reasons, can only count as one person's preference; and if the reasons, when given, are a mere appeal to a similar preference felt by other people, it is still only many people's liking instead of one. For many, however, their own preference, thus supported by their neighbour, is not only a perfectly satisfactory reason, but is the only one they generally have for any of their notions of morality, taste or propriety and is their chief guide in the interpretation of morality. It is this instinctive need for the support of others for their accepted morality that gives rise to distress among traditionalists when one of their own abandon cherished practices.

Men's opinions on what is laudable or blameworthy are affected by all the multifarous causes which influence their wishes in regard to the conduct of others and which are as numerous as those which determine their wishes on any other subject. Wherever there is an ascendant class, a large portion of the morality of the country emanates from its class interests and its feelings of class superiority. The morality between Spartans and Helots, between planters and slaves, between aristocracy and inferiors and between men and women has been for the most part the creation of these class interests and feelings, and the sentiments thus generated react in turn upon the moral feelings of the members of the ascendant class, in their relations among themselves.

The obligation to observe mores

We have already seen that by definition mores, unlike laws, are primarily enforced by social pressures. There may be many occasions when mores could easily be flouted, at least in private without any prospect of effective sanctions. Are there then any effective motives for strictly observing the mores of one's community on those occasions when it would be disadvantageous to the individual to do so? There are motives for the full observance of community mores, even in situations of complete privacy, which would appear to be valid, at least to responsible members of society.

(1) With an overactive press, reprehensible acts may be revealed and the bad example of a pillar of the establishment can weaken the respect of many for rules of behaviour.
(2) The suspicion of contravention in private of what are publicly proclaimed moral attitudes corrodes the moral fibre of a society and upsets members in the group.
(3) Authority within the community depends on the acceptance and observance of the established mores by all members of the community.
(4) The full acceptance of the mores of the community is an important factor in the cohesion of the group.

Particular modes of conduct have their traditional labels, many of which are learnt with language itself. Moral judgement commonly consists simply in labelling the act according to certain obvious characteristics which it presents in common with others who belong to the same group. Some conscientious and intelligent people, however, will carefully examine all the details connected with an act – the external and internal conditions under which it was performed, its consequences, its motive – and since the moral estimate in a large measure depends upon the regard paid to these circumstances, their judgement may differ greatly from that of the man in the street, even though the moral standard which they apply is the same. There is thus in every advanced society a diversity of opinion regarding the moral value of certain modes of conduct (euthanasia, for example). This diversity results from circumstances of a purely intellectual character and from the knowledge or ignorance of positive facts.

Cultural relativity

Enculturation is a process whereby the moral, aesthetic and other personal attitudes are formed by the cultural environment in which the person is immersed.

As soon as one ponders the difference between a European professional and an Australian aborigine, an American tycoon and an Indian yogi, one finds it hard to believe that there is anything basic to the expressions of human nature, although it is the nature shared by all human beings. Such reflection on the profound effects of enculturation easily leads one to the conclusion that what a man is, depends on the society in which he has been brought up.

It might be that enculturation can mould a human being but only within certain limits and those limits are set; either because certain parts of human nature are not plastic at all or because all parts are only moderately plastic. It may be that the need for food and the tendency to grow in a certain way cannot be modified at all by enculturation or it might turn out that every element in human nature can be modified in some ways but not in others. In either case, what a person becomes would depend partly on enculturation and partly upon the nature of the organism being enculturated. Anthropology indicates that within certain natural limits a great many alternative cultural expressions of human society can develop. Human nature makes eating inevitable but what we eat, when we eat and how we eat is up to us. (Cannibalism, while by no means cultured, can be an accepted part of a culture, as in ancient Scandinavia.)

Some think that the discoveries of anthropology have had revolutionary implications for ethics. Many modern authors on the subject tend to give the impression that the only moral obligation is to conform to one's society; that polygamy is as good as monogamy, or that no ethical judgement can be rationally justified. Even anthropologists whose training has made them sceptical of generalities and wary of philosophical entanglements are inclined to believe that the scientific study of cultures has undermined the belief in ethical absolutes. They accept, rightly, that different societies have different mores but then go further, regarding those mores within a society as making an act right or wrong. From this point of view, 'right' simply means according to the mores and 'wrong' means violation of the mores. This analysis of our concept of 'right' and 'wrong' could explain both the imperativeness and the impersonality of obligation. The 'ought' seems to tell one what to do and yet to be more than the command of any individual; perhaps, its power lies in the demands of society. In practice, of course, that means the demands of a particular society in keeping with the culture of that society. In fact, many things that were once thought to be absolute are actually relative to culture. Something is relative to culture when it varies with and is causally determined by culture. Nothing can be both relative to culture and absolute, for to be absolute is to be fixed and invariable, independent of man and the same for all men. In the real world, however, variation is a salient quality of cultures, indicating their relative nature.

General types of action take on specific differences when performed in different societies because those societies have different cultures. It is one thing, for example, for someone from the modern Western world to kill an aged parent. It is quite a different thing for an Eskimo to do such an act. One difference lies in the consequences of the act. In late twentieth-century Western society disposing of old parents allows one to live in greater luxury; to an Eskimo this act may mean the difference between barely adequate subsistence and malnutrition for himself and his family. Can it be accepted then that the nature of this act is culturally relative?

To say that the rightness of an act is relative to the society in which it is performed is not to say that exactly the same act can be both right and wrong. It is because the social context makes the acts different in kind that one can be right while the other is wrong.

This is not the same as saying that the acts are made right or wrong by the mores of society. Our modern Western society rightly disapproves of infanticide, and yet some South Seas societies (and the Greece of Plato's *The Republic*) approve of it; however, it is not this that makes infanticide wrong for Western society and right for some South Seas societies. If infanticide is wrong for the former and seems right for the latter, may it not be, because acts of infanticide have very different consequences in late twentieth-century Western society and in the South Seas?

It appears that the grounds for moral evaluation lie outside the moral emotions since it always makes sense to ask someone why he approves or disapproves of an action. If approving or disapproving made its object morally good or bad, there would be no need for such justification. Thus, the fact that moral emotions are culturally relative does not prove that identical acts or persons can be morally good in one society and morally bad in another.

Obviously the level of scientific knowledge within the culture will influence the outlook on right and wrong behaviour. Lack of awareness of the part played by micro-organisms and ignorance of how they could be controlled could go some way to explaining (but perhaps not excusing) the execution of those who, afflicted with plague, entered a medieval city. So solid was the justification for this practice felt to be, that Aquinas uses it as the basis for his *a fortiori* argument justifiying the burning of heresiarchs and heretics who brought heresy into a community.

An ignorance of genetics may have contributed to the accepted dominance of the male in ancient patriarchal societies. There does not seem to have been a realization within these ancient cultures that there was a vital female element (the ovum) in the production of a person. The womb was regarded merely as a receptacle for the development of the male life-force. Similarly, the previous dominance of the female in very early matriarchates may have been due to a surprising ignorance amongst the primitive hunter-gatherers, of the biology of reproduction. The female was seen as having a magical power to produce new life every now and again. The utter absence of even early stages of ethology contributed to such unhappy judicial situations as the formal execution of animals and, frequently, total indifference to animal suffering.

Simple geography can affect mores as regards rights. Hume, in passing, refers to rights in water but does not put them into an ethical context. Plato goes into great detail on the subject in *The Laws* and in desert cultures discussion of such rights is, literally, 'shooting talk'.

Mores not only determine the conduct of the individuals within a community but their sum total may form a characteristic pattern of that particular community. Whether it was the stratified snobbish society of old Boston:

> 'And this is good old Boston,
> The home of the bean and the cod,
> Where the Lowells talk to the Cabots,
> And the Cabots talk only to God.'
>
> *Toast at a Harvard Dinner*, J.C. Bossidy

or the hedonistic lifestyle of Venice in its heyday:

> 'As for Venice and its people, merely
> Born to bloom and drop,
> Here on earth they bore their fruitage,
> Mirth and folly were the crop;
> What of soul was left, I wonder, when
> The kissing had to stop.'
>
> *A Toccata of Galuppi's*, R. Browning

Education

There is little doubt, given the effective force of mores within a group, that the young are liable to be influenced by any type of education or formation provided within their community. Neither political nor religious bodies have ignored this potential for moulding characters. In *The Republic* Plato stresses the importance of education for the production of the model citizen. The famous, often-quoted saying of Saint Ignatius of Loyola has the ring of truth: 'Give me a boy of eight and I will give you the man' (with an A-level in guilt). But this is not true every time. Even the Jesuits had some spectacular failures, for example Voltaire and Joyce; but even they were influenced by them, although not, perhaps, in the way the Jesuits intended. Following this line of thought, some tend to regard morality as instilled by education, thus regarding it as a purely human construct lacking any objective basis.

It is important to realize, however, that the instilling of information in the process of education does not rob the data of objective truth. Multiplication tables have been instilled into children down the ages; sometimes ignorance of them was removed by the use of brute force (unhappy memories). Such compulsory acquisition of knowledge in no way diminished the reality of such data. The mathematical principles would still be true reflections of quantity in the real world even if no one learnt them. So it could be with ethical principles handed on by education but not created by education.

One topical difficulty in current controversies on ethical themes is the lack of relevant information on specific subjects. Genetic engineering is a case in point. Technology gallops on quicker than consequences can be ethically categorized. Unfortunately, also, would-be leaders in morals either find it difficult to keep up with scientific progress or may be ignorant of the ways of science or do not see the relevancy of scientific fact to the discussion of what is right or wrong. The rules of moral rectitude are seen by some as written in stone, and there is no escape clause allowing us to play God. It is in this area that appropriate education is imperative.

Education in this context is called for on two scores. Rightly there is a call for scientists to be aware of the ethical dimension of their discoveries outside of their own academic circle and the consequences of their activities on the wider world outside. Even more necessary is the need for education in the ways of science for those who would readily pontificate on the rightness or wrongness of the use of any new knowledge (as they inveighed against the use of anaesthetics in childbirth until Queen Victoria hushed the mere males by her example). It is in this ethical atmosphere that education must play a vital role.

It is obvious that, in studying ethics, not only must the indvidual be considered but his position within the society, and the part played by that society in forming the patterns of right and wrong available to him, must be taken into account. In this area ethics comes near to sociology. It is important to distinguish between the two disciplines. Sociology is more concerned with studying the structures of societies as they occur. It is eminently *a posteriori* and probably the better for that. Ethics is obviously *a priori*, based on speculation. When that speculation is intelligent, honest and drawn from valid premises founded in reality, it can be useful in assessing human conduct. It may be a little unfair but an easy method of detection has been suggested for identifying a sociologist. A sociologist blames a crime on everyone except the criminal.

Ethics and law

There has always been a close association of ethics with law, even from the earliest times. Two of the longest works by Plato were the ethical *The Republic* and the legal *The Laws*. The two disciplines coexist in similar territory. If we view the matter in a stricter linguistic mode and emphasize the real distinction between ethics and morals we will find that morals and law are sometimes as one. In the past, certainly, most morality was regarded as having a basis in religious teaching. For many, morality and religion were regarded as synonymous (hence the fascination with the wayward cleric). It should be noted, however, that religious morality is usually law-based, an outcrop from commandments usually regarded as divine in origin. The foundation of much Western morality is in the Bible. It is significant that the most venerable part of that work has been traditionally referred to as the 'Torah', often loosely translated simply as 'The Law'. The same emphasis on the legal aspect of revelation is carried through to the Christian dispensation. The law is not to be destroyed but fulfilled. Even the beatitudes have their sanctions. Here we are concerned, rather, with 'law' in the ordinary sense of the term, associated with the regulations of the various authorities under which we live, whether those regulatory instruments come from Westminster or Brussels – both more prosaic than Mount Sinai.

The relationship of law and ethics is not only a matter of common ground but is more importantly one of mutual support. Ethics has been well-defined as 'exhortation without enforcement'. Thus for general observance even of the most accepted of ethical principles, the law seems essential. On the other hand, law is not self-justifying; except in the case of Draconian legislation it needs moral support in order to be generally acceptable. The law is not an end in itself, nor does it provide ends. It is pre-eminently a means to serve what we think is right.

President Woodrow Wilson admirably summed up this mutual connection between ethics and law:

> 'The law that will work is merely the summing up in legislative form of the moral judgement that the community has already reached.'

The same close relation between morals, referred to in terms of sin, and law is noted in lighter prose, bordering on the flippant. The prose is written by a lady who is, perhaps, no moral philosopher but who is most certainly wise in the ways of the world: 'It ain't no sin if you crack a few laws now and then, just as long as you don't break any' (Mae West). (She even commented authoritatively and from wide experience on the very vexed dilemma of selecting from ethically unacceptable options: 'When choosing between two evils I always like to try the one I've never tried before.')

The law

Law goes a long way back, probably to the mists of prehistory. It appears already in a sophisticated form in the Hammurabi Code of Babylon (*c.* 1690 BCE). In keeping with the thinking of the time, it was given special force by attribution to the deity.

The great legalist, Blackstone (1723–1780), defines law in these words:

> 'Law, in its most general and comprehensive sense, signifies a rule of action . . . it is that rule of action which is prescribed by some superior and which the inferior is bound to obey.'

There are other definitions, for example, 'The body of principles recognized and applied by the State in the administration of justice' (Salmond), and 'Law is a coercive order of human behaviour' (Kelson).

Laws, in the sense that we are dealing with them here, are indubitably the product of humankind, though we may continue to speculate on the source of morality. They are made by legislators, or surreptitiously by judges, or informally by tradition and custom. All law is posited by some society or institution, though not necessarily by a legislature or sovereign.

Law and morality

Some, particularly in the past, saw law, as defined in the previous section, as positive law. Behind these merely man-made regulations, necessary for their support and essential to give them significance, they posited the existence of 'natural law'. This natural law they regarded as legal principles which are valid in themselves without having to be made. They are, therefore, valid at all times and in all communities. According to those who think this way and who, of course, reject relativism in ethics, these legal principles can be discovered by reason. Because of their rational basis they are universal in their application, controlling and limiting positive law.

The consequence of this line of legal and ethical argument is that what purports to be the law of the land is really so only if it is made in ways that agree with the principles of natural law. Indeed it may be held that what is regarded as law can be determined not to be the law after all, no matter what the legislature or anyone else has said, if it is shown to violate natural justice. (Music to the ears of advocates of single issue politics or agitators in direct action politics; but more of politics later.)

This particular doctrine of natural law is an analogue of objectivism in ethics. Indeed natural law would be simply that part of an objectively prescriptive ethics which was specially concerned with the topics with which law commonly deals. This would involve the administration of law, and the making of positive law, taken as including the rule that only what accords with it − either directly expressing it or having been posited in ways that it authorizes − is to be recognized and enforced as law. Natural law itself has sometimes been seen as being intrinsically objectively prescriptive; at other times as deriving its prescriptive component from divine command.

This concept of natural law is a channel through which some of the contents of some morality may be fed into the law, a device by which the positing of the law may be influenced by already posited elements of morality. The outlook which regarded accepted morality and criminal law as mutually interdependent was a basis of the State control by prosecution of deviation from accepted sexual mores. The doctrine also influenced the attitude to divorce and heavily influenced the legal status of women in the past, particularly married women, their property and their rights as citizens. This opinion reinforced a supposed duty of the State to enforce conformity with the accepted true Christian religion and to rid the community of subversive heretics or at least curtail their activity and restrict their facilities for outreach.

Explicit legislation uses such morally loaded terms as 'reasonable', 'harmful', 'wilful', 'wanton', 'malicious' and 'corrupt'. The vagueness of these terms is often resolved in practice in morally determined ways. The first of a long line of laudable factory Acts which culminated in the much-vaunted Health and Safety at Work etc Act 1974 was entitled the Health and Morals Act 1802.

In his work entitled *On Liberty*, John Stuart Mill discussed a topic which has been heatedly debated in legal and moral circles ever since. This dispute concerned the extent to which the law on the one hand should attempt to enforce the normal code of society and to what extent on the other hand, there must be left an area of 'private morality' outside the reach of law. Traditional believers in a supreme natural law saw, of course, no room for discussion on the matter.

A large part of both the criminal and civil legislation enforced by courts at all times and in all states would be regarded by many as accepted morality. Prominent amongst this common material are: prohibition against killing and assault; a demand for honesty, and a respect for the rights and property of others; and a requirement to keep agreements and to contribute in various ways to a community's organized joint purposes. In all such matters some restraints on individual inclinations are needed if people are to live tolerably together. Moral principles, rules, feelings and dispositions are the first line of defence; the formulation and authoritative statement of laws are the second; and the enforement of law is the third. It would seem that sometimes all three are necessary and that the second and third cannot work harmoniously and effectively if not in close agreement with the first. When this topic of whether the law should enforce morality is being discussed, it is not with respect to the central core of morality, or what we might call morality in the narrow sense, that the contenders are arguing. As already indicated, morality in the narrow sense is part of legislation in most nations. The contention is, in practice, only concerned with how far the law should go to back morality in the broad sense – that is, the peripheral areas or those moral tenets about which different religions or moralists themselves dispute. The case of *R. v. Brown and others* (HL. Dec. 1992), known as the Spanner Case, nailed down the point at issue. It resulted in prosecution, conviction and imprisonment of privately performing adult consenting masochists. The debate is complicated by the facts that there are now morally pluralistic societies in many states and because there is often a discrepancy between the morality to which people pay lip-service and that which they seriously subscribe to themselves. The real question, therefore, is whether the morality of one part of a society (e.g. of the Mary Whitehouses or in a different moral field, of the antivivisectionists) should be legally reinforced in its attempt to extend itself to other parts; or whether a morality which enjoys widespread lip-service should be supported by the law against one by which people live but which they are ashamed to avow.

It would seem to be better, where there are in fact divergent moralities in the broad sense, if law confined itself to the task which it shares with morality in the narrow sense – that is, of enabling rival factions as well as competing individuals, to live together by reciprocal limitations of their conflicting claims. Mutual tolerance might be easier to achieve if groups could realize that the ideals which determine their moralities in the broad sense are just that – i.e. the ideals of those who adhere to them – not objective values which impose requirements on all alike.

Perhaps, where people hypocritically profess support for certain rules of behaviour, their bluff should be called by having those rules enforced by law. This, however, would either force resistance to the imposed morality into the open or more probably spread the hypocrisy further so that it infected the machinery of law enforcement as well. A classic example of this process was prohibition in the USA. Experience has shown that corruption is the usual result of an attempt to enforce a morality that enjoys almost universal support on the surface but some considerable part of which is insincere.

The moralist needs the magistrate

Hobbes pointed out the need for legal support for the observance of morality. He speaks of laws of nature; they are, for him, basic moral rules which are unchangeable because the essential outlines of the human predicament do not change. He argues, nevertheless, that they are not unconditionally valid as rules of action. They 'bind to a desire they should take place; but ... to the putting them in act, not always'. One cannot afford to obey these rules unless one has some guarantee that others will do so too. But if one has such a guarantee, then one is obliged to obey them; for obeying them then gives one the best chance of preserving one's life. Consequently, in Hobbes' view, such rules, working merely as moral rules, are not enough. They must be supplemented by the political device of sovereignty. Only if each one knows that these rules will be enforced, that violations of them by others to his detriment will be discouraged by an effective threat of punishment, will he have a good reason for obeying them himself.

Surprisingly, Hume, in spite of his supreme scepticism in matters ethical and his own 'Hume's Law' on the impossibility of going from 'ought' to 'is', speaks of three fundamental laws of nature. For him these were: that of the stability of possession, of its transference by consent, and of the performances of promises.

What about justice?

The main theme of Plato's *The Republic* is justice, which he equates with 'the good'. For Plato the just man was synonymous with the righteous man. For many since those ancient times the term 'justice' epitomized good morals and all that was virtuous.

Justice is a name for certain classes of moral rules, which concern the essentials of human well-being more nearly, and are therefore of more absolute obligation, than any other rules for the guidance of life. Justice consists of moral rules which forbid people to hurt one another, which, of course, includes wrongful interference with each other's freedom. These rules of justice are more vital to human well-being than other maxims which, however important, merely point out the best mode of managing some department of human affairs. It is the observance of the rules which alone preserves peace among human beings. Men have an unmistakable interest in inculcating upon each other the duty of negative beneficence. A person may not always need the benefits of others but he always needs that they should not hurt him.

Justice and law

We have seen that Salmond defines law in terms of justice, in the sense that the law is the practice of justice. For many, the two terms seem almost synonymous but within the legal context there are important distinctions between the two concepts.

Justice can be described as what the law is supposed to produce. The great organizer of Roman law, Justinian (527–565), claims: 'Justice is the constant and perpetual will to render to everyone that to which he is entitled.' This is a wider definition which mainly applies to administrative justice, the type most closely associated with the law. It hints, however, at distributive justice which belongs more to the marketplace or, perhaps, is more commonly lacking therein. Here we are more concerned with it in a judicial setting and may say that justice among men involves an impartial and fearless act of choosing a solution for a dispute within a legal order, having regard to the human rights which that order protects.

It is in the practice of law that the division between the two concepts of justice and law becomes apparent. On occasions, judges, when sentencing a convicted felon, have expressed regret at being unable to impose a heavier sentence than that permitted by statute. Such a judge is indicating, at least in his opinion, a gap between justice and law. In practice the administration of law cannot be isolated from justice. The rigid application of a law, with no consideration of circumstances, may result in injustice. There are good historical developments in this area that illustrate the need of justice to mollify law. The evolution in English legal practice of the notion of equity was as an expression, originally, of the royal conscience. All early Lord Chancellors were clerics and softened the hard edges of the law by dispensing equity in chancery. In ancient Greece and later in canon law, *epieikeia*, which harks back to Aristotle's *Ethics* was a method of softening the law in hard cases by appealing to the 'mind of the legislator' to produce a milder interpretation of the letter of the law.

The ultimate cynicism as regards justice, I suppose, is the adage 'A person is guilty until proved influential'. When Bertrand Russell was attacked by a mob at a pacifist meeting in 1918, pleas to the police to rescue him as a great philosopher, as a world-famous person, fell on deaf ears. The cry, 'He is the brother of an earl', brought an immediate favourable reaction from the police.

Politics and morality

The above heading may strike some as a contradiction in terms. In fact there is a close association between these two topics. Aristotle's definition of man as a political animal sets the whole style of his three works on ethics.

If we can define politics as the general theory of how human communities function and how they can flourish, as I am sure we can, then ethics and politics are by no means strangers one to the other.

There are other more facile definitions of politics; the art of the possible or the persuading of the public to vote for this and support that and endure these for the promise of those. Finally, it is often viewed merely as the gentle art of getting votes from the poor and funds from the rich by promising to protect each from the other. There is little need to describe politics in detail for we are all potential politicians. Robert Louis Stevenson assures us that politics is perhaps the only profession for which no preparation is thought necessary. None of us who work in even a medium-size establishment are untouched by politics, at least in the broad sense and at a lower level. Even within families, at least of the larger size, the art of politics is gained early in life. (As the low man (or rather boy) on the totem pole I can assure you that is very true.) Politics in the broad sense is endemic to any group. The sociologists, of course, have an appropriate phrase: 'group dynamics'. (The basic axiom of group dynamics is: 'nice guys come second'.)

If ethics is the general theory of right and wrong in choices and actions, and what is good or bad in dispositions and interpersonal relations and ways of living, then political activities and aims and decisions come within its scope. The two cannot be kept apart. It would make no sense to confine moral thinking to private life and set up some quite independent principles to determine political values and decisions.

Many of the most controversial moral issues and the ones about which it is hardest for anyone to think clearly and honestly, and on which to take a firm stand, are political ones. Such political issues include questions about changing or preserving economic and social structures, and about conflicts of interest between organized groups within a State or between States or races; and even when one has chosen what seem to be laudable goals, questions about the methods one may use to pursue them, how to defend legitimate but threatened interests (acceptance of the notion of a just war) and how to vindicate rights that have been violated. Similar problems come up in somewhat different forms for private citizens, for those working in and through political movements or influential organizations, and for statesmen who act on behalf of nations or, perhaps, of supranational institutions.

The choice of political goals belongs with views about the good life for human beings. Since there will always be divergent conceptions of the good, a good form of society must somehow be a liberal one. It must leave open ways in which different preferences can be realized (room for the carnivore as well as the vegetarian). Tolerance should be a key word of any serious political movement. A good form of society must be able to accommodate and regulate differences and will neither try nor pretend to eliminate them.

Caution is paramount in this dangerous area. Political and economic problems are genuinely complicated. There can be no single change or number of changes, however radical or catastrophic, which would put everything right. It is an error, though an attractive and inspiring one, to suppose that there is some one evil – capitalism or colonialism – the destruction of which could bring about Utopia. There are extreme forms of injustice and exploitation which can give rise to disastrous civil, national and interracial wars but even the very means used to remove injustice and exploitation can on occasions create a worse situation. Such bleak prospects have not deterred those involved in moral philosophy from being involved in social reform. Edwin Chadwick, who was The Secretary of Bentham (the apostle of utilitarianism), was responsible for changes in social welfare with his Poor Law Amendment Act 1834.

On a much larger canvas and over a greater segment of time with much more disastrous results for many billions of the earth's population, Karl Marx (1818–1883) propagated his dialectical materialism. It was a heady brew of both moral and political philosophy with its roots in the abstruse metaphysics of Hegel (1770–1831).

Reference

Mackie, J.L. (1990) J.L. Mackie concurs with the notion that there is a close association between an accepted morality and the society in which it is found. *Ethics*, p. 109 *et seq.*, Penguin.

Part II

Ethics and Animals

Chapter 7

Human Attitudes to Animals

Applied ethics

Part II is not concerned with ethics *per se*. It is hoped that ethics as such has been adequately reviewed in Part I. Part II is intended to throw light on the basic material relevant to a proper grasp of the arguments most frequently presented in discussions on animal use. It presents knowledge of the ongoing interaction between humans and animals. An understanding of this process is of use in appreciating the various opinions and attitudes which fuel the controversies about our relationships with animals. Part II can be regarded as constituting an informed background to 'zoological ethics'.

The following material deals with a specialized area of applied ethics. To that extent it is a commentary on the application of ethical principles to real-life situations. Although the expression 'applied ethics' has a modern ring to it, traces of this approach to moral philosophy, bringing it closer to morality, as popularly understood, are to be found in the past. In *The Republic*, Plato confronted such practical issues as the treatment of women and the conduct of public officials. Lucretius discussed the moral implications of philosophical attitudes to death. Both Augustine and Aquinas speculated on the notion of a just war and the absolute evil of lying. Hobbes, with the civil war a recent reality, wrote on the moral basis of civil obedience. Hume drew on Seneca in his discourse on the justification for suicide. The Utilitarians were deeply involved in practical social reforms, particularly Bentham. John Stuart Mill dealt copiously with the moral aspects of capital punishment, liberty and the status of women in society. Many modern moral philosophers tended to be more theoretical but C.E.M. Joad wrote on political and social issues and was involved in the 1933 Oxford Union debate on patriotism. Bertrand Russell was deeply involved in the moral disputes of his day, especially those concerning nuclear warfare.

In this century, prominent philosphers such as A.J. Ayers tended to limit themselves to the study of the nature of morality and the meaning of moral judgements. This pursuit constituted 'meta-ethics'. This term denoted that they were not actually taking part in ethics but were engaged in a higher level study about ethics. In the early part of the century, under the influence of the writings of ethicists like G.E. Moore, normative ethics came to the fore. Normative ethics concentrated on a study of the general theories about what is good and bad, right and wrong.

The move towards the serious consideration of applying ethics to the moral problems of real life began to loom large in the middle of this century as the dogmatic sway of religion over the opinions of many began to decline. The American civil rights movements, attitudes to war, as the Vietnam battlefields came into living rooms through television, together with student activism, drew philosophy professors into the discussion of the moral issues of equality, justice, war and civil disobedience. Moral philosophy was inveigled by the media to become practical.

The founding of the journal *Philosophy and Public Affairs* (New York 1971) heralded the coming-of-age of applied ethics.

Due to a lack of precedents in the rapidly expanding field of research, progress and changing situations in the living sciences, bioethics developed to meet a growing demand for moral guidance in this field. Mary Warnock, a philosopher, was appointed by the Government to chair the Committee of Inquiry into Human Fertilisation and Embryology. In various countries philosophers are called upon to play a part in committees on the use of medicines, on programmes of research and on the use of animals for experimentation. In Victoria, Australia, it is a legislative requirement that medical experiments involving human embryos must be approved by a committee which includes 'a person holding a qualification in the study of philosophy'.

Most material appearing under the title of applied ethics tends to be specific in nature. This naturally follows from the fact that once one begins to apply ethical principles in practice, they are bound to be in connection with a specific controversy such as that on euthanasia, population control, etc. In such disputes the question of the status of ethical judgements falls into the background. What is important to the protagonists is that their professed opinion is established as reasonable, or at least emotionally acceptable. They argue, if possible, from widely accepted premises; or they attempt to convince their audience by concentrating on exposing the inconsistencies in the arguments of their opponents; or by pointing out the arbitrary distinctions made by defenders of the contrary point of view. On occasions the polemics can descend into blatant arousal of tear-jerking emotional responses.

All animals are equal

I think the following material is a good and relevant example of applied ethics in discussions of topics of public concern. This introduction is not intended to confirm the validity of the arguments used. The usefulness of this sample is to illustrate the dialectical form occurring in applied ethics and particularly in the discussion of a topic of the greatest relevancy. The special value of this material is that it is based on an article by Peter Singer, himself a most ardent protagonist of the worth of applied ethics (Singer 1992).

Singer's primary contention is that we should extend to other species the basic principle of equality that most of us recognize should be extended to all members of our own species.

Singer immediately attempts to deal with a most frequently occurring form of attack on the suggestion that all animals are equal. The form of polemic he has in mind is the old stand-by, the *argumentum ad absurdum* which aims at eradicating traces of degrees within categories – an approach which only accepts black and white and conveniently ignores the fact that reality is an infinity of greys. The *argumentum ad absurdum* is superficial but it is immensely popular and can be extremely effective. This fallacy is often purveyed by those who lack logical subtlety and are incapable of perceiving the delicate distinction which occurs between the push and the shove.

In fact in the past, the supposed outlandish notion of animal rights was used to parody, along the lines of the *argumentum ad absurdum*, the case for women's rights. When Mary Wollstonecraft, a forerunner of later feminists, published her *Vindication of the Rights of Women* in 1792, her ideas were widely regarded as absurd, and they were satirized in an anonymous publication entitled *A Vindication of the Rights of Brutes*. The author of this satire (actually Thomas Taylor, a distinguished Cambridge philosopher) tried to refute Wollstonecraft's reasonings by showing that they could be carried one stage further. If sound when applied to women, why should the arguments not be applied to dogs, cats and horses? The arguments seemed to hold equally for these brutes; yet to hold that brutes had rights was manifestly absurd; therefore the reasoning by which this conclusion had been reached must be unsound, and if unsound when applied to brutes, it must be unsound when applied to women, since the very same arguments had been used in each case.

Although a slight but essential deviation from the main flow, the drift of the argument used by Thomas Taylor is to be deplored and could be regarded as bringing philosophy itself into disrepute. It is reminiscent of the sentiments noted by Tennyson. He was not expressing his own sentiments as regards the appreciation of womankind: he was reflecting an extreme manifestation of male chauvinistic attitudes.

> 'He will hold thee, when his passion
> Shall have spent its novel force,
> Something better than his dog,
> A little dearer than his horse.'

Locksley Hall, Tennyson

There has been discrimination throughout history affecting women, based on a difference of sex, and on the fact that they were outside the dominant group. This pattern of behaviour is analogous to the speciesism that Singer and others so vehemently condemn when applied to animals. We do not have to go too far back in history to find blatant instances of this type of lack of concern for those outside the 'in-group'. In 1954 Commander G.H. Hatherill (Scotland Yard) made the following statement: 'There are about 20 murders a year in London and many not at all serious; some are just husbands killing their wives' (Hatherill 1997). This is an analogous type of speciesism rampant.

It is worth noting that Plato, in his seminal work on ethics *The Republic* (381 BCE), is adamant that women should be treated equally with men. In fact the only discrimination he would tolerate was as regards apparel or the lack of it during athletic pursuits in the gymnasium. He argued forcefully for equality for women even though it was against the customs, or *ethos*, of his time and society.

The case for equality between men and women cannot validly be extended to non-human animals. Women have a right to vote because they are just as capable, if not more so, of making rational decisions, as men are. Dogs, on the other hand, are incapable of understanding the significance of voting, so they cannot have the right. The significance of this line of argument can be illustrated by the fact that any serious discussion of the right to vote will be concerned with the age (taken as indicative of maturity and political awareness) of contenders for the vote.

Continuing this theme, it might be said that men and women are similar beings and should have equal rights, and that non-humans are different and should not have equal rights. No doubt the differences between humans and animals must give rise to some differences, in the rights that each can have. Recognizing this obvious fact need not be a barrier to extending the basic principle of equality to animals. The differences between men and women are equally undeniable, and the supporters of Women's Liberation are aware that these differences may give rise to different rights. Many feminists hold that women have the right to an abortion on request. It does not follow that since these same people are compaigning for equality between men and women they must support the right of men to have abortions too. Since a man cannot have an abortion, it is meaningless to talk of his right to have one. Since a pig cannot vote, it is meaningless to talk of its right to vote. There is no reason why either Women's Liberation or Animal Liberation should get involved in such nonsense.

The extension of the basic principle of equality from one group to another does not imply that we must treat both groups in exactly the same way, or grant exactly the same rights to both groups. Whether we should do so will depend on the nature of the two groups. The basic principle of equality is equality of consideration, and equal consideration for different beings may lead to different treatment and different rights. It has been said, perhaps rightly, that it is inequitable to treat the unequal equally.

The proposition claiming equal treatment for all, even if that 'all' is limited to all human beings, brings to light many complicated philosophical difficulties. Humans come in different shapes and sizes, they have different moral capacities, different intellectual abilities, different amounts of benevolent feelings, differing sensitivity to the needs of others, different abilities to communicate and different capacities to experience pleasure and pain. In short, if the demand for equality were based on the actual equality of all human beings, we would have to stop demanding equality; it would be an unjustifiable demand.

When we talk about the moral demand for equal treatment of human beings, however, we are usually speaking in terms, not of individuals as such, but of the right to equal treatment of different races and sexes. This is so because from the mere fact that a person is black or is a woman we cannot infer anything else about that person. The racist claims that his group is superior to others. Although there are differences between individuals, some individuals in the despised group are invariably superior to some indiviuals in the supposed superior group in all the capacities and abilities that could conceivably be relevant. For example, a person's sex is no guide to his or her abilities, and so it is unjustifiable to discriminate on the basis of sex.

The fact that humans differ as individuals, rather than as races or sexes, is a valid argument against those who would defend systems such as apartheid. The existence of individual variations that cut across the lines of race and sex, provides no defence against a more sophisticated argument which undermines the case for equality. This type of argument can appear in the form of a claim that the interests of those with IQ ratings above 100 should be preferred to the interests of those with IQs below 100. If we tie our moral principle of equality to the factual equality of the different races or sexes taken as a whole, we would have no basis for objecting to the kind of inegalitarianism based on IQs.

In the case of racism or sexism, however, there can be no absolute guarantee that abilities and capacities really are distributed evenly without regard to race and sex. There seems to be certain measurable differences between both races and sexes. These differences only become apparent when it is averages which are being considered. We do not, however, know how much of these differences are really due to the different endowments of the various races and sexes, and how much is due to the environmental differences that are the result of past and continuing discrimination. It would be dangerous to claim that all differences arise from environmental influences and so reject the possibility of the lack of any specific ability in a particular race or sex being genetic in origin. Such an assumption could make it more difficult to condemn racism or sexism in the future if the genetic base of specific abilities should become established beyond reasonable doubt. It is not wise to tie crucial moral arguments to scientific theories, however well received. They have been known to change. He who is wedded to the present is doomed soon to be widowed.

Equality is a moral ideal, not an assertion of fact. There is no reason for assuming that a factual difference in ability between two people justifies any difference in the amount of consideration we give to satisfying their needs and interests. The principle of the equality of human beings is not a description of an alleged actual equality among humans; it is a prescription of how we should treat humans. Jeremy Bentham incorporated the essential basis of moral equality into his utilitarian system of ethics in the formula: 'Each to count for one and none for more than one.'

This principle of equality implies that our concern for others ought not to depend on what they are like or what abilities they possess; however, precisely what this concern requires us to do may vary according to the characteristics of those affected by what we do. It is on this basis that the case against racism, sexism, etc. ultimately rests. It is in accordance with this principle that speciesism is also to be condemned. Singer argues that if possessing a higher degree of intelligence does not entitle one human to use another for his own ends, how can it entitle humans to exploit non-humans? Singer adopted the term speciesism from Richard Ryder.

The principle of equal consideration of interests had been presented by some philosophers in the past but it was rarely recognized that this principle could be applied to other species as well as to our own. Bentham was one of the few who did realize this. He wrote:

'The day may come when the rest of the animal creation may acquire those rights which never could have been withholden from them but by the hand of tyranny. The French have already discovered that the blackness of the skin is no reason why a human being should be abandoned without redress to the caprice of a tormentor. It may one day come to be recognized that the number of the legs, the villosity of the skin or the termination of the os sacrum, are reasons equally insufficient for abandoning a sensitive being to the same fate. What else is it that should trace the insuperable line? Is it the faculty of reason? But a full-grown horse or dog is beyond comparison a more rational, as well as a more conversable animal, than an infant of a day, or a week, or even a month, old. But suppose they were otherwise, what would it avail? The question is not, Can they reason? nor Can they talk? but, Can they suffer?'

(Bentham 1789)

In this passage, Bentham points to the capacity for suffering as the vital characteristic that gives a being the right to equal consideration. The capacity for suffering – or more strictly, for suffering and/or enjoyment or happiness – is not just another characteristic like the capacity for language, or for higher mathematics. The capacity for suffering and enjoying things is a prerequisite for having interests at all, a condition that must be satisfied before we can speak of interests in any meaningful way. Singer points out that it would be nonsense to say that it was not in the interests of a stone to be kicked along the road. A stone does not have interests because it cannot suffer. Nothing that we can do to it could possibly make any difference to its welfare. A mouse, on the other hand, does have an interest in not being tormented, because it will suffer if it is.

If a being suffers, there can be no moral justification for refusing to take suffering into consideration. No matter what the nature of the being, the principle of equality requires that its suffering be counted equally with the like suffering, in so far as rough comparisons can be made, of any other being. If a being is not capable of suffering, or of experiencing enjoyment or happiness, there is nothing to be taken into account. This is why the limit of sentience (using the term as a convenient, if not strictly accurate, shorthand for the capacity to suffer or experience enjoyment or happiness) is the only defensible boundary of concern for the interests of others. To mark this boundary by some characteristics like intelligence or rationality would be to mark it in an arbitrary manner.

Singer's line of argument uses the analogy of racism. The racist violates the principle of equality by giving greater weight to the interests of members of his own race, when there is a clash between their interests and the interests of those of another race. Similarly, the speciesist allows the interest of his own species to override the greater interests of members of other species. The pattern is the same in each case. Singer goes on to drive home his arguments more forcefully.

In eating animals we treat them purely as means to our ends. We regard their life and well-being as subordinate to our taste for a particular kind of dish. The term 'taste' is used deliberately as it is claimed that the consumption of meat is purely a matter of pleasing our palate. Singer denies that there can be any defence for eating flesh, based on nutritional needs. It is argued that we could satisfy our need for protein and other essential nutrients far more efficiently with a diet that replaced animal flesh by soya beans, or products derived from soya beans, and other high-protein vegetable products. Singer supports his stance by pointing to relative efficiencies of protein production:

'In order to produce 1 lb. of protein in the form of beef or veal, we must feed 21 lb. of protein to the animal. Other forms of livestock are slightly less inefficient, but the average ratio in the US is still 1:8. It has been estimated that the amount of protein lost to humans in this way is equivalent to 90% of the annual world protein deficit.'

(Lappé 1971)

Singer pursues further the argument concerning meat-eating. It is not merely the act of killing that indicates what we are ready to do to other species in order to gratify our tastes. The suffering we inflict on the animals while they are alive is perhaps an even clearer indication of our speciesism than the fact that we are prepared to kill them. In order to have meat on the table at a price that people can afford, our society tolerates methods of meat production that confine sentient animals in cramped, unsuitable conditions for the entire duration of their lives. Animals are treated like machines (Harrison 1964; Singer 1975).

The animal machine converts fodder into flesh, and any innovation that results in a higher 'conversion ratio' is liable to be adopted. It has been said that cruelty is acknowledged only when profitability ceases. Since none of these practices caters for anything more than our pleasures of taste, our practices of rearing and killing other animals in order to eat them is a clear instance of the sacrifice of the most important interests of other beings in order to satisfy trivial interests of our own.

Singer turns his attention to the most controversial topic concerning the use of animals – animal experimentation. He sees the same form of discrimination against other species in the practice of experimenting on animals. In the past, arguments about vivisection have, all too often, been put in absolutist terms. Would the abolitionist be prepared to let thousands die if they could be saved by experimenting on a single animal? (Back to the *reductio ad absurdum*.) The way to reply to this purely hypothetical question is to pose another: would the experimenter be prepared to perform his experiment on an orphaned human infant, if that were the only way to save many lives? (Singer talks in terms of an orphan to avoid the complication of parental feelings, although in doing so he claims he is being over-fair to experimenters, since the non-human subjects of experiments are not orphans.) If the experimenter is not prepared to use an orphaned infant, then his readiness to use non-humans is simple discrimination, since adult apes, cats, mice and other mammals are more aware of what is happening to them, more self-directing and, so far as we can tell, probably as sensitive to pain, as any human infant. There seems to be no relevant characteristic that human infants possess that adult mammals do not have to the same or a higher degree. Someone might try to argue that what makes it wrong to experiment on a human infant is that the infant will, in time and if left alone, develop into more than the non-human. However, one would then, to be consistent, have to oppose abortion, since the fetus has the same potential as the infant, indeed, even contraception and abstinence might be wrong on this ground, since the egg and sperm, considered jointly, also have the same potential. In any case, this argument still gives us no reason for selecting a non-human, rather than a human with severe and irreversible brain damage, as the subject for experiments.

The experimenter, then, shows a bias in favour of his own species whenever he carries out an experiment on a non-human for a purpose that he would not think justified the use of a human being at an equal or lower level of sentience, awareness, ability to be self-directing, etc. No one familiar with the kind of results yielded by most experiments on animals can have the slightest doubt that if this bias were eliminated, the number of experiments performed would be a minute fraction of the number performed today.

Singer berates philosophers for perpetuating a third and subtle form of speciesism. He thinks that philosophy ought to question the basic assumptions of the age. Thinking through critically and carefully, what most people take for granted is the chief task of philosophy. Philosophy does not always live up to this historic role. Philosophers are human beings and they are subject to all the pre-conceptions of the society to which they belong. Sometimes they succeed in breaking free of the prevailing ideology; more often they become its most sophis-ticated defenders. Most philosophers do not challenge the preconceptions about our relations with other species. Those who do tackle problems that touch upon the issue, reveal that they make the same unquestioned assumptions as most other humans. What they say tends to confirm readers in their comfortable speciesist habits.

It is significant that the problem of equality, in moral and political philosophy, is invariably formulated in terms of human equality. The effect of this is that the question of the equality of other animals does not confront the philosopher, or student, as an issue in itself. This is an indication of the failure of philosophy to challenge accepted beliefs. Some philosophers have found it difficult to discuss the issue of human equality without raising, in a paragraph or two, the question of the status of other animals. The reason for this is that if humans are to be regarded as equal to one another, we need some sense of 'equal' that does not require any actual descriptive equality of capacities, talents or other qualities. If equality is to be related to any actual characteristics of humans, these must represent some lowest common denominator, pitched so low that no human lacks them. But then the philosopher comes up against the catch that any such set of characteristics which covers all humans will not be possessed only by humans. In other words, it turns out that in the only sense in which we can truly say, as an assertion of fact, that all humans are equal, at least some members of other species are also equal, that is, to each other and to humans.

Singer justifies his estimation of philosophers by referring to *The Concept of Social Justice* by William Frankena (Frankena 1962). Frankena opposes the idea of basing justice on merit, because he sees that this could lead to highly inegalitarian results. Instead he proposes the principle that:

> '. . . all men are to be treated as equals, not because they are equal, in any respect, but simply because they are human. They are human because they have emotions and desires, and are able to think, and hence are capable of enjoying a good life in a sense in which other animals are not.'
>
> (Frankena 1962)

What is this capacity to enjoy the good life which all humans have, but no other animals? Other animals have emotions and desires, and appear to be capable of enjoying a good life. We may doubt that they can think but what is the relevancy of thinking? Frankena goes on to admit that by 'the good life' he means 'not so much the morally good life as the satisfactory life', so thought would appear to be unnecessary for enjoying the good life; in fact to emphasize the need for thought would make difficulties for the egalitarian since only some people are capable of leading intellectually satisfying lives, or morally good lives. This makes it difficult to see what Frankena's principle of equality has to do with simply being human. Every sentient being is capable of leading a life that is happier or less miserable than some alternative life style, and hence has a claim to be taken into account. In this respect the distinction between humans and non-humans is not a sharp division, but rather a continuum (shades of pantheism) along which we move gradually, with overlaps between the species (chimps and babies?), from simple capacities for enjoyment and satisfaction, or pain and suffering, to more complex ones.

Faced with a situation in which they see a need for some basis for the moral gulf that is commonly thought to separate humans from animals, but can find no concrete difference that will do the job without undermining the equality of humans, philosophers tend to waffle. (This is surely just a topical application of the 'Truman Law': If you can't convince them then confuse them.) They resort to high-sounding phrases like 'the intrinsic dignity of the human individual'. They talk of the 'intrinsic worth of all men' (note 'men') as if men had some worth that other beings did not possess. Even the Bible has some telling comments: 'You are worth more than any number of sparrows' (Luke 2:7). Some philosophers will talk in terms of human beings as ends in themselves or posit that everything other than a person can only have a value *for* a person.

Singer traces the idea of a distinctive human dignity and worth back to the humanists of the Renaissance, although a thousand years previously Protagoras spoke in terms of 'Man being the measure of all things'. The renaissance humanist Pico della Mirandola, in his *Oration on the Dignity of Man*', based human dignity on the idea that man possessed the central, pivotal position in the 'Great Chain of Being' that led from the lowliest forms of matter to God Himself. When we accept that humans are no more than a small sub-group of all the beings that inhabit (but in the case of humans also dominate) our planet, we may realize that in elevating our own species we are at the same time lowering the relative status of all other species. Once we ask why it should be that all humans, including infants, mental defectives, psychopaths, Hitler, Stalin and the rest, have some kind of dignity or worth that no elephant, pig or chimpanzee can ever achieve, we see that this question is as difficult to answer as our original request for some relevant fact that justifies the unequal treatment of other animals *vis-à-vis* human beings. High-flown talk about intrinsic dignity and moral worth only takes the problem back one step, because any satisfactory defence of the claim that all and only humans have intrinsic dignity would need to refer to some relevant capacities or characteristics that all and only humans possess.

Attitudes to animals

When the Under-Secretary of State at the Home Office, David Mellor, introduced the second White Paper (1985) on proposed legislation to control the use of animals in research, he said: 'One of the tests of a civilized society is its treatment of animals.' If this statement is correct, and there is no reason to think otherwise, some primitive societies may have been more civilized than those which followed them and than some which exist at the present time. Works by anthropologists indicate that some early cultures displayed a closer relationship between man and the other animals. A greater closeness to nature may have inspired a feeling of kinship with animals, even with wild animals, which did not exclude respect, indeed reverence, for the animals they hunted. It must be admitted, however, that not all cultures in the past had a predominantly benign attitude to the treatment of animals.

Marina Warner, in her Reith Lecture of 1994, stated:

> 'Few Elizabethans would have considered themselves kin to a crocodile, or thought of adopting an endangered species to prevent its extinction. In Elizabeth I's time, a courtier, bespattered with blood foaming from the lips of a bear at a bear-baiting session, rejoiced in the sport. The early French rationalist René Descartes arrived at the firm analysis that an animal was merely a machine: natural but lacking a soul.
>
> As we all know, our evolutionary proximity to the apes caused horror in the last century. Adam had been Lord of the Creation in the Bible, and named the beasts; now he was merely one of their kind. The peacock no longer existed simply to delight his eye, or the pig to fill his belly.'
>
> (Warner 1994)

But let us return to earlier days. In hunting cultures the interdependence of humans and animals demanded that an intimate knowledge of the behaviour and characterisitcs of prey animals be acquired by the hunter. Obviously in those primitive conditions the lifestyle of the animal and that of human beings was not so marked. The dens developed by animals and the nests built by birds could be seen as similar to the caves or coverings acquired by humans. The forming of trails, the marking of one's territory, the calling and signalling to one another, even mating rituals, could be perceived as reflecting human activity. It is little wonder that in some cultures, like those of the North American Indian, other creatures could be regarded as lesser brethren. In such situations, in the face of awesome natural phenomena, any supposed supremacy of mankind could pale into insignificance. With their acquired skills and use of tools some tribes may at the most have seen themselves as *primus inter pares* (first among equals) in respect to other animals. Primitive man could have been more struck by the similarity between himself and the beasts rather than have been aware of the differences.

This identification with other animals certainly surfaced early on in the development of the 'totem' – the association of a tribe or clan with a particular species of animal. The honouring of the totem-pole gave material expression to this acceptance of other creatures as associated with humans. Not only in many early cultures were other animals accepted in this way as equals but, to a certain extent due to the honour given to the totem-pole, they began to be worshipped. Some animals no doubt were regarded as being in some ways superior to man, for example the fox for its cunning, the lion for its courage, the gazelle for its speed and the cat, no doubt, for some good reason. These attitudes do not belong only to prehistory or the dim past. Even in a sophisticated and technological civilization such as that of ancient Egypt, the cat as well as other animals were exalted beyond humanity into the realm of the divine and were worshipped as deities.

This primitive relationship was not without its tensions. Hunting cultures needed to cope with the anxiety of getting sufficient animals to keep the tribe fed. Yet there must have been a certain angst affecting the psyche of those involved in hunting and killing creatures which they regarded as a sort of kin or even reverenced as symbols of their own community. Lacking any special theological basis for separating humans from other animals, the projection of inner attitudes on to animals was as natural as the imputation of subjective awareness on to other members of their own family. One of the most ancient expressions of the acceptance by humans of their 'togetherness' with other animals, in fact a readiness to empower other animals, still visible in Eurasia and the Americas alike, is a ritual attitude towards animals. The 'bear ceremonialism' still found among the Paleosiberian Ainu is not merely continuous around the world in the northern hemisphere but goes back to the caves of southern Ice Age Europe. The Ainu completely anthropomorphize the bear, raise and suckle it with human mothers, treat and speak to it like a human, and call it father; in this circumpolar cult, the bear is totemically oedipalized.

Somewhat less complete and dramatic, but even more widespread, is the ritual attitude of hunters towards their kill. If humans live off the lives of animals, they are concerned that these animals be reborn, be fertile and be plentiful for the hunter. Thus the plains hunter placed the feet of a slaughtered buffalo at the four corners of a rectangle, addressed the spirit of the dead buffalo and adjured it to live anew and come back in the flesh of a live buffalo again. This bone-magic was prevalent also in Asia.

The earliest leaders of ancient communities were probably shamans to whom special power over animals was attributed. In Greek mythology the charismatic figure of Orpheus fulfils this role. The close association of man and animals is clearly perceived in the Greek cult of Dionysus. The acceptance of animals as part of human society was even more marked in ancient Egypt. One of the earliest truly historical documents extant (2800 BCE) bears an image of a bull prefiguring the worship of Apis, the sacred bull. Other bulls were worshipped as well, as was Hathor, the sacred cow.

This veneration of animals was no deviation from the norm. The modern Eskimo showed reverence and paid respect to the seal he slayed and was about to eat. Totemism was not solely a Red Indian phenomenon. It was primarily a system in which different groups of primitive society were given the name of a particular animal species, like a scout pack. It classified humans by means of a classification of animals. The human group was regarded as having a relationship of a practical kind with its totem. Even the sophisticated religion of Mithraism, the one near-successful challenger to Christianity in the Roman World, presented the close association between man and animal – peaking in the horrific Taurobolus. This was in stark contrast to the gentler notion of the Lamb of God. The identification of animal and man in early religious settings was by no means always favourable to animals. The cruel ritual of the scapegoat was not unique and most ancient religions revelled in numerous and bloody sacrifices.

Religious and legal attitudes to animals

Religious attitudes

Christian moralists drawing inspiration from the Bible have tended to be negative in their approach to man's obligations in respect to animals. In Genesis, man is portrayed as master of the beasts, naming them as if they are all his property. In Psalm 8:8, sheep, oxen, the beasts of the field, the birds of the air and the fishes of the sea are portrayed as under his feet. The Old Testament is not completely insensitive to animal welfare: 'muzzle not the ox that treads the corn' (Deuteronomy 25:4). The Talmud, a later collection of Judaic teaching, emphasizes the need to show kindness to animals. It is stipulated that an owner of an animal must be capable of properly providing for it. The Koran shows the same concern for the welfare of animals. Eastern religions, some with a fundamental pantheistic philosophy which implies a continuum of life forms, have always showed consideration for animals. The sacredness of the cow to the Hindu is proverbial and a similar benign attitude to beasts occurs in Buddhism. In the opinion of many Westerners, the Jains may have carried solicitude for even the lowliest members of the animal kingdom to extremes.

Most Christian teachers, like Augustine, taught that a community of mutual obligations could not include animals. The Christian approach was confirmed by Aquinas who pointed out that men are the agents of God, animals are their instruments. Animals are divinely provided for use by rational creatures as they see fit. Hence there is nothing wrong in man making whatever use of animals he chooses. Cruelty to animals can only be condemned on the grounds that it might lead to cruelty to humans or that some psychological harm might come to the perpetrator of the cruel act. This approach continued to represent the opinions of moral theologians through to the present century (Davis 1941).

Legal attitudes

The legal attitude to animals has usually been concerned mainly with possession. Even within the Decalogue, those original basic laws, one only of the ten is concerned with animals: 'Thou shalt not covet thy neighbour's house . . . nor his ox, nor his ass' (Exodus 20:17). This epitomizes much of later legislation dealing with animals – the protection not of the animal itself but the protection of the property rights of its owner. In the *Institutes of Justinian* (AD 532), a basic authority of Roman law, the only material concerned with animals deals with how they can be acquired and how long possession of them may be sustained or how such ownership can be lost (Book II,

Title I, 12–16). Later additional legislation on animals tended to be concerned with the damage they might cause and with their trespass on land. Even from early times, on occasions, the law turned its full fury against offending animals – a goring ox was to be stoned (Exodus 21:28). A full account of such legal sanctions can be found in *The Criminal Prosecution and Capital Punishment of Animals* (Evans 1987).

The first laws intended to protect animals begin to appear in the West in the nineteenth century, e.g. Martin's Act 1822. Even the main Act protecting animals in this century, the Protection of Animals Act (1911), displays a bias towards ownership. Under this Act only domesticated or captive animals are protected.

It is only towards the end of this century that a more caring and sophisticated aspect of animal legislation developed. The Diseases of Animals Act 1950 was designed to control animal diseases, mainly those that occur amongst agricultural animals, and was of economic intent. The Agriculture (Miscellaneous Provisions) Act 1968 instigated Codes of Recommendation for the welfare of animals. By 1981 the emphasis had changed from disease to health in the Animal Health Act 1981. A further advance towards concern for the animal as such, is hinted at in the Animal Health and Welfare Act 1984.

Awareness of the need to protect those animals who are not owned by someone was evident in the introduction of such legislation as the Badgers Acts (culminating in the Protection of Badgers Act 1992 which even brought Brock's abode within legal restraints). Legal protection of many wild animals was introduced by the Wildlife and Countryside Act 1981 and 1984. Enlightment was slow to develop on the international front. The Endangered Species (Import and Export) Act 1976 embodied the Convention on International Trade in Endangered Species of Fauna and Flora.

All law on animals tends to be not only speciesist but also elitist. This follows from the very nature of the animal world itself where creatures appear to be arranged in ascending and descending orders. This is most obvious in the operation of the Animal (Scientific Procedures) Act 1986 where special consideration must be given as regards the use of, for example, cats, dogs and primates in research. It was in this area of animal experimentation that more recently legislation has begun to come to the fore, even outside the British Isles. As long ago as 1450, Leonardo da Vinci had talked in terms of future legislation to control the use of animals in experiments but his prediction took centuries to be fulfilled.

Well-meaning and well-written Conventions may be in place but that is not proof that consequent legislation has been enacted nor does it imply equal observance by all the signatories. Apart from what may be regarded as divine law, all legislation is human in origin and can only be enforced by humans. It is not surprising, therefore, that law tends to be anthropocentric and is not so orientated towards our 'younger brothers'. After all, 'animals can't sue'.

Philosophical attitudes to animals

Considering the ready acceptance of slavery by Greek philosophers and later Christian indifference to the slave trade, it can be presumed rightly that few would have, in the past, been outraged by the use of animals in experiments. Aristotle summed up the accepted view on animals in terms such as: 'plants exist for animals and animals exist for man'.

According to Descartes (1596–1650), there are two crucial differences between humans and animals: the latter cannot form statements by which they may make known their thoughts and they do not act from knowledge, only from the disposition of their organs (*Discourses* Part V). Like Aristotle before him, Descartes believed animals to have no capacity for reason and, along with the rest of the class of machines into which animals were relegated, could not even feel. Voltaire (1694–1778) ridiculed Descartes's idea that it is in virtue of speech that a living being can be said to have the faculties of thought, feeling and memory. Faced with the same stimuli, argued Voltaire, animals exhibit much the same behavioural patterns as humans. Hume (1711–1776), in this matter as in most others, opposed Christian tradition in his reasoning:

> 'No truth appears to me more evident than that beasts are endowed with thought and reason as well as man.... In performing goal-directed actions, animals like men, are guided by reason and design, and from the similarity of their external actions to our own we can deduce the similarity of their internal or mental actions.'

Kant (1724–1804), in good Christian tradition, regarded duties to animals as merely indirect duties to mankind.

Schopenhauer (1788–1860) criticized the Cartesian idea that animals are not self-conscious and have no ego. In his work *On the Basis of Morality* he states:

> 'If any Cartesian were to find himself clawed by a tiger, he would become aware in the clearest possible manner of the sharp distinction such a beast draws between its ego and its non-ego.'

He emphasized, along with Voltaire and Hume, that all evidence pointed to the similarity and not the difference between human nature and animal nature.

Personal attitudes to animals

Throughout the ages and in the present day, most humans have developed their own individual pattern of relationships with animals, for example:

- The care of the farmer, stockman, even the cowboy, etc. for their beasts as assets and sources of energy for work.
- The complex attitude of the hunter to his livelihood.
- The pride of the exhibitor in the outstanding qualities or beauty of the animal which she or he owns.
- The emotional attachment to a favoured pet.

- Admiration of the ingenuity and magnificence of certain animals.
- Amusement at the performances of animals; unfortunately, sometimes as figures of fun as in a menagerie or circus.
- At the worst, gratification of sadistic tastes, e.g. dog fights.

More on speciesism

The term 'speciesism' is not always regarded as respectable among research workers. It tends to be viewed askance in keeping with the dialectical mode of the dialogue of the deaf. It is, however, a topic which needs to be addressed positively. It will not just go away of its own accord.

This theme has been fully explored in the second section of this chapter entitled 'All animals are equal'. This slogan has been reiterated and exaggerated by Ingrid Newkirk of PETA (People for the Ethical Treatment of Animals) with her rallying cry: 'A rat is a pig, is a dog, is a boy.'

It behoves us here merely to consider the nature of speciesism and some salient points concerning it. The essence of speciesism can be summed up in the phrase: 'the boundary of my group is the boundary of my concern'. A natural corollary of this in the past, when from Aristotle to Descartes the accepted attitude to beasts could be well-expressed in the phrase 'Vive la différence', was an unrestricted use of animals for whatever purpose suited man. Porter claims that there exists among many research workers the inarticulated acceptance that they are justified in giving priority to the needs of humans above those of other animals, particularly in respect to the health and survival of humankind. This accepted attitude is a direct practical expression of speciesism (Porter 1986).

The difference implied by speciesists between humans and other animals is not as widely nor as dogmatically defended as it used to be. As far back as 1831, Marshall Hall, a leading physician and physiologist, had spelt out his principles demanding due and grave consideration be given to decisions on the use of any animals in research. His sentiments were by no means universally reflected in the attitude of the majority of scientists in his century even though his principles were reiterated in *The Lancet* in 1847. There were some however, among the great and the good, even in scientific circles, who did not regard animals as outside their concern and they called loudly for the protection of the animals being used in experiments. Darwin, Huxley, Jenner, Owen and the Presidents of the Royal College of Physicians and Surgeons signed a petitition demanding control of animal experimentation by law.

In the twentieth century, even up to a few decades ago, the differences between humans and other animals, justifying their use in any way appropriate in research, were taken for granted by many in the scientific community. There was little evidence of soul-searching amongst active practitioners of animal experimentation. Some voices of concern were raised on behalf of experimental animals; Russell and Burch for example, and the members of UFAW (Universities Federation for Animal Welfare). Other bodies, such as the Littlewood Commmittee in 1965, drew the attention of workers in the field to the consideration that should be given to the use of animals in research. In this 'end of the century', however, there does seem to have developed a greater awareness of the needs of animals, an acceptance of obligations to the animals we use and less inclination to regard them as mere 'tools' of research – a phrase which at one time may have been used without any compunction by some in the research community.

Many more workers in research now regard animal life as more akin to that of humans. Evidence of this I think can be seen in the prominence given in animal units to the provision of environnmental enrichment or enhancement for laboratory animals. This is surely an indication that those using animals are viewing them much more as individuals, akin to ourselves, rather than material for experimentation.

In fact the similarity of other animals to ourselves is the critical factor in animal experimentation. If they were not analogous to us, then extrapolation – the primary process in research – would lack a factual basis. The closer the animal is to us, for example a primate species, the greater will be the validity of any extrapolation from a procedure performed on that species. However, the overall similarity to humans of the species used will not always be the most relevant factor. For example, where pigs are used in the development of transplant techniques, the reason why the pig is chosen is because in that instance the particular feature involved is most similar to the corresponding feature in humans. In short, it is the close similarity between ourselves and animals which is the essential basis for the usefulness of animal experimentation.

It would seem paradoxical to use animals in experiments because they are so like us, yet treat them in other ways as a completely different type of creature, without any claim on our concern. It is that compassionate 'concern' for the creature outside the group which obviates the undesirable effects of speciesism. Just as it is ruthless 'exploitation' which marks the activity of the speciesist.

Nature, in its rich variety, is blatantly speciesistic in the sense that everywhere we look in the animal and plant world there is an abundance of differing species. Not only are there myriads of species wheresoever life occurs but inevitably these species are divided into subspecies and these in their turn are split into strains and varieties. Diversity is the very texture of life. Such distinctions are not always benign: struggle is the very warp and weft of life. The predator–prey relationship is a salient feature of the reality of living. Even the most dedicated animal lobbyist cannot campaign for both the saving of the whale and of the krill at the same time. Unfortunately, it is 'dog eat dog' out there.

The existence of species, even the conflict between species, in nature does not justify humans, as rational animals, to abuse other creatures for their own human benefit. No doubt humans have done so in the past but of course they also, and to an even greater extent and in a more cruel way, abused their fellow humans. We lingered long enough on the evil of slavery. Most of us now would roundly condemn such exploitation. Such exploitation was regarded as acceptable because it was the exploitation of those outside the group and therefore outside the concern of that group, just as animals being outside of our species could be considered beyond our concern.

The exploitation of 'breeds beyond the law' has a long history. As far back as AD 69 the Emperor Vespasian attempted, in the guise of an interest in science, to ascertain the specific gravity of the water in the Dead Sea by immersing Jewish prisoners beneath the waves by means of varying weights attached to their bodies (Josephus *c.* AD 90). The victims were not Roman citizens. They were outside the boundary of the accepted group and so beyond concern. This was quite in keeping with the teaching of Aristotle, that slaves – and the survivors of Vespasian's experiments would become slaves – had no rights. I am sure all right-minded people would agree that they should have had rights. Even Pasteur, many centuries later, did not scruple about the use of Russian serfs or Siamese peasants in experiments involving real infection (*Spectator* 1892). Experimentation on *untermenschen* (subhumans) was commonplace in the setting of the concentration camp. It has been suggested that some clinical trials unacceptable in the industrial nations of the West have taken place in Third World countries. It has been argued that such trials are of great benefit to such patients who have no other available alternative modes of health care. A use of human organs for transplants, not always from volunteers but, perhaps, even from arranged executions, has been reported in the media. In the past, the classic experimental animal for toxicity testing, i.e. the royal taster, was obviously of a lower class and by no means of blue blood. The above facts may seem irrelevant to a discussion on the use of animals in research. They have, however, undertones of speciesism, a difficult and sensitive topic in this area.

Species élitism

The word 'élitism' means 'a favourable selection out of a particular group'. Grading of non-human species appears in the Animals (Scientific Procedures) Act 1986. The very definition of 'protected animal' in the Act is selective, initially embracing only vertebrates. Then by a Statutory Instrument, an Order in 1993, it became more blatantly élitist. Among the octopoda, only the vulgar were favoured. It may be a moot point in law whether the squid, a fellow cephalopod, is better off taking its chances under the Protection of Animals Act 1911, if it is captive, than being given legal status under the 1986 Act.

In Danish law it is stipulated that lower (a questionable term among animal-lovers) animals are to be preferred for experimental purposes. Few, except extremists, would question the rationale of some legal distinctions to be found in animal law. In short, species are, in fact, specifically different.

The biological continuum

Absolutely contrary to speciesism is a belief in the unity of all life. This pantheistic notion, that all beings are as one with God, has been much more common in Eastern religions and therefore Eastern cultures than in Western ones. Those who hold by this philosophical approach to reality claim that all animals, including humans, must be treated equally. In some cases the results of such beliefs can be surprising. Drivers in Katmandu face stiffer penalties for running into cows than they do for hitting a human. The custom of the devout Jain to have a servant preceding him to brush away any insects he may crush with his step is amazing. The keeping by the Jains of animals until they die naturally even though suffering tremendously is also surprising.

Concern shown to animals in Western cultures is not so marked and probably does not arise from religious or philosophical concepts, but may sometimes be unusual. There are lawyers in the USA that specialize in pet custody cases, purely, so they say, for the pet's benefit. It is crucial, these legal eagles claim, that the pet goes to the separating spouse that will spend the most quality time with the animal (Channel 5 1998). From another direction, in a case reported from South Africa in 1985 in the *Daily Telegraph* an injured black woman was kept waiting while a stabbed police dog was rushed to a vet. In another surprising example, a tortoise was flown from the Galapagos Islands to Florida for medical treatment. No such facility was available for any humans on the Galapagos Islands (BBC2 1994).

The extreme interpretation of the teaching of the unity of all life is that no species must be regarded as expendable nor should one species be abused or exploited by another. Unfortuately, such benignity does not exist in nature, for 'nature is a hanging judge'. The slightest misjudging of the movement of a predator can spell the death of an unwary prey. One good effect of a moderate acceptance of a biological continuum has been efforts to preserve endangered species. A reluctance to harm any creature, however unpleasant, can lead to a strange respect for unique genetic patterns and the questioning, for example, of the complete eradication of the smallpox virus. However, the retention of the smallpox virus, at least by the USA and Russia up to the present (i.e. 1998), is hardly being done out of respect for this lowly life form.

The more extensive our impact on the natural world, the more need there is for ethical restraint at the interfaces between people, animals and nature. Hopefully in the future, animals will fall less under our domination and move further within the scope of our concern. This will facilitate a more acceptable form of symbiosis between humans, animals and nature.

There is an essential difference between animals and humans under experimentation. Humans can effectively withhold consent. They can take the researcher to court if he or she goes beyond his or her remit, and even claim compensation. Animals cannot even complain in any meaningful way.

Though some animal activists may argue that speciesism is peculiar to modern man, there is abundant evidence to the contrary. Laws both ancient and modern certainly classified animals as property at the absolute disposal of the human owner.

Anthropomorphism

This is the attribution of human traits to other beings, both celestial and terrestrial. This term is often used as an immediate jibe, by purists in science, especially behaviourists, against any author applying to animals, even in a broad sense, characteristics associated with humans. To be accused of being anthropomorphic in the living sciences is to be damned as being unscientific in the extreme. Not to be

anthropomorphic in some situations is to be unreal in the extreme. As a man –
anthropos – it is difficult not to think in an anthropomorphic way. We must look out
on the world using our own thought patterns based on our own nature. We have no
other option. We must, however, not completely project our own nature on to
outside objects. Many regard anthropomorphism as a fallacious attempt to bridge a
gap between human and non-human characteristics. It is dismissed as an irrational
relic of primitive human awareness of reality. A logical fallacy would only arise if we
attributed human traits to the sort of thing which could not possibly bear them. It
would certainly be logically fallacious to attribute cleverness to Tuesday or alertness
to a theorem. No one, however, objects to attributing traits which we normally
attribute to human bodies or biological processes to animal bodies or biological
processes. Indeed, built into animal research is a presupposition of anthropomorphism: the assumption that many human traits are portrayed in some relevant
fashion in animals.

While accepting the biological and physiological common ground of both
humans and animals, some still reject anthropomorphism as a fallacy when it implies
the existence of similar mental traits in humans and animals. A fallacy would indeed
be present if we knew for certain that animals were not the sort of things to which
mental predicates could be applied. There is no such total certainty. No rational
person would apply the term 'good-natured' to a day of the week, but many sane,
rational and intelligent people in most cultures and during most historical periods
have applied mental-state terms to animals. It is possible that they have been wrong
in so doing but it is certainly not a fallacy unless one can prove that such terms cannot
sensibly be applied to animals.

It is not the people who impute pain to animals who are anthropomorphic; they
have good evolutionary, physiological and behavioural reasons for doing so. Relevant details will be produced later in this text. It is rather those who deny that animals
suffer pain on the grounds that their behaviour during affliction does not exactly
mirror human reactions, who are anthropomorphic. Who but someone guilty of the
grossest anthropomorphism would expect expressions of animal feelings to be precisely like ours? A cow in pain could hardly be expected to cry 'Oh dear, dear me, it
does hurt.' Animals do show unique pain behaviour. It does not happen to be human
pain behaviour. Why should it be? Signals of distress to conspecifics are bound to
differ according to whether the victim is gregarious or solitary, predator or prey. If
this were not so, messages for help could jeopardize the safety both of the sufferer and
the would-be assistant. We would expect the behaviour of the animal in pain to be
appropriate to its *telos* – the unique evolutionary determined, genetically encoded,
environmentally shaped set of needs and interests which characterize the animal in
question – the pigness of the pig, the dogness of the dog, etc.

From the dictates of experience and common sense, those who deal a lot with
horses are aware that a tightening of the palpebral (eyelid) muscles indicates great
agony. This would mean nothing to the person who is expecting the whole range of
human pain behaviour from the horse. I had a conversation with a scientist, an expert
in the way of fish. Though he by no means denied that it could be a fact that fish felt
pain, he rightly commented that there was no way of ascertaining what the exact

nature of such pain might be. He posited that the behaviour of the fish, pulling on the hook and so apparently increasing the pain, indicated that the sensation experienced by the fish differed from that which would be felt by humans in similar situations. This form of argument is akin to the punter claiming that race horses have no dread of Beecher's Brook since some of them keep on attempting to jump it even when the jockey is no longer aloft. There is much still to be learnt about how animals experience reality, either as regards pain or pleasure. An uncritical anthropomorphic approach is definitely unjustified, but a cautious use of anthropomorphism in the form of speculative probes may be a useful method of exploring animal awareness. After all, *anthropos* is an animal as well.

A summary of human attitudes to animals

Human–animal relations are kaleidoscopic, forever changing and never completely predictable. As we near the end of the millennium one attempted prediction seems to have fallen somewhat short of reality:

> 'By the year 2000, man will have learned to manufacture all the animal protein he needs and will no longer have to be dependent for sustenance on the animal kingdom. Through genetic control, man will be able to produce superior pets, combining the qualities of two different species, a dog–cat animal companion, for example. This animal will then be truly looked upon as man's junior partner who will accompany him on his space odysseys. Man will have learned how to communicate with his animal companions, and the latter in turn will be able to convey more fully and accurately their wants, desires, hopes and aspirations. Man will learn how the animal perceives his world and his relationship with man. The animal companion also will help man to communicate with the world of the unseen, the world of parapsychic phenomena.'
>
> (Levinson 1974)

Truly we have not got that far and we only have 16 months to go. I doubt we will get there by 2000. We may be heading that way. A Texan millionaire has paid researchers at A and M University in Texas $5 million to clone his pet dog, Missy (BBC1 1998).

Human attitudes to animals have varied immensely down the ages. There has been fear, awe, veneration, affection, use and unfortunately abuse of animals by humanity in different times and different places. It would be extremely difficult to portray these divergent relationships in any detail or with any accuracy. As Elias Canetti so rightly commented: 'History talks too little about animals.'

References

BBC1 (1998) *The News* 6.15 PM 24 August. British Broadcasting Corporation, London.
BBC2 (1994) Television programme 8.00 PM, 17 July.

Bentham, J. (1789) Refer to the material on Bentham in the references at the end of Chapter 2.

Channel 5 (1998) The sample anecdote given was one among many in the Channel 5 TV programme *Leeza* (11.10 AM, 24 August) which illustrate what was referred to above by Davis as 'false sentimentality'.

Davis, H. (1941) 'Animals have no rights: they can give us nothing freely nor understand our claims. We have no duties of justice or charity towards them, but as they are God's creatures, we have duties concerning them and the right use we make of them. In the treatment of animals we may not give way to rage or impatience, nor invade our neighbour's right of ownership in them, nor may we give way to cruelty in the treatment of animals, nor wantonly misuse or abuse them, for this disposes us to dull the fine edge of pity and to be cruel to human beings.

'The contrary tendency of lavishing affection on beasts – not wrong in itself – may lead, and often does lead, to the neglect of one's duty to a neighbour in need, and to an altogether false sentimentality.' H. Davis S.J. *Moral and Pastoral Theology*, Vol. II, p. 258, Sheed and Ward, London. Davis, true Thomist as he was, based this common sense view firmly on the *Summa Theologica* of Thomas Aquinas.

Evans, E.P. (1987) The almost esoteric work on animals in court has already been referred to: Evans' *The Criminal Prosecution and Capital Punishment of Animals*, Faber and Faber, London.

Frankena, W. (1962) Frankena's attitude to animals is regarded by Peter Singer as typical of the human elitism of many philosophers. William Frankena develops his concept of being human in his article 'Social Justice' in *The Concept of Social Justice* (ed. R. Brandt), Englewood Cliffs.

Harrison, R. (1964) An ardent advocate for animal welfare, Harrison backs his condemnation of intensive farming with examples in his book *Animal Machines*, London.

Hatherill (1997) This extraordinary, and now surely politically incorrect, statement was published in the *Bibliophile*, Catalogue 153, July.

Josephus, F. (*c.* 90) This ancient example of indifference to those outside the accepted group is graphically described in *The Jewish Wars*, Book VII in the *Works of Flavius Josephus* translated by William Whiston, William P. Nimmo *et al*.

Lappé (1971) The impressive statistics were produced in *Diet for a Small Planet*, pp. 4–11, Friends of the Earth/Ballantine, New York.

Levinson (1974) These daring prophecies were given in a speech, 'Forecast for the Year 2000', at a *Symposium on Pet Animals and Society*, on 31 January at the Zoological Gardens, London.

Porter, D.G. (1986) David G. Porter wrote a very balanced article on the ethical dimension of the use of animals in research in *Nature*, **356**, 101.

Singer, P. (1992) Much of the material in the early part of this chapter uses material from Peter Singer's seminal article 'All Animals are Equal'. The article appears in a valuable book *Applied Ethics*, pp. 215–228, Oxford University Press, Oxford. Peter Singer edited this work himself in the series *Oxford Readings in Philosophy*.

Singer, P. (1975) Peter Singer makes his case for concern for animals in his work *Animal Liberation*, New York.

Spectator (1892) 10 September.

Warner, M. (1994) The attitudes of humans to animals was the theme of the 4th Reith Lecture by Marina Warner, Feb., BBC television.

Chapter 8

Animal Rights

'Cub right is the right of the Yearling.
From all of his pack he may claim
Full-gorge when the killer has eaten;
And none may refuse him the same.'

The Law of the Jungle, R. Kipling

Introduction

Ronald Lee and Clifford Goodman were both sentenced to three years' imprisonment at Oxford Crown Court (24 March 1975). They had been convicted of causing £50 000 worth of damage to laboratories. 'I ask for justice for all animals', said Ronald Lee, a former trainee solicitor. The militant wing of the animal rights movement had, it believed, its first political prisoners, its first martyrs for the cause.

The plea for justice, not just for consideration, for care, nor for concern, dramatically highlighted a modern but controversial issue – the question of animal rights. Although, to many, a novel idea, the notion has been accepted in many circles. Some undergraduate colleges in the USA and at least one veterinary school (Colorado State University) now offer courses in animal rights. These developments stem from writings such as those by Peter Singer. Singer developed the notion of 'equal consideration of interests', first expounded by Jeremy Bentham. Bentham had argued that it was as illogical to put human above non-human as it was to put white skin above black. Singer developed this theme as a demand for an 'equality of consideration' for all animals (Singer 1974).

Some contenders in this controversy point out that if animals are excluded from the class of right-holders, the very young and the mentally retarded must also be excluded. Among others, Tom Regan thinks that these groups of human beings do have rights and so then animals should also have rights (Regan 1986a). Some audacious opponents of animal rights do not concede that it is obvious that babies and the mentally retarded have rights and so they have no difficulty in excluding animals from the class of right-holders.

Recent arguments in this area have focused on the question of interests. The protagonists of animal rights claim that as animals can be shown to have interests, they can be said to have rights. It is dubious, however, if there is any essential inference from 'having interests' to 'having rights'.

For most philosophers in the past the notion of animal rights would not have made any sense. There are those who would say that to assert that some animals have rights leads to nonsensical conclusions, for example that plants and stones have rights as well. Even without going to such extremes as raising issues regarding vegetation or minerals, moot points can arise within the animal kingdom. Which animals could claim rights? Is the worm-killing blackbird morally culpable? Was the arraigning of the sparrow fully jusified because the right to life of cock robin had been usurped? Are animals empowered to claim rights from other animals? At what level on the evolutionary scale do animals become right-holders?

Dr Tom Regan, Professor of Philosophy at North Carolina State University, attempted to deal with these strong challenges based on the argument of *reductio ad absurdum* (Regan 1986b). He acknowledges that he would not extend rights to an amoeba which he regards as merely a 'stimulus response mechanism'. He seems to regard the critical point at which animal rights become relevant, to be the point when we can say we are dealing with an animal that has a 'unified psychological presence'. These are animals, like dogs, which he claims have 'a biography and not just a biology'. Here he considers himself in tune with Darwin, who believed that animal minds differ in degree and not in kind. Regan states that many species of animals, like humans, have a richness of psychological presence in the world. That he is unable to draw a clear line through the species, above which line this 'unified psychological presence' begins to be found, he does not regard as a weakness in his argument. He refers to the 'bald man fallacy' which indicates that it is not necessary to know precisely how many hairs a man has on his head, or perhaps rather more correctly how many he lacks on his head, to be able to decide that the said gentleman is in fact follicularly challenged. Equally, we do not need to know exactly which animals qualify for rights, in order to know that some do.

Many writers have entered this arena arguing that there is no reason to deny that animals can be the proper subjects of rights. They see the right to life and a right not to be caused suffering as inextricably linked and as such possessed by animals.

On the other hand, for some the concept of rights only has meaning by reference to human society and therefore animals cannot be within the community of right-holders. The traditional approach to this debate can be summed up by the crisp statement: 'Rights and duties are essential one to the other; since animals do not have duties, neither do they have rights.' It was regarded as not possible to ascribe rights to animals since man, animals and plants do not share mutual obligations.

The nature of rights

Before we are lost in a welter of conflicting and even irrelevant arguments on the issue of animal rights, it would be appropriate to try to define 'a right'. It is presumed that the connotation of the term 'animal' is clear, although the extension of the term, as regards those species to which rights may be attributed, is far from definite as must be already apparent. A working and acceptable definition of a right could take the form: 'A right is the power to claim what is due.' That power draws its force from law in the case of legal rights, from morality in the case of moral rights, and from the state of things in the case of natural rights. 'What is due', implies that someone owes something to the holder of the right. In refusing to fulfil this obligation to the right-holder, the defaulter is acting unlawfully, immorally or against the natural order of things according to whether it is a matter of legal, moral or natural rights.

The word 'due' is akin to the word 'duty'. Duties and rights are closely associated: two sides of the one coin. A right implies a duty on the part of someone and so it would seem that if there is no corresponding duty there can be no right. As there is universal silence on the duties of animals, it may be asked: how can they have rights?

The necessary connection, however, between rights and duties is not self-evident. Many who approach this question from a religious stance, particularly Christians, tend to deny rights to animals yet talk of humans having duties towards animals. Such duties are to avoid cruelty to animals and to show kindness towards them. Is this a case of duties without rights? Although rights and duties usually exist in tandem, if the situation is closely examined it is seen that the right resides in one individual and the duty resides in another – an arrangement which lends itself to the acceptance of rights and duties as separate entities. Furthermore, in practice a beneficial effect can accrue to a third party distinct from the one holding the right and the one owing the duty. It does not necessarily follow that, because we have duties or obligations, animals have rights to those duties. It is important to distinguish between obligations *to*, or duties *to*, and obligations *about*, or duties *about*. This, perhaps for some, is an oversubtle distinction; however, it can be illustrated by the following example. Georgina promises Jasmine that she will look after Jasmine's aged mother while Jasmine is on holiday. It is then Jasmine and not Jasmine's mother who possesses certain rights. These would be moral rights if based on a promise, or even legal if they had entered into a contract. Although it is Jasmine's mother who stands to benefit by Georgina's performance, the obligation is *to* Jasmine *about* Jasmine's mother. It is Jasmine who holds the right to the performance of this service. She alone can claim it. Jasmine's mother receives the benefit of the service but has no right to claim it.

The nature of 'right' can be further elucidated by comparison with a similar term – 'privilege'. A privilege is gained by indulgence, by favour. A right can be demanded in justice and in some cases sanctions can be called into play to enforce the claim. An apt illustration of the relative connotation of the two terms springs to mind. David Mellor, Parliamentary Under-Secretary at the Home Office in the crucial period around 1986, pointed out to the British Veterinary Association Congress that: 'The use of animals for experiments is a privilege, not a right.' He added a very significant rider which we could all take to heart: 'To abuse this privilege or take it for granted is unforgivable.'

An important aside

With the above rider in mind, it would be appropriate to deviate to consider what is certainly due from us to the animals we use in research and to whom so many who have reaped the benefits of modern medical science, owe so much. Let us leave aside for the moment the subtle philosophical and legal niceties of the exact meaning of rights and the controversial issue of whether animals have rights or not. Let us look at what really matters: the care of the animals with which we have the privilege of dealing. The pattern of that care was outlined admirably by Professor Brambell in association with the Farm Animal Welfare Council in 1979. They are the five freedoms. The relevancy of these ideals are by no means restricted to any one group of animals. They should be the shibboleth of any animal establishment. They are the flip side of what some might like to regard as animal rights.

(1)   Freedom from thirst, hunger and malnutrition by ready access to fresh water and a diet to maintain full health and vigour.
(2)   Freedom from discomfort by providing a suitable environment including shelter and a comfortable resting area.
(3)   Freedom from pain, injury and disease by prevention or by rapid diagnosis and treatment.
(4)   Freedom of normal behaviour by providing sufficient space, proper facilities and company of the animal's own kind.
(5)   Freedom from fear and distress by ensuring conditions which avoid mental suffering.

A few practical comments

These principles are not intended to be regarded from afar in the abstract. They must be fulfilled in the variety of the details called for in the practice of good animal husbandry appropriate to each species being cared for. A few hints might not be out of place. (The following points (1)–(5) correspond to the five animal rights previously listed.)

(1)   This calls for the checking of valves in automatic watering systems or frequent provision of fresh water in clean bottles. The emptying of food hoppers of stale food and the monitoring of diets.
(2)   This calls for efficient environmental temperature control adapted to the species being used. Even an increase of a few degrees Celsius can cause maximum distress to the sensitive rat. Bedding, the essential micro-environment of many laboratory animals, needs to be changed regularly and frequently; a build-up of ammonia is neither good for man nor beast.
(3)   There may be a little irony here where the animals are being subjected to regulated procedures. What is being called for is the use of every means possible to reduce whatever pain may be involved. As the people who have the most contact with the normal animal, animal technicians are best placed to detect abnormality arising from injuries or disease. It is incumbent on them, therefore, to use all their skills and in many cases natural gifts to protect the animal from further suffering by appropriate action which may involve calling the vet. No doubt in the wild, animals get sick and die of disease but they do have escape distance. In an enclosed full animal room, protection from infectious diseases which could run rampant must be provided by efficient barrier systems. Sterilization is a necessary practice for the proper maintenance of animal health within any animal facility. Animals outside captivity will avoid injury if they

can, apart perhaps from a suicidal lemming. Hence it behoves those who are responsible for equipment used for animals, to make sure that it is safe; for example, that cages washed in strong disinfectants are properly rinsed.

(4)   What is being called for here is not inspired by a sentimental anthropomorphism but by hard-headed stockmanship based on an insight into the natural needs of the specific animal. In the early 1980s there was consternation in primate units. Some captive monkeys were afflicted with marmoset wasting syndrome. The provision of larger cages, equipped so that the monkeys could properly exercise their muscles, alleviated this potentially fatal affliction. Except for the lone hamster, the Greta Garbo of the animal world, animals require the company of their conspecifics and should not be deprived of it for any long period of time, particularly guinea pigs. To talk of a miserable solitary cavy is tautological.

(5)   What is required here is an awareness of the structures within animal groups. Animals are hierarchical; they have a pecking order. Thoughtless mixing of animals can lead to fighting, injury, fear and even death. Foresight may be called for to avoid such mayhem. It is not unknown, for example in the case of mice, for a solitary individual, in the haste of cleaning many cages, to be accidentally transferred to the next cage. If they are mature males, not only the new boy on the block but other innocent bystanders unable to escape from the cage will suffer accordingly and not just mentally but even fatally.

Apart from any discussion of animal rights, it would seem to be beyond dispute that there is a moral obligation on any person who, for his own purposes, for example for gain, deprives any animal of the above five freedoms, to provide for any resulting deficiency in the animal's well-being. Left to its own devices an animal will strive often successfully to cater for its own needs. If by our use, for our benefit, we deprive an animal of the facilities to satisfy its own natural needs, surely we are morally obliged to make up whatsoever that animal lacks due to our use of it.

What rights could animals have?

If the existence of animal rights is conceded, it may with justification be asked: what are those rights? How has a widespread ignorance of them lingered down the ages? Who conferred them and with what authority? Are they analogous with human rights? Animal rights campaigners tend to be coy about these consequential questions, tending to dismiss them as trivial details, insignificant in the presence of their high ideals. It might, with justification, be asked if 'right' is the *mot juste* for what the campaigners are advocating. As Professor Joad (1891–1953) was wont to say: 'It depends on what you mean by rights.'

The most widely known and most easily understood rights are legal rights. Salmond, the learned jurist, defined legal rights as 'an interest recognized and protected by the law, respect for which is a duty and disregard of which is a wrong'. In the light of this definition, talk of animal rights seems out of place in the absence of clear legal statements on the topic, either in the UK or abroad. Few, however, would regard rights as solely legal. We talk of rights outside a legal context. When the justice of legislation is questioned, as was done in the case of apartheid, or when legal reform is called for, appeal is made to rights beyond the law – moral rights. If it were not taken for granted that there are rights outside and indeed above the law, by which the law itself can be judged, such an appeal would be to non-existing entities.

These moral rights are on a higher level than legal rights. For most people down the ages, these higher obligations drew their force from religious authority. Outside the orbit of moral theology the notion of moral rights had its basis in conscience, in personal awareness of correct behaviour or in a sense of duty (shades of the categorical imperative of Kant).

Moral rights, though less clearly defined, are more enduring than legal rights. Some legal rights which are more or less now universally accepted, for example the right to property, were in the past denied by many legislative systems to some sections of the community. In spite of such legal attitudes there is evidence that reformers considered such rights, as the right to property, existed for all people, whether granted by law or not. The foundation of such claims to rights could not have been based on laws that did not then exist but they were regarded as moral rights. Under such moral pressure, legislation like the Married Women's Act (1882), transformed these presumed moral rights into legal rights.

Natural rights are even more ambiguous than moral rights. Their vagueness has not excluded them from the arena of controversy on animal use and abuse. Natural rights appear to arise from the nature of things as they are or as they are thought to be by the proponents of specific natural rights. A famous historical exposition of such rights can be found in the Declaration of Rights associated with the French Revolution: 'Man is born free ...'. This implied a right to freedom arising from the innate nature of man. Can similar natural rights be argued for, on the basis of the nature of animals? The nature of many animals implies the need to roam and the power to adjust to their environment. Are they also 'born free' and so inherit an analogous right to freedom?

A case for animal rights may be made by positing that since animals exist, their existence proves that they have certain needs, and therefore interests and intrinsic worth and ecological significance. This does not imply that animals have the same status as humans nor that all rights are absolute and inviolable; rather that animals should at least be accorded consideration. Such consideration should be based on their physical, emotional and social needs.

The main spring-board of the argument against animal rights is a presumed essential distinction between human beings and other members of the animal kingdom, a presumption which was prominent from the time of Aristotle in the fourth century BCE until well after the time of Descartes in the seventeenth century AD. This proposed crucial distinction is associated with human rationality which was regarded as unique to our species.

There is a long tradition attributing rights only to rational beings yet no intrinsic logical connection can be derived from the definition of either rights or rationality. In practice one need not be an active, moral and rational agent in order to have rights. Rights are not denied to infants or comatose patients. One might suspect, and rightly so, that there may be some so-called 'dumb beasts' who qualify more highly in the rationality stakes than some human beings. Concern by some birds with egg clutch-size may be regarded as goal-directed behaviour. This form of awareness, and action consequent upon such awareness, has in the past been assumed to be specifically human. Our growing knowledge of animal behaviour of this type, fudges a little any clear distinction between rational animals and the rest of the animal kingdom. Further evidence which frays somewhat the traditional demarcation between ourselves and the other animals continually appears as research progresses. Experiments at the University of Oklahoma's Institute of Primate Studies indicated that certain specially-brought-up chimpanzees were competent to some degree in the sentence functions of language. It is unproven that only a being that can give linguistic expression to thought has the power to think. Various forms of non-linguistic animal behaviour may be taken by some as indicative of thought. Unfortunately there is no way, even if we grant that animals can think in some form, we can ascertain that they can think reflectively, or have thoughts as such.

However much these involved arguments might edge some animals towards being accepted as quasi-rational creatures, it is of little consequence. Animals are fully adapted for autonomous existence. In the face of life's challenges they have proved themselves to be as adequate as human beings are in similar circumstances. It appears unfair to reject claims concerning rights for animals with arguments based merely on the doubtful lack of the specific quality of the ability to think.

Arguments pertinent to animal rights

The attribution of natural rights

The most basic and limited form of rights to animals is, perhaps, the easiest to justify. It can be argued that natural rights of animals arise from the knowledge that animals do have certain interests and needs which are part of their intrinsic nature, independent of the needs, interests and worth that we place upon them. Animal rights may arise from the awareness that we, as their stewards, are obliged to treat them appropriately with regard for their intrinsic nature. We would thus be obliged to give them sufficient freedom to allow realization and expression of their nature, and satisfaction of their needs.

In what form could such basic rights, as natural rights would necessarily be, be expressed? A right to a natural life – not to be massacred indiscriminately? A right to well-being according to their nature – to live their life in keeping with their capacities and their needs? To be immune from wilfully inflicted suffering? We might concede that there are such rights but that they are not absolute. It may be posited that they could be overridden for the good of nature as a whole or in keeping with the human perception of what is good for nature as a whole.

The attribution of moral rights

Moral rights of animals, if the notion is allowed for, would be less vague than the more easily conceded natural rights already mentioned. Moral rights imply a much higher type of personal obligation on the part of an individual. There is a certain *quid pro quo*, a give-and-take element involved. A commensal or symbiotic relationship could constitute a platform for mutual obligations. Human use of animals may be regarded as putting human beings under an obligation to their animal servants. One might regard the unsolicited gift from a friend as putting oneself under an obligation. The benefits which we receive from the animals which we press into our service are far from unsolicited. They are more akin to benefits received from employees. Few moralists would deny that a profiteer had obligations to those whom he exploited. This implies corresponding rights on the part of the exploited. This was a sensitive topic in moral theology. One of the four sins crying to Heaven for vengeance, was defrauding a labourer of his wages. Before we are carried away, let me stress that this is not a wage claim for laboratory animals. In passing it may be noted that primate sympathizers in Holland set up a monkey trade union (Channel 4 1993). What is being considered here is merely that there could be a moral obligation wheresoever there is an exploiter–exploited relationship. If someone benefits from another's labour or property, a debt may accrue which morally cannot be ignored; akin to what is referred to in legal jargon as a quasi-contract.

The debt of mankind to animals is accentuated by need. The need is on the human side. Animals roamed the earth without humankind for millions of years. Even today, animals live full independent lives far from human habitation. There have been civilizations without a written script, even human communities without the wheel. However, there are no records of any culture that did not use animals for food or work or transport or even for fighting other groups of humans. Animals still loom large in modern civilization; in sport, entertainment, food and research. We owe them much. Does not owing imply rights on the part of the creditor?

Such moral rights could be more clearly defined and imply more serious obligations than mere natural rights. From the arguments advanced in their defence, it would seem that moral rights could only pertain to animals associated with humans. In practice, legislation, particularly in this country, has underpinned concern for animals by forbidding unnecessary cruelty to domestic animals (Protection of Animals Act 1911); by directing that the health of animals must be provided for (Animal Health Act 1981); by regulating the transport of animals to avoid discomfort (Transit of Animals (General) Order 1973); and by stipulating details as regards their welfare (Animal Health and Welfare Act 1984).

It may be argued that animals in the wild do not give each other rights but their situation differs from what occurs when they interface with human beings. In the absence of humans, natural mechanisms operate to control their behaviour and regulate their numbers for the good of the entire ecosystem. However, because human beings exploit animals and alter ecosystems, rights for animals may need to be elaborated as ethical guidelines or as moral restraints. A Declaration of Animal Rights cannot be expected from animals because as British Rail printed in bold type in their pamphlet on animal transport: 'ANIMALS CAN'T COMPLAIN'.

The attribution of legal rights

Legal rights are based on explicit man–made law. They frequently come into existence as the result of legally recognized contracts. Although some arguments supporting the existence of natural and moral rights for animals may be acceptable, there
seems to be no justification for positing legal rights for animals. They can neither sue
nor be sued and except in some eccentric courts, not only in the Middle Ages, they
have been considered beyond the reach of prosecution.

The full–blown agreement – the legal contract – is not the only source of legal
rights. In tort an injured person may have the right to claim damages without any
prior agreement. The right is no weaker for the lack of what lawyers call 'a meeting
of minds' (*consensus ad idem*). In the vast field of law concerned with trusts we
encounter rights conferred on beneficiaries without either agreement or knowledge.
Equitable obligations and corresponding equitable rights are created and even
contingent interests may be conferred on non-existing persons (for example, the
first-born of a favoured son, as in the Perpetuities and Accumulations Act 1964
section 3). If rights, albeit equitable but which can be enforced by the courts, can be
associated with the unbegotten, is it then logical to completely deny the association
of rights with living creatures merely because they lack rationality? Further, in
constructive trusts which are said to express the conscience of equity, obligations may
be imposed, as has already been hinted at, on a constructive trustee, without any prior
agreement or even knowledge on the trustee's part; consequently, rights are
endowed on the constructive beneficiary. In the context of such legal arrangements,
a preconceived notion of rights in law as solid, clearly defined and easily ascertained
interests, tends to fray at the edges.

This diversion into trust law is not completely irrelevant as regards animals. In
English law a trust for the benefit of animals in general (but not for the good of any
individual animal) is accepted as a charitable trust (*Re Wedgwood* 1915). This means
that where such a trust exists, and there are now many, someone is bound to carry it
out. There is an obligation implying a right on the part of the beneficiaries, i.e. the
animals.

Reference to law and legal rights for animals may seem a little far-fetched as
regards animal rights. In practice, however, as we have already seen, it has been the
legislator rather than the moralist who has shown the greatest amount of concern for
the animal. Since Martin's Ill-treatment of Horses Act 1822, there has been an
increasing amount of law concerned with the well-being of animals. It must be
granted that much of the early law concentrated on animals useful to man but the
scope of law beneficial to animals has spread in such statutes as the Wildlife and
Countryside Act 1981, to cover non-captive animals.

References

Channel 4 (1993) 7.00 PM 29 January.

Regan, T. (1986a) This case for animal rights is forcefully argued by Regan in his article 'The
Rights of Humans and Other Animals', *Acta Scandinavica*, **554**, 33–40.

Regan, T. (1986b) Regan emphasized his support for animal rights in *The Case for Animal Rights*.

Singer, P. (1974) A fuller exposition of this theme of equal consideration for all animals was presented by Peter Singer in *Philosophic Exchanges*, Summer, **1**, No. 5.

Chapter 9

Benefits to Animals from Human Activity

'O Mary go and call the cattle home
And call the cattle home,
And call the cattle home,
Across the sands of Dee.'

The Sands of Dee, Charles Kingsley

Domestication

The beginning of domestication of animals belongs to the dim past of prehistory. It may have even been initiated by animals themselves; by the more comfort-loving wolves coming in from the cold to benefit at a safe distance from the warmth of the caveman's fire. In the warmer climes of Africa the rat-loving cat may have seen a marked advantage in hanging around human grain stores, thus providing a service of economic value to the harvesters. In whatsoever manner this symbiotic relationship was initiated, it was well-established before history began. Clear evidence of the domestication of animals appears on and in all early human records, whether of stone or papyrus. Larger animals such as cattle already feature as an important part of the human scene in the earliest hieroglyphics. Even the earliest and most primitive extant legislation protects the ownership of animals. Some animals, for example the dog and the cat, may have been predisposed to domesticity on account of 'delayed adulthood' (Budiansky 1992).

There is no doubt that humans have reaped great benefits from bringing animals into their home but equally the advantages to the domesticated animal have been numerous; indeed, one could say without fear of contradiction, tremendous. The coop, the paddock and most of all the herdsman brought a form of protection to animals completely lacking in the wild. The constant fear of predators endured in the wild by their prey has been alleviated by domestication; a little-mentioned privilege of the laboratory mouse. Without doubt, the greater survival potential accorded by their domestic status has benefited billions of animals through the ages and extends to numerous species.

Even the provision of a humble shelter for our animal associates has been a welcome protection from cold, rain, wind and sun for beasts which would otherwise be exposed to great extremes of weather and might easily perish from such hardship.

The alleviation of thirst has also been a great boon to the kept animal in many parts of the world.

Further advantages to beasts arising from their domestication by man involve nutrition. A regular supply of food, regardless of the season, is an amenity unknown to the animal in the wild, as is the provision of food in times of sickness or old age. The quality of the food provided (e.g. tins of gourmet food for the discerning feline) is in a different dimension from that of debilitated prey or wild berries. Not only have special diets been produced for the improved well-being of our animals but ideal crops have been developed to provide the food most appropriate for particular species of farm animal. However, there has been a dark side to the provision of fodder, BSE for example.

Because of the great economic importance of domestic animals to any nation, legislatures have shown an interest in their protection. Laws have been enacted to ensure the welfare of these animals. There have been numerous such statutes issued in the UK; for example the Agriculture (Miscellaneous Provisions) Act 1968 and its accompanying Codes of Recommendation, leading on to the more legally binding The Welfare of Livestock Regulations 1994.

By selective breeding, conducted for their own gain, humans have produced improved models of the wild animal: larger or faster, more intelligent, more productive, or more adapted to a particular purpose. It can hardly be argued that this is always a disadvantage to the animals themselves. It could be claimed that it enhances the quality of their life. It certainly increases their worth, which should bring increased care for an asset of value.

Nevertheless, there may be some hesitation in accepting new departures in the field of animal production involving genetic manipulation. The Dutch Parliament (1993), took the bull by the horns, and allowed Herman to go forth and multiply. Herman, the world's first transgenic bull, carries a modified version of the human gene for lactoferrin. No doubt there will be a continuing ethical dialectic about this momentous decision taken on the advice of the Agriculture Minister of the Netherlands but great benefits are hoped for from this and other such procedures in the future. In this case, milk from Herman's daughters could be a source of human lactoferrin to fight human infections, particularly the gut infections common among patients with AIDS. The benefits are not all one-sided: the lactoferrin gene could protect Herman's daughters from suffering with mastitis. There seems no limit to progress in this area of animal production.

The most important story in the media about animals in 1997 was the cloning of Dolly, the sheep, at the Roslin Institute, by nuclear transfer technology from an adult cell. In April of 1998 Dolly gave birth to a lamb, Bonnie. This birth followed a natural mating with a Welsh mountain ram. Dolly is not only able to breed normally but various physiological measurements indicate that she is normal in every way. A government grant this year, 1998, helped to improve the precision of genetic modification using nuclear transfer. One immediate benefit is the facilitation of the production of therapeutic proteins, such as Factor IX for haemophilia B, in the milk of ruminants and rabbits. The developing technology will offer a faster, more efficient method of producing the founder animals for flocks of transgenic livestock, because it permits a wide range of precise genetic modifications to be made (RDS 1998).

In July 1998, there were claims that Japanese scientists had been able to progress in cloning techniques so as to successfully produce cattle by these means. This development of genetic manipulation of animals may seem far removed from the homely rustic image of Farmer Giles with one or two cows or the romantic Wild West of the cowboy and his herd or the shepherd watching his flocks by night, but each of those emotive scenes was in its own way an interference with the natural state of animal life. They brought varying benefits to the animals involved. It is going beyond the evidence to claim that these modern technical advances will not be advantageous to future animals, strange though the processes may seem.

Domestication has been a long, enduring, variable and in some ways a successful form of symbiosis.

Veterinary medicine

The development of veterinary medicine is surely the most apparent benefit to animals from their contact with humans and the advantages have not been confined to those animals possessed by humans. The ministering services of veterinary surgeons and the therapeutic drugs developed in research are frequently made available to animals, particularly in wildlife hospitals and sanctuaries.

It is with respect to pets and domestic animals that research has produced an abundance of medicines and vaccines. On the farm, cattle, pigs and sheep are healthier and many more of their young survive to maturity. Not long ago a hill farmer could lose more than half of his young lambs and sheep through various diseases. Now there is a good range of effective and safe vaccines and medicines to prevent such losses.

Antiparasitic drugs are now available and antibiotic drugs are widely used for many infectious diseases of animals. It has been estimated that new treatments preventing dehydration have saved each year about 100 000 calves in Britain alone. Most antibiotics used as veterinary medicines, such as penicillin, were developed for humans but it is difficult to imagine how a small animal or farm veterinary practice could manage without them.

The list of vaccines for animals which have been developed by research is indeed impressive. These vaccines have been the result of both animal experimentation and *in vitro* procedures, such as that which produced a distemper vaccine by the use of tissue culture. It is estimated that 100 million animals have been saved by anthrax and cattle plague vaccines.

Transport

As the human race has spread over the globe it has taken its animals with it. Various benefits have accrued to these animals from the new terrain and climates in which they found themselves. Animals themselves, independent of nomads, have hitched rides with human travellers. A classic example is the rat which, with the help of humans, has proliferated throughout the known world. Such free transport, while often beneficial to the animals involved, has not always proved advantageous, as in the case of rabbits transported to Australia.

Conservation

It is only more recently that human provision for the welfare of wild animals has come into practice on any large scale. Previously, the main concern with animals in the wild was that of the hunter for his quarry. Legislators reflected the interests of hunters and fishermen in a large array of Game Acts. These laws controlled the population of wild animals for financial reasons and on economic grounds.

A more enlightened and less anthropocentric approach to all animals has now developed. Many species of animals have become protected and this protection is unrelated to their use by or association with human beings.

On the international front, the demand to preserve rare species has been guaranteed by a convention. Many nations now honour this Convention on International Trade in Endangered Species of Wild Fauna and Flora (CITES) which has become part of the law of many countries (cf. Endangered Species (Import and Export) Act 1976).

It is not often realized that indirectly many wild animals, especially in the UK, have been saved from dreadful diseases such as rabies by wise quarantine controls dating back to the time of King John (1167–1216).

Finally, not only have human beings preserved various species from extinction but it could be argued that many more animals have come into existence than would have done had humans taken no interest in breeding them. If to be is better than not to be and to be alive is something desirable in whatsoever form it takes, then no doubt the human race has proved to be, if not always benevolent, at least beneficial to animals.

Dependency of animals in general

Much more so now than in the past, with the emergence of the global village, all life forms are becoming increasingly interdependent. Environmental variations engendered by humans can at least indirectly affect various forms of animal life. Reduction in the number of krill in Antarctica can affect whale populations over a far wider area. In fact, the survival of some species may depend completely on human activity. This indirect dependence of some forms of animal life on the behaviour of human beings should not be ignored.

The modern 'Chaos Theory' gives food for thought and suggests that we ought to consider carefully how even small projects may adversely affect the natural environment on which all animals depend. Consequently, there are many wild animals which depend for their well-being and survival on human activity or the lack of it, whether it be nuclear explosions, dam constructions or similar human ventures.

It is by looking at those animals more closely associated with us that the dependency of some animals becomes more apparent. The prolonged process of domestication of animals has created a whole class of creatures who are programmed to dependency. Many animals, such as sheep, may prove inadequate for life in the wild. In the case of turkeys, our special selection methods have produced, in practice, a flightless bird and in some cases the size of the male turkey has been so increased that mating would crush the female unless an appropriate saddle were provided. In these circumstances there is little doubt that such animals depend on humans for survival.

Any captive animal, by reason of its captivity, in some way becomes dependent on its keeper. Captivity invariably involves some restraint on an animal which means that the kept animal will in some way be rendered incapable of attending to all its own needs, necessarily depending on others to provide them. The more stringent the restriction, the greater the ensuing dependency.

The dependency of animals in research

It is sufficient here to outline the general areas of dependency especially associated with animals kept in animal houses. The details of provision for the welfare of these animals belong to animal husbandry. In general, animals used for experiments depend on the laboratory staff for attention to such necessities as:

- a regular supply of uncontaminated water;
- sufficient space for freedom of movement;
- adequate provision of food of the right kind in keeping with both their metabolic and dietary needs;
- freedom from fear of threats within their surrounds;
- freedom from aggression, even from their peers or mates from whom they may be unable to escape;
- freedom from annoyance, arising perhaps from the employment of incompetent workers;
- freedom from danger of injury due to the negligence of technicians or others working in the unit;
- freedom from disturbance from such sources as noise or improper lighting;
- freedom from inappropriate temperature or humidity;
- freedom from offensive smells resulting from poor ventilation or inadequate hygiene;
- freedom from stress;
- freedom from boredom;
- health care;
- avoidance of all unnecessary suffering including the reduction, as far as possible, of any pain;
- a comfortable micro-environment constructed from materials suitable to the animal and similar to that animal's natural habitat;

- a degree of social access or privacy according to the preference of the species;
- facilities for or performance of grooming, especially where the specific need arises from the conditions in which the animal is kept. This may involve clipping of claws, etc;
- outlets for the expression of various specific natural instincts;
- provision of death with the least amount of distress, particularly if that death has been hastened by the work in which the animal was involved.

In the case of such specialized animals as gnotobiotes, necessarily retained within isolators, the dependency of the animal on its carer increases enormously. The life of these animals is dependent on an emergency generator on permanent stand-by. Without the constant guarantee of continual air changes within their confined quarters, laboratory animals kept in isolators would be in danger of dying through shortage of oxygen.

Another area in which there is a complete dependence of animals on their handlers is transport. This activity, perhaps most of all because of the inevitable noise involved which is magnified within containers, may be one of the most traumatic experiences ordinarily endured by animals. The emotive response to the transport of calves (1995) indicated the public awareness of the suffering which, if there is not due care, can arise in the movement of animals. For the alleviation of any hardship or discomfort in transit the animal is completely dependent on all the humans concerned with the operation. This is such a serious matter that the Home Office will not permit the transfer of an animal used for experiments without specific permission.

The responsibility for some animals

This responsibility is a direct consequence of the dependency of animals upon humans. That such a responsibility exists is obvious but it may be ignored or even forgotten. Such a responsibility arises naturally once someone takes an animal under their protection in any circumstances. A cliché but nevertheless valid is the aphorism, 'a dog is for life not just for Christmas'.

A corollary of the principle stated in the previous section could read: the greater the dependency, the more serious the responsibility. Such responsibility for the animals with which one is involved may vary greatly. The responsibility to supply milk to a roaming hedgehog who visits your garden on a regular basis in order to supplement his natural diet is hardly to be compared to the responsibility of a research worker to the caged rat he is using. Between these two extremes there are many degrees of responsibility for the animals which people own. In some cases the practical expression of this responsibility has become idealized and has even acted as an example for inter-human relationships, for example the shepherd and his flock. Although this may not always be a realistic picture of agricultural life, it indicates that the notion of the need to care for the animals that depend on us, goes a long way back.

We have already considered the needs of the dependent animal; the responsibility of those in charge of animals is to meet all those needs in full according to the circumstances and in keeping with the extent of their commitment to the animals involved.

In the case of animals used in research this is a most serious reponsibility and is of course a 24-hour commitment. There is also a duty to anticipate emergencies which may cause hazards from which, because of the conditions in which laboratory animals are necessarily kept, the animals would be unable to escape.

The details of how the various responsibilities to animals are met is a matter of stockmanship and animal husbandry. The essential features of these duties, as regards animals in research, are now enshrined in well-thought-out Codes of Practice: the Code of Practice for the Housing and Care of Animals used in Scientific Procedures 1989 and the Code of Practice for the Housing and Care of Animals in Designated Breeding and Supplying Establishments 1995.

There is no doubt in law about the existence of responsibilities towards animals. In the 1989 Code of Practice specific functionaries are named as being responsible for laboratory animals:

> 3.4. Responsibility for the care of laboratory animals which are involved in or held for scientific procedures falls to:
>
> (i)   the personal licence holder who is responsible for all animals submitted to procedures under the terms of his or her licence;
> (ii)   the animal technician;
> (iii) the named animal care and welfare officer;
> (iv)   the named veterinary surgeon (or, in exceptional circumstances, another suitably qualified person) who monitors and advises on the health and welfare of the animals;
> (v)   the project licence holder;
> (vi)   the holder of the certificate of designation.

It is obvious that the authorities see the relationship to the laboratory animal, on the part of those dealing with it, very much in terms of 'responsibility'.

Finally, we must never lose sight of the fact that the dependency of an animal is usually the result of human interference with its *modus vivendi*. It is logical, therefore, to demand that whosoever is consequently associated with the animal is responsible for any need arising from that interference and is morally bound to supply what is wanting to the well-being of the animal resulting from its loss of freedom.

References

Budiansky (1992) Budiansky presented a clear exposition of his view on domesticity of animals in a television programme, BBC2, 8.00 PM, 27 July.

RDS (1998) The basic facts produced here were taken from the *Research Defence Society Newsletter*, July, 2. I am indebted for many of the topical facts used in this work to the comprehensive reporting, characteristic of the RDS newsletters.

Chapter 10

Animal Awareness and Pain

'Nothing begins, and nothing ends,
That is not paid with moan:
For we are born in other's pain,
And perish in our own.'

Daisy, Francis Thompson

Introduction

The term 'awareness' is used to include the various means whereby a creature has knowledge of what is happening to it and around it as well as the means by which it recalls past stimuli and anticipates future events. The main categories of the complex phenomenon associated with the thought processes involved in awareness are consciousness and memory. The specific role of memory is the recall and recognition of former states of consciousness. It is important in this context because memory can either mollify or intensify the awareness of suffering. The physiological bases of these forms of awareness as also the biological nature of pain lies outside the scope of this text and are amply dealt with elsewhere. Here we are more concerned with the ethical implication of the existence of such awareness amongst animals and the need to minimize any possible adverse effects on animals for which we may be responsible.

The presence of awareness is fundamental to concern about the supposed suffering and pain of other creatures. Moral concern for others is cogent only on the presumption that others have subjective experiences, that we can more or less know them, that their subjective states matter to them more or less as ours matter to us, and that our actions have major effects on what matters to them and on what they subjectively experience. If we genuinely did not believe that others felt pain, pleasure, fear, joy, etc., there would be little point to moral locutions or moral exhortations. Morality supposes that the objects of our moral concern have feelings.

The presumption of feeling is a necessary condition for moral concern but it is not the only condition. One must also believe that the feelings of others warrant our attention. For most of us, the realization that others, human or non-human, experience negative feelings in the same way that we ourselves do, is enough to generate a stance of moral concern; it is irrelevant whether that moral concern arises out of rational self-interest (Hobbes), innate sympathy (Hume), or a sense of a rational requirement to universalizability (Kant). Whatever its supposed source, that concern is the basis of moral conduct and the justification for sympathetic behaviour.

Doubts about animal consciousness

Consciousness is the summation or totality of sensations and a correlation of these sensations by the organism involved in them. It is, therefore, something more than mere neural activity; rather, it is a full interpretation of neural activity.

In the past, consciousness has, by some, been attributed solely to humans. This denial of the existence of consciousness outside the human species supported the opinions of such as Descartes who thought that animals did not suffer. A belief of this kind did, of course, remove the need for any concern for animal suffering in circumstances such as their use in research.

The literature on the use of animals in research contains abundant material on the arguments about animal consciousness because consciousness was not only associated with feelings but was regarded by some as the specific quality which rendered an individual a person, that is, one having rights.

Bernard Rollin deals with this matter in great detail, often refighting old academic battles. He, rightly, realized that the existence or absence of consciousness in a creature is crucial to whether that creature can suffer or not. In short, concern for animal welfare turns on the presence of consciousness in animals. Though crudely put, the old adage, 'Where there's no sense there's no feeling', has a certain validity, and its consequences have ethical relevancy (Rollin 1989).

Some biologists and psychologists, particularly behaviourists, called into question the existence of consciousness in animals. The behaviourists tended to avoid references to consciousness, regarding it as an unscientific concept.

There is no doubt that vital activity can occur without consciousness. Physiological experiments and pathological lesions prove that in our own and in other organisms the mechanism of the nervous system is sufficient, without the intervention of consciousness, to produce muscular movements of a highly co-ordinate and apparently intentional character. The acceptance, however, of some unconscious activity does not directly obviate the supposition of the presence of consciousness.

Behaviourism went further than merely attempting to pass off most of the apparent signs of consciousness in animals as highly complex reflex actions. Behaviourists, for example Watson (1878–1958) and Broadbent (1926–1993), went further and undermined the notion of consciousness itself. They viewed statements about consciousness as uncertain since such statements were concerned with what was private rather than public. This placed it in an area not amenable to study relegating it to virtual non-existence. Consciousness ceased to be a legitimate object of scientific enquiry. When behaviourists talked in terms of positive and negative reinforcement, reward or punishment, they did so in terms of their effects – positive reinforcements being those which increase the probability of a particular behaviour, negative reinforcements those which decrease it. For the behaviourist, the common-sense idea, that stimuli like electric shocks and rewards of food are negative and positive reinforcers because they evoke good or bad feelings respectively, is operationally meaningless and scientifically irrelevant. Within this climate, studies of the mental states of animals would appear wholly out of place.

Acceptance of animal consciousness

There are obviously degrees of awareness, even in the same individual at different times, for example a 'brown mood' or 'on a high'. Thus the level of consciousness which can be attained by various animals differs from species to species. By no means is the same quality of consciousness posited of the snail and the gorilla. Often the evidence of consciousness, particularly higher levels in animals, is anecdotal. This does not mean that it is false but it does imply that critical appraisal should be employed in each case from whatever source it comes, whether it is a little old lady from Worthing-on-Sea or a Professor of Zoology at Cambridge. Among scientists and laity alike there has always been a common-sense acceptance that some animals possess a consciousness akin to our own. Darwin, for example, did not see an essential distinction between the consciousness possessed by humans and some other animals. He regarded the occurrence of consciousness to be in the form of a continuum parallel to evolutionary progress.

The behaviourist W.K. Estes wrote:

> 'Conceptions of learning and cognition couched in terms of mental processes did not begin to grow to the stature of formal theories until the recent relaxation of the hold of behaviouristic thinking. Only in the last few years have we seen a major release from inhibition and the appearance in the experimental literature on a large scale of studies reporting the introspections of subjects undergoing memory searches, manipulation of images, and the like.'
>
> (Estes 1975)

The new cognitivist approach did result in the tentative restoration of animal consciousness as legitimate subject-matter for psychology. Once consciousness came back as a valid object of study it was difficult, for evolutionary reasons, to restrict it to human beings. It has been shown that purely psychological stresses, like exposure to a new environment, can generate greater physiological stress responses than something clearly physical like heat. So it is clear that talk of stress involves covert reference to an animal's experience or consciousness or mental state to make it coherent and plausible.

Clearly, common sense and ordinary language have traditionally extended the presumption of mentation to animals. This ordinary practical attitude existed without any direct reference to any speculative notions of anthropomorphism. Probably the major reason for this popular attitude was because it worked. By assuming that animals feel and have other subjective experiences, we can explain, predict and control their behaviour. Why check a dog if he is not aware of the sanction? Why does a dog drool and beg for scraps if they don't taste good? Why do animals scratch if they don't itch? Common sense continued to accept the presence of animal consciousness whatever might be indicated by scientific ideology or behaviourist orthodoxy. Behaviourists themselves thought in this way in their ordinary moments and acted accordingly at home and in relation to their own pets.

Animal thought

Thought belongs within the whole area of mentation, i.e. mental activity, which also includes such processes as imagination, memory and learning. Thought is the production of ideas, the forming of universal concepts as opposed to simple individual images. John Locke taught that this ability was possessed only by humans, though he claimed that other animals had other forms of awareness: 'Brutes abstract not, but they perceive and remember.'

Opinions in support of the notion that animals think, do not intend to imply that some higher primates, other than humans, are capable of highly abstract speculative thought; rather, they suggest the presence of simple forms of reasoning and primitive types of learning. Jennings demonstrated the existence of learning at the level of the protozoa. This, by no stretch of the imagination, could be confused with thought but it might indicate the phylogenic continuity of mentation. It is, of course, only among higher animals that reference to animal thought can have any meaningfulness. Human thought is intimately connected with the activities of the human brain. Other vertebrate animals as well as ourselves have very complicated brains. In some cases those brains appear to be physically very much like our own. This suggests that what goes on in animal brains has a good deal in common with what goes on in human brains; indeed laboratory experiments on animal behaviour provide some measure of support for this suggestion (Jennings 1919).

Walker, a notable writer on criminal subjects, deals with the most prominent and long-lasting argument against the ability of animals to think – the fact that they cannot talk.

> 'There remains the great fact that men do and animals do not use language. Washoe, the splendidly named Nim Chimosky, and other hard-working primates have signalled with gestures, tokens and by pressing buttons. But their utterances have no real grammar. Animals do not talk to themselves as children do and they show no interest in speech or in any form of communication that is not tied to an immediate reward, whether it be food or a tickle. But it seems clear that animals do not just respond instinctively to what they perceive. They rely on memory and seem to make use of schemata, mental maps of their environment and of objects as identical through time, in guiding their actions and movements. Perhaps the proneness of primates to mimicry gives an insight into their mental processes.'
>
> (Walker 1983)

A practical adaptation of mentation occurs in learning. Many animal activities, whether the useful herding done by the sheepdog, the complex enacting of the choreography of dressage or the amusing antics in the circus, are clear indications of the learning skills of animals. Experiments conducted in the 1950s challenged the behaviouristic dogma that learning proceeds incrementally by repetition, and reintroduced the notion of one-trial learning, something already accepted by common sense and associationists like Hume. Furthermore, any farmer can tell you that it takes only one shock to teach animals not to touch an electric fence.

The universality of pain

Pain is perhaps one of the most vivid forms of awareness. Pain and similar forms of experience are at the heart of any ethical discussion of the use of animals in research. The essence of legality in the use of animals in research is 'regulated procedure', the essential feature of which is the avoidance of 'pain, suffering, distress or lasting harm'. Every one knows by experience what pain is. There is no concept whose objective existence has been so empirically and universally established yet all direct knowledge of it is necessarily subjective and any clear definition of it proves elusive. One working dictionary definition of pain is an adverse sensation experienced when the body is injured or afflicted in some way. In a scientific setting, pain is associated with such nociceptive systems as sensory, motor and memory systems. In this context it may be defined as an adverse sensory experience caused by actual or potential injury which is accompanied by protective somatic and visceral reactions and induces changes in behaviour including social behaviour which can be specific for an individual animal (UFAW 1989).

Pain and suffering are rampant in nature. The slightest mistake in life or an inadvertent exposure to infection on the part of any creature can bring immediate, inevitable and dire consequences, even death.

A major relationship in the existence of most species is that of prey and predator – nature is red in tooth and claw. This may be reminiscent of the pessimistic philosophy of Schopenhauer but he was one of the first among the philosophers to claim that animals shared (the privilege of?) awareness of suffering with us. He argued vigorously, as we have seen, against Descartes's opinion that animals could not feel pain. Schopenhauer's thoughts, however, did not concentrate solely on suffering; he claimed that he had observed his dog, called World-Soul, seeking a mechanical explanation for the mode of operation of some new curtains.

Animal pain

In the past, doubt may have been expressed about the fact that animals felt pain. It was probably, in practice, more a matter of ignoring the existence of pain amongst animals and being indifferent to animal suffering. In fact there is no justification for the Cartesian assumption that animals have no feelings. Descartes must have sat in a coach, heard a coachman crack his whip and experienced the reaction of the horses to an anticipated unpleasant experience.

The mechanisms responsible for pain behaviour are remarkably similar in all vertebrates. Anaesthetics and analgesics control what appears to be pain in all vertebrates and some invertebrates. The biological feedback mechanisms for controlling pain seem to be remarkably similar in all vertebrates, involving serotonin, endorphins, enkephalins and substance P. Endorphins have even been found in earthworms. The existence of endogenous opiates indicates that animals are capable of feeling pain. They would hardly have neurochemicals and pain-inhibiting systems identical to ours and hardly show the same diminution of pain signs as we do if their experiential pain was not being controlled by these mechanisms in the same way that ours is.

The Institute of Medical Ethics Working Party (in 1987) decided that an animal can feel pain if it meets the following criteria:

- Receptors sensitive to noxious stimuli are present in functionally useful positions on or in the body.
- The brain contains structures analogous to the human cerebral cortex.
- Nervous pathways link receptors sensitive to noxious events and the higher brain.
- Receptors in the central nervous system, especially the brain, are activated by opioid substances, implicated in pain control.
- Painkillers modify the response to noxious stimuli and are chosen by an animal given access to them when the experience is unavoidable.
- The animal responds to noxious stimuli by avoiding them or by minimizing the damage to its body.
- The animal's avoidance of noxious stimuli is relatively inelastic. The response is largely unchanged irrespective of how much the animal is rewarded for a particular behaviour.
- The animal's response to noxious stimuli persists and it learns how to associate neutral events with noxious stimuli.

A self-evident argument

The many similarities between animals and humans in anatomical and chemical pathways of pain perception are used to justify the validity of the use of animals in research for the benefit of man. Therefore, conditions which are painful in humans should be assumed to be painful in animals until behavioural or clinical signs prove otherwise.

Is it worse for animals?

Undoubtedly, because of the numerous marked specific differences between other animals and humans, it must be granted that the type, quality and degree of pain will vary. It may not, however, always necessarily be of less intensity for the animal. Specific factors may moderate or intensify the suffering caused by pain in animals. For humans, a greater awareness of the future does indeed give that biting edge to the anticipation of pain – the dentist's waiting room syndrome. This temporal dimension of pain may be lacking in the total pain experience of animals. Animals probably live more in an eternal present. On the other hand, if animals are not as mentally aware as we are, they can have no such palliatives as: realizing a small jab prevents more pain, knowing the pain will soon pass, tolerating the pain for a greater good, or the power to concentrate the mind on higher things. If they are less rational than us, are they perhaps, therefore, more sentient? Do they feel more intensely? These suggestions arise merely from personal speculation but I do not seem to be a voice completely alone.

On a more philosophical level, Spinoza, who attempted to present ethics in a mathematical mode, pointed out that understanding the cause of an unpleasant sensation diminishes its severity, and that by the same token, not understanding its cause can increase its severity. Common sense readily supports this conjecture; indeed, this is something we have all experienced with lumps and even more so with suspected heart attacks which turn out to be indigestion. There may be reason then to believe that animals suffer more severely than humans, since they have no grasp of the cause of their pain. Furthermore, even if they can anticipate, they have no ability to anticipate the cessation of pain which is outside their normal experience; this could be particularly true in the case of animals used in experiments, especially of an unusual kind. There is certainly evidence of animals becoming aware of impending pain. For example, in the presence of someone who has treated them cruelly they will display signs of anticipating an assault: they will attempt to take action to avoid a repetition of the experience by trying to escape or by attacking their tormentor.

Response to pain can be divided into a sensory-discriminative dimension and a motivational-effective dimension. The former is concerned with locating and understanding the source of pain, its intensity and the danger with which it is correlated; the latter with escaping from the painful stimulus. If animals cannot deal intellectually with danger and injury as we might do, by understanding its source and possible intensity, their motivation to flee as a compensating mechanism must be correlatively stronger than ours. If that urge is frustrated, they could possibly feel the hurt more than we would do.

Measuring pain

The measurement of pain is of scientific importance and involves technical skills. The specific topic, i.e. the assessment of pain in animals, is copiously dealt with in the appropriate literature (e.g. Morton & Griffiths 1985; UFAW 1989; LASA 1990; and Manser 1992). There are also more specialized works available as regards the various species and are worth consulting on the subject. It is sufficient here to briefly note some aspects of this vital aspect of animal welfare and the use of animals in research.

The Littlewood Committee (1965), having researched the subject in depth reported that, 'It is not as a rule possible to assess degrees of real pain in animals'. Dr J.D. Rankin, former Chief Inspector at the Home Office, told a symposium: 'There is no way in which we can measure severity; it is and can only be a subjective assessment' (Rankin 1982).

We have progressed somewhat from that position. To quote from UFAW:

> 'Since a wide variety of biochemical, physiological and behavioural parameters must be considered and since adequate statistical analyses of the relative

importance of each are not available for each species and type of pain, the overall assessment of welfare in individual cases can only be treated as a value judgement [shades of Karl Popper and ethics] based upon the experience of those presented with the task.'

(UFAW 1989)

No doubt a gradation in the degree of pain, distress or suffering can be recognized. At one end of the spectrum there is trivial and momentary pain, such as that evoked by a simple injection. There is also trivial distress and discomfort, for example the restraint involved in clipping a dog's claws. This trivial and short-lasting procedure is acceptable and requires no treatment other than a humanitarian approach. However, technical incompetence or undue repetition could escalate the degree of suffering to one that would be considered moderate or even severe.

At the other end of the spectrum there is severe pain which has been described as 'that produced by procedures to which normal humans would not voluntarily submit without appropriate analgesia or anaesthesia'. Such pain could result from extensive tissue injury or with certain malignant tumours. Severe distress, on the other hand, might be that associated with conditioned helplessness experiments, or with deprivation of food and water or social contact for long periods.

In between these extremes there is a grey area that is more than trivial yet less than severe, a moderate pain band which often may be relatively long-lasting.

There are certain features of possible animal suffering which should be considered before embarking on a project involving regulated procedures:

- What is the animal's capacity to experience events that might damage it or shorten its life?
- What is the animal's response to being kept in laboratory conditions?
- How adequate are the facilities for recognizing suffering in the animal and dealing with it if it occurs?
- If it is taken from the wild, what is the animal's response to capture, transport, quarantine and acclimatization?
- What is the effect on the wild population of its removal? (The use of the horseshoe crab was hailed as a great breakthrough in the use of alternatives; it replaced rabbits in pyrogen testing but the practice depleted the ranks of the horseshoe crab.)

Professor D.B. Morton was a pioneer in the detailed appreciation of the extent of animal pain and suffering. In his article, written in conjunction with P.H.M. Griffiths (Morton & Griffiths 1985), he gave details of the various signs indicating pain, distress or discomfort in experimental animals of the more common species. He explored the relationship between signs and degrees of pain, distress and discomfort. The UK Co-ordinating Committee on Cancer Research (UKCCCR) gives the following guidance on this matter:

'Before assessing the severity of any regulated procedure on the well-being of an animal it is essential that the observer is familiar with the normally accepted behaviour, anatomy, physiology and environmental requirements of the species used, for example growth rate, dietary intake and microbial status. Particular attention should be paid to those body systems most likely to be affected by the procedure. Appropriate assessment techniques will include: evaluation of the overall clinical condition, including appearance, posture, body temperature, behaviour and physiological responses; assessment of food and water intake and changes in body weight.'

(UKCCCR 1988)

The UKCCCR also provides illustrations of a more specific nature regarding procedures in cancer research:

'No precise quantitative guide can be given as to the acceptable upper limit of tumour burden, since the adverse effects on the host will depend on the biology of the tumour, the site and mode of growth and the nature of associated treatments. However, tumour burden should not usually exceed 10% of the host animal's normal body weight. In tumour therapy experiments with adult rodents, it is recommended that weight loss should not normally exceed 20% of the host animal's body weight at the commencement of the experiment.'

(UKCCCR 1988)

Such a complex problem as measuring suffering can never be fully resolved to the satisfaction of everyone. The difficulties inherent in such a project were highlighted in an article in *LASA Newsletter*:

'A current "burning issue" for people working with laboratory animals concerns the difficulties of assigning procedures to the severity bands – mild, moderate and substantial. John Finch made an initial attempt to deal with this problem producing a clinical signs appendix based on the "generic" signs of pain and/or distress in rodents and rabbits. This has now been expanded and refined by Tony Buckwell and the product was greeted with initial enthusiasm by technicians, licensees and members of the Inspectorate. Tony has produced a less refined listing of clinical signs for the dog but does point out that it is less easy to obtain agreement for these animals.'

(LASA, 1992)

Although specifically concerning rodents and rabbits, the following classification produced by Tony Buckwell is a good indication of how levels of animal suffering can be assessed (see Table 10.1)

Within the context of the Animals (Scientific Procedures) Act 1986 the gradation of pain is accepted and provided for in the setting of the three bands of severity: mild, moderate and substantial. The frequent references in both legislation and relevant literature to the paramount duty to avoid severe pain presumes not only the existence of animal pain but the possibility of assessing it.

Table 10.1   Classification of suffering in rodents and rabbits.

Mild	Moderate	Substantial
	Weight loss	
Reduced weight gain.	Weight loss of up to 20% of bodyweight.	Weight loss greater than 25%.
	Reduced food and/or fluid intake	
Food and water consumption 40–75% of normal for 72 . hours.	Food and water consumption less than 40% of normal for 72 hours.	Food and water consumption less than 40% for 7 days or anorexia (total inappetence for 72 hours).
Partial piloerection.	Bristling (or 'staring') coat, marked piloerection.	Bristling (or 'staring') coat, marked piloerection, with other signs of dehydration, such as skin tenting.
Subdued but responsive – animal shows normal provoked patterns of behaviour.	Subdued – animal shows subdued behaviour patterns, even when provoked. Little peer interaction.	Animal unresponsive to extraneous activity and provocation.
Hunched – transient.	Hunched – intermittent.	Hunched – 'frozen'.
Vocalization – transient.	Vocalization – intermittent, when provoked.	Vocalization – 'distressed' unprovoked.
	Pallor of eyes, nose, ears and foot pads.	Pallor and animal feels cold when handled.
	Oculo-nasal discharge	
Mild or transient.	Persistent.	Persistent, copious.
	Altered respiration temporary or intermittent, abnormal breathing pattern.	Laboured respiration.
	Tremors	
Transient.	Intermittent. Convulsions intermittent. Prostration, transient (of less than 1 hour duration).	Persistent. Convulsions persistent. Prostration, prolonged (of more than 1 hour duration).
		Self-mutilation.

Hedonism in practice

In the past there was little concern in philosophy with the phenomenon of pain as such, even though hedonism surfaced early, for example in the teaching of Epicurus (341–270 BCE). The essence of hedonism – the notion of pleasure (in the best possible taste, of course) as 'the good' to be sought at all cost, as desirable in itself – was the theme of the poems of Lucretius (96–55 BCE). He, indeed, implied that the ideal of pleasure extended to animals in so far as he regarded concern for the welfare of animals as laudable. The principal rivals to the Epicureans, the Stoics, did not ignore the existence of pain but delighted (if that is the right word for the stiff-upper-lip brigade) in their ability to meet suffering without flinching. Later Christian philosophers concerned themselves with suffering in their attempt to provide a half-way acceptable answer to the problem of evil – the difficulty of the existence of evil, such as suffering, in the creation of an all-good and all-powerful creator.

On the topic of suffering, the great pessimist, Shopenhauer, seemed to revel in his teaching that life was a series of afflictions – a veritable vale of tears. Vivid displays of outright rejection of hedonism have appeared, particularly in religions and especially in the East. Devotees seem to wallow with great satisfaction in the endurance of pain. These trains of thought and ascetical practices displayed a readiness to regard pain as acceptable if not as something good, implying a complete rejection of hedonism which logically demands the avoidance of pain.

Hedonism was revived and became respectable in modern times, not perhaps unexpectedly in England. In the utilitarianism of Bentham, the undesirablility of pain was given an equal status with the desirablility of pleasure. It is this stress, in utilitarianism, on the imperative to avoid pain that makes it an ideal ethic in which to work out widely acceptable premises in discussions on painful experiments on animals. The primary utilitarian principle 'the greatest happiness of the greatest number', comes into play in such debates, modifying the imperative to avoid all pain. That the imperative to avoid pain was not absolute was fully accepted by Bentham, himself a committed carnivore. We have in this type of ethics an ideal matrix for the forming of valid arguments concerned with the cost–benefit balance which is crucial to proper interpretation of the European Convention on Animal Experimentation (1986) and is central in every application for a project licence.

It is not only common-sense utilitarianism that lends itself to a rational but humanitarian approach to animal experimentation. The more idealistic philosophy of Albert Schweitzer, while being hedonistic in outlook as regards all creatures, allowed for the possibility of pain in our dealings with animals. One of Albert's dicta was: 'Avoid hurting sentient creatures whenever possible.' The telling phrase, 'whenever possible', allows for situations in which suffering may be a feature in animal–human relations.

Acceptability of pain

Pain is the greatest disadvantage of using animals in research because of the distress caused to the animal. There is also a scientific reason for avoiding pain in the use of animals in research; that is, the reactions which it is intended to observe can be distorted by pain due to the high stress factor involved. In spite of these considerations many will concede that a certain amount of pain is acceptable to advance our knowledge, particularly as regards medicine. This reflects human attitudes to pain throughout human history. For example, some pain was used as a distraction to relieve greater pain in barbaric operations; the use of pain, sometimes grotesque, was employed as an instrument of law and order; and it was not only in Sparta that endurance of pain was used as a method of character formation.

In fact, pain is not all bad; it has its positive uses. It is functionally a warning signal indicating internal and external danger. Children whose pain mechanism is defective have a low survival rate. Pain also operates in the context of penalty/reward mechanisms involved in the process of learning in both animal and man.

It must be stressed that in spite of the fact that pain has been regarded as an acceptable part of reality, most of us strive, and rightly so, from humanitarian motives to avoid inflicting pain on animals. This is particularly true of many involved in research. The corollary of such an attitude is that whatever pain is involved in the use of animals is not only controlled but restricted as much as possible. Pain is only tolerated in these conditions when it is considered objectively to be a cost worth paying. The abundant benefits of scientific research using animals down the centuries, and particularly in this century, which have accrued to animals and humans alike, seem to justify such cost. Perhaps we can accept the proposition that we may hurt a little in an attempt to help a lot.

Concluding words on the subject of pain

There is so much that is still unclear about pain, particularly its relative severity, since no relevant precise scale of measurement exists. Perhaps, in the future, science, the salient achievement of which has been to measure practically everything exactly, ought to seek to establish a unit of pain, a 'dol' for example, so that assessment of suffering may become a practical and meaningful procedure.

Our concern for animals in practice should go far beyond mere exclusion of pain where possible. Not only should we be concerned with their welfare in a narrow sense but should strive to provide a comfortable existence for the animals we use. Environmental enrichment or enhancement attuned to the species involved should be provided so that the individual animal can achieve an enjoyable fulfilling life within the necessary limits of captivity and the purpose for which the animal is being kept.

The provision of such facilities would generate in the animals an interest to remain alive as long as such a satisfying life would endure. This implies that animal life is of value in and of itself. Should we then question the morality of killing animals even painlessly? Perhaps pain should not be the major factor to be considered in our concern for animal well-being. Certain interests are of higher priority to animals than pain. Animals will chew off limbs to escape from traps, implying that desire for freedom or for life itself takes priority over the avoidance of pain. In some cases an animal will choose sexual contact at the cost of pain.

References

Estes, W.K. (1975) Estes had been the prize pupil of the committed behaviourist, B.F. Skinner. His appraisal of the situation has special significance, in view of the way he puts it in *Handbook of Learning and Cognitive Process*.

Jennings, H.S. (1919) This early exploration of the existence of animal thought appears in his book *Contributions to the Study of the Behaviour of the Lower Organisms*.

LASA Newsletter (1992). LASA, December.

LASA Working Party (1990) The assessment and control of the severity of scientific procedures on laboratory animals. In *Working Animals*. LASA Working Party Report, Vol. 24, pp. 97–130.

Manser, C.E. (1992) *The Assessment of Stress in Laboratory Animals*, RSPCA, Horsham.

Morton, B.B. & Griffiths, P.H.M. (1985) Guidelines on the recognition of pain, distress and discomfort in experimental animals and an hypothesis for assessment. *Veterinary Record*, April.

Rankin (1982) This observation, in keeping with the thinking of the Littlewood Committee and published in their report, was made at a *Symposium on Laboratory Animals*, Zoological Gardens, London.

Rollin, B.E. (1989) Rollin has been the leading champion for recognition of animal consciousness. He drives home his message in his book *The Unheeded Cry*, Oxford University Press, New York.

UFAW (1989) A useful and comprehensive approach to the assessment of animal suffering has been published by the Universities Federation for Welfare in *Guidelines for the Recognition and Assessment of Pain in Animals*, Association of Veterinary Teachers and Research Workers, Potters Bar.

UKCCCR (1988) This pamphlet deals with the topic of humane end-points and provides specialized, useful and practical comments on assessment of pain in animals. The full title is *UK Co-ordinating Committee on Cancer Research Guidelines for the Welfare of Animals in Experimental Neoplasia*, The Medical Research Council, London.

Walker, S. (1983) Walker deals with the often repeated jibe that 'animals don't talk therefore they don't think', in his book *Animal Thought*, Routledge and Kegan Paul.

Part III

Ethics, Animals and Science

Chapter 11

The Controversy

'Both read the Bible day and night,
But thou read'st black where I read white.'

The Everlasting Gospel, William Blake

Introduction

The dictum of Elias Canetti (b. 1905), 'history talks too little about animals', is unfortunately very true; however, there are, even if somewhat isolated, historical references to their use in research. Ancient biblical narrative, for example, refers to the story of the use of a dove to monitor flood abatement. In a more historical context we learn that, in Alexandria in the third century BCE, Erasistratus was using animals to study bodily functions. It was not until much later, during the Renaissance, that censure of such activity seems to have appeared. Leonardo da Vinci (1452–1519) predicted that one day experimentation on animals would be judged as a crime. At that time such an opinion was very much a case of *Athanasius contra mundum* (a lone voice). The prevailing attitude to animals in the West, throughout the last two millennia had been coloured by Aristotelian and Scholastic philosophy. As regards animals, the teachings of Aristotle and the Scholastics were summed up by Descartes: 'Animals do not speak, therefore they do not think, therefore they do not feel.' Such an opinion tended to justify the using of animals for whatever purposes humans saw fit. Such a stance could be given biblical backing (Psalm 8:8).

An early, most outspoken critic of the use of animals in experiments was Dr Johnson (*c.* 1758). In 1796, a Mr Feltham wrote widely propagated articles on 'the rights of animals'. Feltham was a precursor of the prolific propaganda which has appeared since and continues to appear.

Dr Johnson was expressing a concern for the plight of animals – a concern which was beginning to emerge among some members of English society. An official scrutiny of the treatment of animals was initiated in 1781 and by 1786 a licensing of slaughterhouses was instituted. An Act to directly protect some animals from cruelty appeared in 1822 in the form of the Ill Treatment of Horses Act (Martin's Act). In the same period (1824), concern for animals took a more organized form in the shape of the body we know as the RSPCA. It was an offshoot of the Animal Friends Society and prosecuted scientists under a new more extensive animal protection Act entitled the Cruelty to Animals Act 1835.

Marshall Hall had published his principles of animal experimentation in 1831:

'We should never have recourse to experiment in cases in which observation can afford us the information required.

No experiment should be performed without a distinct and definite object and without the persuasion that the object will be attained and produce a real and uncomplicated result.

We should not needlessly repeat experiments, and cause the least possible suffering, using the lowest order of animals and avoiding the infliction of pain. We should try to secure due observation so as to obviate the necessity for repetition.'

(Hall 1831)

An early convert to the antivivisectionists was Charles Bell, who had been using animals to investigate the spinal nerves, at the same time as the great French neurologist, François Magendie, around about 1832. As the nineteenth century progressed, opposition built up in some quarters to the use of animals in research, and not only from outside the scientific community. Darwin complained that the thought of painful experiments made him sick and kept him awake at night. This was no idle remark. He, together with Thomas Huxley, Jenner, Owen, the President of the Royal College of Physicians, the President of the Royal College of Surgeons and other eminent scientists, signed a petition indicating the need for legislative control of animal experimentation. In 1871 the British Association for the Advancement of Science and the British Medical Association issued guidance for would-be experimenters on the use of anaesthetics wherever possible, the need for proper facilities and the avoidance of operations to demonstrate known facts or to acquire manual dexterity. There was also concern in the political arena. In a letter on animal experimentation, Mr Disraeli expressed concern in response to Queen Victoria's anxieties for sensible legislation on vivisection.

The mounting concern produced a Royal Commission on the subject in 1875. With surprising rapidity this official body was responsible for positive legislation in the form of the Cruelty to Animals Act 1876. This was the first piece of full-blown legislation to permit painful experiments on animals for specific purposes and under certain conditions.

The twentieth century has witnessed continual attempts to add more stringent controls to this early legal venture, or even to achieve the complete abolition of animal experimentation. One of the first cases to test the tolerance of the new legislation was when Wellcome Laboratories applied for Home Office registration to conduct animal experiments. Their application made in 1896 was not successful and so another application for registration was made in 1900. It was considered that Wellcome Laboratories, being a commercial enterprise, could only be registered if the pillars of the medical profession condoned the move. The Royal College of Physicians, the Royal College of Surgeons and the Pharmaceutical Society opposed the registration. The opposition seemed so powerful that Wellcome's agents abroad were instructed to investigate local laws and regulations relating to animal experimentation. This investigation revealed few restrictions in Europe or the USA, and Wellcome discussed moving the laboratories abroad, property near Milan being the preferred site. The Home Office wisely recognized the economic threat of taking such work abroad, and invited Wellcome to again submit the application. It was this call for a 'level playing field' across Europe which alarmed the Government, particularly in the face of prohibitive Private Members' Bills, and was to inspire the move towards a European convention on animal experimentation. The Wellcome Physiological Research Laboratories were registered on September 1901. In 1905 this precedent was used successfully by Brady and Martin, a small medicine firm in Newcastle. They also argued that their registration was needed to deal adequately with American and German competition in the trade in medical products.

Progressive though it was, and unique in the world, the 1876 Act did not satisfy the animal lobby. Reforms were being demanded and a Royal Commission in 1906 was set up to look at possible amendments. It deliberated over a long period, issuing an important report in 1912. It added the special conditions concerning the use of curare (a muscle relaxant used in surgery) and recommended that an impartial body be set up to monitor the application of the 1876 Act. This Advisory Committee was established in 1913.

In 1945, after three years deliberation, an unofficial committee, set up by a number of scientific societies, issued a report on the use of animals in research. They called for a national advisory committee on laboratory animals. Their vision eventually evolved as the now defunct Laboratory Animals Centre.

In 1963 a Departmental Committee on Experiments on Animals was chaired by Sir Sidney Littlewood. In 1965 the *Report of the Departmental Committee on Experiments on Animals* was presented to Parliament but was of no great consequence. The real danger to the progress of research came from various Private Members' Bills proposed to Parliament during the 1970s. Bills proposed by Lord Willis in 1972, Douglas Houghton in 1972 and Peter Fry in 1979 would have gravely handicapped the use of animals in research. In 1979 a more scientist-friendly Bill was put forward by Lord Halsbury. These expressions of desire for new legislation galvanized the Government into action. In 1980 the Home Secretary invited his Advisory Committee on Animal Experiments to study the framework of legislation to replace the 1876 Act, with particular reference to the proposals before the Houses of Parliament and the Council of Europe. A Council of Europe committee of experts began work in January 1978 on a draft convention for the protection of animals used for experimental and other scientific purposes. The Government was prepared to accept and sign the convention and legislate accordingly. Although practically complete in 1981, the full acceptance of the convention was delayed until 1986 because of a controversy concerning the insertion of a need to fix humane endpoints. As soon as the convention was in place in March 1986, the UK Government speedily produced the required law in May 1986. Literature from antivivisectionists continues to loom large in the mailbags of most Members of Parliament (Barley 1997).

The involved

So much is heard in the media about those who oppose the use of animals in research that it may be appropriate to first consider those groups which put forward arguments in support of animal experimentation. Pioneers in the field of medical research such as Harvey and Lister not only defended the use of animals but vigorously promoted animal experimentation. Darwin, who deplored some forms of animal experimentation, testified to the Royal Commission in 1875 that he thought a ban on animal experimentation would be 'a great evil'. It was in this scientific tradition that leading academics formed groups to present the case for the legal use of animals in research.

The Research Defence Society

This prominent society was established in 1908, under the leadership of Stephen Paget, to counteract the concerted efforts of diehard reformers to influence the Royal Commission (1906–1912). It has done valiant work ever since. It monitors, on behalf of researchers, developments in the law. By its publication, *RDS News*, it provides relevant information to researchers. In latter years it has launched a forceful poster campaign designed to form public opinion in favour of research.

Far from merely regurgitating dry statistics, its presentation of facts is often attention-catching. In July 1994 it published interesting figures on animal use. For example, in 1991, 3.24 million animals were used in research in the UK. In the same year 693.2 million animals were killed, note killed, for food in the UK (see Table 11.1).

Table 11.1 Breakdown of animals killed for food in 1991.

Type of animal	Number killed (millions)
Chickens	607.0
Turkeys	33.5
Sheep	20.0
Pigs	14.2
Ducks	10.0
Rabbits	5.0
Cattle	3.5*

*A 1992 figure.

These figures would indicate that in a human population of 60 million, 11.5 animals were eaten per person and only 0.05 animals per person used in research. Most of those were rodents, in fact 75% of them, that is about 2.43 million. The average number of rodents exterminated by rodent extermination operators per annum is 8.65 million as against about 2.43 million used in research.

The relevancy of these figures was enhanced in a Channel 4 television programme (11/5/94) which presented the following statistics. The normal person in the UK eats in their lifetime: 6 cows, 36 pigs, 36 sheep and 750 chickens. That is apart from those with a more exotic palate who may indulge in the occasional game stew or even the odd slice of ostrich. I think the point is made that, in spite of ethical anguish over the use of animals in research, the man at the table causes more havoc among animals with far less comment and for a far less exalted purpose than the alleviation of suffering of both man and animal.

A more recent and less prominent service being supplied by the Research Defence Society (RDS) is support for research workers who need assistance in court cases. In 1994 the RDS Legal Defence Fund helped Professor Colin Blakemore to sue for libel in *Blakemore* v. *Coleman*.

It must be stated that RDS propaganda does not go unchallenged. The National Anti-vivisection Society (NAVS) claimed hip replacements as a triumph of 'progress without animals' whereas the RDS rightly advertised it as the result of techniques practised on dogs, sheep and goats. The NAVS claimed that the circulation of the blood was a non-animal discovery. The RDS rightly proclaimed it as the work of Harvey in St Bartholomew's Hospital in 1628, using about 40 different species.

The International Council of Laboratory Animal Science (ICLAS)

ICLAS is a world organization which helps to develop the use of laboratory animals for scientific and medical research. It is increasing its international information campaign in the face of growing activities by animal pressure groups. ICLAS is concerned that the validity of well-conducted and well-controlled experimentation, essential for cancer research and drug trials, is being seriously challenged by increasingly active movements.

The Universities Federation for Animal Welfare (UFAW)

As a scientific animal welfare society, UFAW occupies a somewhat ambivalent position and seeks to improve the welfare of experimental animals by cooperating in a practical way with those who work with them. It aims to create an atmosphere of sanity, objectiveness and intellectual honesty in which the very difficult ethical problems that arise can be discussed dispassionately and without the excitement and invective with which the subject has come to be associated. The *UFAW Handbook* has been described in a court of law as the Bible of animal technology. UFAW does not approve of all the procedures described in its literature. It hopes that as knowledge accumulates, alternatives will increasingly replace the use of animals and more humane techniques will be continually developed.

The Committee for the Reform of Animal Experimentation (CRAE)

CRAE was formed in 1975 by Lord Houghton, Richard Ryder of the RSPCA and Clive Hollands, and exhibits a more positive and dynamic attempt than the previous groups to reduce as far as possible the use of animals in research.

Fund for the Replacement of Animals in Experimentation (FRAME)

FRAME was founded in 1968 and, although coming from a scientific background, has tended, under the leadership of Dr Michael Ball, to emphasize the need to move away from the use of animals in research.

The European Centre for the Validation of Alternative Methods (ECVAM)

This arm of the European Commission is the new thrusting body concerned with implementing the three Rs (i.e. reduction, refinement and replacement).

The Dr Hadwen Trust for Humane Research

The trust is another body which is active in pursuit of viable alternatives to animals in research.

Other societies

There are societies involved in animal work which, though not pressure groups as such, are deeply concerned with the welfare of animals in research and have contributed greatly to the well-being of laboratory animals. They are, for example:

- the Association of the British Pharmaceutical Industry (ABPI);
- the British Laboratory Animal Veterinary Association (BLAVA);
- the Institute of Animal Technology (IAT);
- the Laboratory Animals Breeders Association (LABA);
- the Laboratory Animal Science Association (LASA).

The concerned

There are some groups dedicated to animals which are concerned primarily with animal welfare but admit some need for animal experimentation.

The Royal Society for the Prevention of Cruelty to Animals (RSPCA)

The RSPCA is a long-established animal society, whose roots go back as far as 1824, and has a membership in excess of 20 000. In spite of internal conflicts, it still officially tolerates the use of some animals in experiments. It has a representative on the Animal Procedures Committee.

The Scottish Society for the Prevention of Vivisection

This society was established in 1911 and indulges in political lobbying to limit the use of animals in research. It gained prominence when its leader, Clive Hollands, chaired Animal Welfare Year in 1976.

Activists

By far the largest proportion of pressure groups in this area of conflict are opposed to the use of animals in research. They vary in the ferocity of their opposition. The Humane Education Society concentrated on lectures in schools but later broadened its scope under the title of Earthconcern. The Animal Rights Militia, on the other hand, are given to the use of explosives. The following are some of the more prominent among a whole galaxy of groups.

British Union for the Abolition of Vivisection (BUAV)

BUAV was established in the 1880s. It has a membership of about 16 000 and has contacts with over 120 animal rights groups. It has a large staff and runs its own newspaper.

Animal Aid

Animal Aid was founded by a teacher, Jean Pink, in 1977, as a non-professional group to fight on all fronts and to oppose all forms of vivisection. It has about 11 000 members.

Co-ordinating Animal Welfare

Established in the late 1970s, Co-ordinating Animal Welfare links the various radical organizations. The intention is to mobilize all animal activist groups. It has a membership of about 300.

Animal Liberation Front (ALF)

The Animal Liberation Front, with roots in the hunt saboteurs movement, is not above putting rat poison in Mars Bars, favours direct action and advocates the liberation of pets. It dates from 1976 and boasts about 2000 supporters.

Animal Rights Militia

The Animal Rights Militia is a shady organization which has claimed responsibility for letter bombs.

People for the Ethical Treatment of Animals (PETA)

PETA is unusual in that it is not home-grown. It claims to be the world's largest animal rights pressure group. Founded in America in 1980 it has opened offices in Amsterdam, Hamburg and London (1994). PETA intends to target specific companies who carry out animal testing.

The Justice Department

The Justice Department is thought to be under the auspices of ALF which may act as an umbrella organization for various active militant units. Their speciality is the letter bomb.

Practical consequences (security)

Although the majority of antivivisectionists are sincere and law-abiding people, there is, as is obvious from the preceding section, a small minority who resort to vandalism and other criminal activity. The *RDS News* of October 1994 published a list of outrages against research establishments and research workers, associated with the Justice Department:

> Campaign: 30 mousetrap devices.
> 22 poster tube bombs.
> 19 video cassette box bombs.

These are only selected samples of attacks of one organization over a specific period.

There is little doubt that the danger from extremists is real. It follows that there is a serious moral duty on all designated establishments to be concerned with the safety of their staff. The details of security hardly belong in this text. Suffice it to say that all involved in research should be properly warned, and carefully instructed in the need for caution and awareness. There is a need to scrutinize all new staff and visitors as well as goods coming on to or near the premises. Surveillance equipment needs to be in place and liaison with the local constabulary is essential.

It is worth mentioning that it is not only staff that are at risk from activists; animals also may be in danger. The released laboratory animal could be a helpless, endangered creature. For example, not so long ago in East Anglia pet cats suffered from attacks by mink which had been released in an animal liberation operation.

A similar catastrophe resulted from the exploits of the Animal Liberation Front in August 1998. A total of 3000 mink released by them from a fur farm in the New Forest caused havoc among wild birds and killed owls in a bird sanctuary. It was interesting to see numerous mink returning to the erstwhile place of their capitivity. It was evident from scenes witnessed on television that some of the released animals were seeking readmission.

As a response to these extremist forays, the RDS has done valiant service in recording for the benefit of scientists the various assaults on the research community. It is an ongoing battle. These recent events in 1998, no doubt soon to be superseded by other attacks on people and property, illustrate the constant menace to those working to advance medical and other sciences. Their list of recent events is as follows (RDS 1998):

(1) 18 April: Large (800) and aggressive demonstration at Hillgrove Farm laboratory animal breeders.

(2)   24 April (World Day for Laboratory Animals), peaceful demonstrations:
- 30 at Huntingdon Life Sciences in Occold, Suffolk.
- 20 at Shamrock Laboratory primate suppliers, near Shoreham.
- 20 at RDS office in London.
- 30 at Pfizer pharmaceutical company, Sandwich, Kent.
- 20 at Quintiles contract research company in Ledbury.
- 10 at B & K Universal laboratory animal breeders near Hull.
- 12 at Astra Charnwood pharmaceutical company in Loughborough and at Harlan UK, Belton.

(3)   25 April: Large aggressive (300) demonstration in Cambridge which visited the University Downing Site and Wellcome/CRC building; 20 windows were smashed at the biochemistry building; 27 demonstrators were arrested. This demonstration then joined up with a larger (400) road protest demonstration for a rally.

Demonstrations of this type are not new. The Brown Dog Affair had all the elements of later displays of opposition to animal experimentation, including infiltration. In 1902 two Swedish students at the London School of Medicine for Women initiated an exposé of the use of animals in research. The diaries of these two ladies, Lind-af-Hageby and Leisa Shartau, were later published as *The Shambles of Science*. The main feature of their revelations was an experiment on a brown dog without, they claimed, proper anaesthesia.

The professor involved sued Stephen Coleridge, General Secretary of the National Antivisection Society (NAVS), for libel. Professor Bayliss won his case but NAVS had got what it wanted – huge publicity.

And there's more. Louisa Woodward, a prominent antivivisectionist, commissioned a bronze statue, in the form of a drinking fountain, commemorating the brown dog 'done to death' in University College. The statue was unveiled at Battersea in 1906. In the following year, minor skirmishes and full-blown riots occurred, involving clashes between police and medical students attempting to destroy the statue. Eventually the statue was removed in 1910. Protest marches and a court case followed to try to reinstate the little brown dog but the statue was destroyed in 1911. Due to agitation on the part of the NAVS and the BUAV (British Union for the Abolition of Vivisection) a replacement statue was unveiled by the GLC in Battersea Park in 1985. A full and most interesting account of this whole affair has been published (Mason 1997).

For many, this aggressive opposition to the use of animals in research appears as a British phenomenon. However, there are other parallels. Magendie (d. 1855), a leading French neurologist of his time, met a lot of resistance to his use of animals; even his own wife and daughter were among the ranks of his adversaries. Although action against vivisection did once appear to be more prevalent in this country, this is becoming less and less the case. The following is a list indicating the proliferation, throughout the world, of attacks by the Animal Liberation Front:

- 1973 United Kingdom
- 1979 USA, Netherlands

- 1980 France
- 1981 Canada
- 1982 Australia, Switzerland
- 1983 Germany, Malta, South Africa, New Zealand
- 1984 Ireland, Denmark
- 1985 Sweden
- 1987 Italy, Austria, Spain
- 1992 Israel
- 1994 Poland
- 1995 Finland
- 1996 Norway

Aggressive, official governmental action against the use of animals in research is not unknown. In the early 1930s the Nazis passed laws banning vivsection in Bavaria and Prussia. In August of 1933 Hermann Göring announced an end to the unbearable torture and suffering in animal experiments and threatened to commit to concentration camps those who thought they could treat animals as inanimate objects. The ideal, if not the sanction, was indeed praiseworthy. The elimination of torture, of animals as well as humans, is something devoutedly to be wished for. We will see later that the goal of diminishing and alleviating the suffering of animals in research is the whole thrust of the application of our 1986 Act and the introduction of the Ethical Review Process. The above Bavarian and Prussian legislation was not an isolated gesture. The Nazis hosted an international animal protection congress in 1934. Animal protection was made by them a university major topic in 1938. With friends like that, what need is there of enemies? (Rowan 1992).

Disadvantages of using animals in research

The primary and most compelling reason for not using animals in research is simple: it might hurt them. The possible causing of pain, suffering, distress or lasting harm to any animal is undesirable. As will be discussed later, reasons may be produced which would satisfy people that in certain circumstances such hurt, as long as it is not a hurt too far, and if justified, may be acceptable. However, there are other very marked disadvantages of using animals in experiments.

Scientists agree with antivivisectionists that it is not desirable to use live animals in experiments. Scientists differ from antivivisectionists in accepting the need for animal experimentation although the scientist is more aware of the practical disadvantages of using animals. The following quotation from a Medical Research Council source in *Conquest* (RDS publication) makes the point.

> 'I think that people should clearly understand that no one in his right mind in laboratory practice wants to use animals if this can possibly be avoided. They are unreliable, subject to all sorts of biological variations and difficulties, particularly those arising from disease. They are also very costly to maintain and the money expended could well be used for other purposes.'

In the early 1970s, the then Minister of Education and Science, Margaret Thatcher, stated: 'The Government's view is that scientists always prefer alternatives where available for reasons of humanity, economy and convenience' (Hansard).

The following types of disadvantages, apart from the obvious one of suffering, are among the difficulties associated with the use of animals in research.

Cost

It may be a mercenary consideration but it is a most telling argument against the use of animals in research. As a budget-holder of an animal unit for nigh on 20 years, it is one of the few subjects upon which I can write with a little authority. Costs incurred, for example, in the use of gnotobiotic animals can be astronomical. An example from the 1980s illustrates well how money can be saved by the use of alternatives.

> For certain export tests, obligatory under law, sheep were used and the examination of each sample cost £50. A bench test was adopted, which was previously not acceptable internationally, with considerable saving in sheep (the most important factor), as well as staff time and money. The cost of each test came down to £1.

Intrinsic dangers

Bites and scratches are a constant hazard in animal work and some large animals can cause serious injury. The health hazards associated with zoonoses can prove fatal and cannot be ignored. Laboratory animal allergy (LAA) is now an industrial disease and is a serious matter. Career prospects of young research workers can be easily jeopardized by reactions to fur, feather and various body fluids.

Extrinsic dangers

The danger of violence against staff and their property as a real possibility has already been mentioned. Irksome restraints are consequent upon the strict security needed to counter these threats.

Variations

Accurate calculations are crucial for the production of valid results from any experiment. Calculations vary in complexity in relation to the number of variables involved. Variables associated with experimental animals, for example age, heredity, health, status, stress, etc., are more numerous and unpredictable than the corresponding parameters involved in other techniques such as cell culture. Some of the variables can be, and are, obviated but only with great effort and high costs.

Distortion

The ideal model for biological research would be an average normal unstressed animal. An average animal, almost by definition, does not exist in the real world. Such an animal is the creature of statistics – out of data by equation. The normal is determined in relation to extremes; it is more an ideal projection than a real animal.

Pain and stress are most potent forces tending to distort the characteristics of an experimental animal. The animal under experiment has a specific status which is well described as a 'dramatype'. There are, of course, real physiological phenomena underlying this distorting 'dramatype'. These are, for example: increased secretion of adrenalin which raises the blood pressure, heart rate and the breakdown of glucose; violent muscular contractions which cause a more rapid breakdown of the energy store of biochemicals; hyperventilation which increases the carbon dioxide in the blood which tends to alkalinity; increased metabolic rate and temperature which cause other changes in enzyme reactions. One cynic once commented, not perhaps seriously, but correctly in a technical sense: 'It's useless giving animals tests – they panic and give the wrong answers.'

Analogous argument and extrapolation

The argument from analogy, probably the weakest form of logical argument, is based on the similarities found in two different subjects and progresses from these recognized similarities to posit other similarities. In analogy, it is not a matter of comparing like with like. It is a matter of comparing part like with part like.

The many similarities to be found in the anatomy and physiology of varous species can be used as a basis to presume that the way in which, for example, a drug acts in the body of one species will be similar to the way it acts in another species of animal. The more similar the two species, the more valid the conclusion that the drug will initiate the same reaction in each species.

Results based on analogy are arrived at by the process of speculation known as extrapolation. It is on the proper operation of this process of extrapolation that the validity of knowledge gleaned from animal experimentation depends. Many species of animals are similar but none are identical, otherwise they would not be separate species. The most assiduous extrapolation from numerous experiments using morphine on many other species could not predict the dramatic effect of this drug on cats. The development of, for example, penicillin could have been very adversely affected if it had depended on guinea-pig trials. Likewise, the history of the use of thalidomide may have been different had there been more meticulous extrapolation involved in its research and had it been tested on a greater variety of species.

An indication of the importance of concentration on the method of extrapolation rather than depending on crude presumptions of analogy based on apparent similarities is illustrated by the usefulness of tissue culture. There are several instances where the extrapolation from human tissue culture to other human beings is more reliable than from whole animals to humans since in this method the species difference is eliminated. Tissue cultures react to most viruses affecting humans, whereas many species of laboratory animals are insensitive to a number of viruses. In short, mice are not men nor vice versa.

The importance of direct relvancy of every detail of research using an animal model for proper extrapolation has been emphasized by the Animal Procedures Committee. Their *Annual Report for 1989* (HMSO 1989) noted that while strychnine-induced convulsions had been used as an experimental model for epilepsy, it was known that the mechanism of convulsions produced by strychnine differed from the seizures which typically occur in epilepsy. The use of strychnine to simulate epilepsy could not therefore be justified. The extrapolation was not valid and the relevant licence was withdrawn.

Distaste

Experiments on animals usually demand that the animal is deprived of its freedom, is kept in a cage or even restrained. Operations may be part of the experimentation. No caring human being can be responsible for such a scenario without feeling reluctance to cause distress to a fellow creature. There is not only the distasteful task of disposing of carcasses but the ending of the life of any animal disturbs sensitive and caring technicians and scientists.

On a much lower level – sewer level, in fact – animal units bring their own special problems of waste disposal. It is not without reason that the unofficial symbol of the animal technician is a scraper.

Obligatory use of animals in research

Because there is some concern among researchers about strict legal restraints on the use of animals and there is so much intensive lobbying by animal activists to increase legal control of animal use or even to achieve total legal abolition of animal experimentation, one tends to ignore the fact that there are legal demands for the use of animals in research. Some politicians speak with a forked tongue on the matter; supporting the aspirations of the activists while echoing trade union demands for more stringent safety tests of suspect substances on animals.

The legislation demanding the use of animals for testing possibly hazardous substances has existed for some time. It includes, for example:

- Public Health Act 1936
- Agriculture (Poisonous Substances) Act 1952
- Medicines Act 1968
- Control of Pollution Act 1974
- Health and Safety at Work etc. Act 1974
- Biological Standards Act 1975
- Consumer Safety Act 1978
- Food Act 1984.

Sentiment

Sentiment is a universal human phenomenon which, like other basic reactions of living creatures, is difficult to define precisely. It may be described as thought or reflection coloured by emotion. Sentiment influences opinions, such as moral judgements, by basing decisions on feelings and emotions rather than on reason and logic – frowned upon perhaps in the groves of Academe, but valid motivation in daily life. Humans are not mere computers. We share the rich appetites of vibrant life with the rest of the animal kingdom. We are motivated by complex forces which reflect reality more closely than does cold intellectual speculation. Sometimes sentiment is derisively dismissed as mere sentimentality, implying a quality associated with a person of weak moral fibre, easily swayed, who forms passing opinions without any solid basis.

Human sentiency, as opposed to sentimental indulgence, may be acceptable as a valid basis for moral judgements. The humane feeling of animal technologists, and not a spurious moral outrage, does and will continue to maintain the care and welfare of laboratory animals. Human sentiency should be realistic. Life has evolved integrally. Life and death maintain one another. Medical students may faint in the course of witnessing their first operation but this hardly implies any moral condemnation of the surgeon. The experience merely overwhelms the trainees. They will become habituated to the situation but this process by no means blunts their moral sensitivity nor diminishes their caring nature. Sentiment, as an expression of the emotional influences on our behaviour, is an essential element in the human condition. It serves a purpose throughout life to attune us to our surroundings and helps in the choice of mutually beneficial relationships. Rarely are partners chosen on a statistical basis but rather for sentimental, and patently valid motives, albeit subconscious. Even the most sceptical of philosophers, Hume, in his *Enquiry* talks in terms of a 'sentiment of humanity' as being a potent force in the development of morality. The most famous maxim on this subject is the saying of Blaise Pascal, in his *Pensées*: 'The heart has reasons of which the head knows nothing.' This may be seen as a highly charged poetical flight of fancy from an eminent philosopher but in fact Pascal was more famous as a mathematician (for instance, if you lose positive pressure in an isolator you are talking 'pascals').

Sentiment and animal use

In discussions on any matter of import, as contention increases emotions are aroused and sentiment then tends to play an even more prominent role in the controversy. In debates on the use of animals, sentiment is often to the fore even at the beginning of the polemics and is often the main basis of contention throughout the dialectics. The sick child and the fluffy bunny will crop up at some time in the argument so as to forcefully drive home each contender's claim.

Any attempt to produce a poll on opinions in this area needs to be carefully constructed. Names of some species of animals will elicit sympathy and a consequential condemnation of their use in research, for example cats, dogs, rabbits or horses. The names of other species are not so favourably evocative, for example rats, mice, snakes or any creepy-crawlies. Likewise, automatic reactions to the suggestion of using animals in the search for a cure for cancer, a highly emotive term, will usually attract a positive response. Any mention of association of animals with cosmetics can bring forth a knee-jerk reaction. Usually there will be no room for reflection on what cosmetics include, for example soap and toothpaste which need to be safe if they are to be allowed to come into close contact with delicate infant skin. The mention of tender baby skin can strike a different note of persuasion, however.

Sentiment is reprehensible if it is misinformed, inconsistent and illogical. Uninformed sentiment is often selective and even counter-productive. Examples of inadequate expressions of sentiment are not uncommon. For instance, antivivisectionists found themselves apologizing to a butcher for daubing his house, by mistake. The intended target, a scientist, lived next door.

Britain's cats kill approximately 100 million small birds and mammals every year. A survey carried out by Professor Robert May, a researcher at Princeton University in America, studied the hunting instincts of 70 well-fed domestic cats in the Bedfordshire village of Felmersham. The village has twice the average cat population with a cat to every four houses. Over the year the cats brought home 1090 'prey items': 535 mammals, 297 birds and 258 unidentified furry objects. Among the victims were 22 species of bird and 15 of mammals, the most common being woodmice, sparrows and field voles.

Allowing for the fact that there are about six million cats in the UK, Professor May estimates that about 100 million birds and small mammals are killed each year by the well-fed feline population.

It appears, however, that the population of Britain are largely unconcerned by this mass slaughter of innocents and yet are, by contrast, deeply concerned by the loss of animal life in the laboratory, the numbers of which pale into insignificance compared to the havoc caused by the Great British Tabby.

In the same vein, another tragic but relevant fact is that, of 90 000 pigeons in a race from Nantes to England, 80 000 perished (*Spectator* 1997).

Public relations

Just as the accounts of the vicious activities of violent pressure groups demands attention to security, so consideration of the crucial role of sentiment in the animal controversy calls for attention to public relations.

The dialogue of the deaf

Most popular literature on the use of animals in research appears to be antagonistic to animal experimentation and often unfortunately aims to shock rather than inform. It is only of late that propaganda favourable to the use of laboratory animals has been presented in a popular way; in such forms as the Research Defence Society posters or in Animals in Medicines Research briefs. Unfortunately, even the paper conflict seems to reflect what may often be detected in this controversy; that is, that the contenders seem to be so convinced by their own arguments that they see little need to take into account the contentions of their opponents. One side loudly bemoans the maltreatment of defenceless animals in research while on the other hand scientists rightly proclaim the wonderful benefits which have accrued to both humans and animals from the use of laboratory animals.

It is a *sine qua non* (a necessary condition) of any discussion, to listen carefully to and address the reasons of a protagonist if the beginnings of agreement are to emerge. The alternative is the sterile dialogue of the deaf which perpetuates and fossilizes differences. Such a 'dialogue of the deaf' is the greatest obstacle to the resolution of any controversy.

Conflicts cannot, within a free society, be done away with but it is desirable that they should be conducted in a relatively peaceful way. All those involved in conflicts should understand what the contention is about and think clearly and reasonably about it. It is risky if, instead, they are content with a view which may, indeed, include partial truths but which is made substantially false by over-simplification – reality, when human judgements are involved, is invariably complex. It may seem easy to provide all the answers if you only know half the questions. Unfortunately, oversimplification is often rhetorically more effective (a half-truth like a half-brick is much easier to throw) and may help the contender to acquire and exercise authority. Fruitful discussion is easier if the opposing parties not only understand each other's arguments but appreciate the motives and the moral basis on which they rest.

Notoriously, the same activities look very different from opposing points of view. Whom one party sees as a terrorist gunman another sees as a fearless freedom fighter; or more aptly, whom one sees as a power-crazed scientist another sees as a dedicated pioneer of medicine. Debate between parties who see the issues only in such polarized terms is not likely to be fruitful. A first step is made when both sides see that there are points of view from which each of the rival descriptions make some sense. A second, harder, but necessary step is made if they can each see some force in the opposing point of view – that is, give some weight to the values and ideals that underlie the aims of their opponents. Without such *rapprochement*, conciliation is unattainable and the divide widens.

In arguments about laboratory animals, certainty is often more prominent than truth; the two terms are by no means synonymous. When associated, they are often in inverse proportion. Those who are certain may feel that they can dispense with the need for factual support for their opinions. Ardent belief has always been sufficient to produce unquestioning conviction. In the presence of such mind-sets, reality can become irrelevant. An antivivisectionist leaflet proposed that:

> 'Only a fool would attempt to suggest that public health has benefited from animal experiments in the field of psychology; therefore, we will not have to deal with the fear sometimes felt by the public for their own health if we seek to outlaw this area of research.'

With this complete refusal to consider facts, the antivivisectionist *Liberator* develops the flawed argument:

> 'We believe that the press – always out for sensationalism and a new angle – will be able to utilize the fact that the experiments are so foolish and that public money is being spent in this area whilst it is clearly so desperately needed by the NHS.'

> (*The Times* 1983)

The fully committed draw support from one another, intentionally ignoring any outside influence or sources of reasonable doubt. Fervent mutual support of 'right thinking' easily results in a complacent conviction of invidious righteousness.

It is essential that personal views be broadened if any accord is to be arrived at in a controversy. In the absence of a meeting of minds, discussion withers, the extreme views of the activists flourish, and the unfortunate violent consequences which we have mentioned occur. Violence is not just the repartee of the illiterate but also of the ignorant. That ignorance must be dispelled by the widespread dissemination of the true conditions and the immense achievements of animal experimentation presented in such a way that it deals with reasonable objections. Publicity of an abundance of relevant information is paramount. Against logic there is no armour like ignorance; let that ignorance be dissipated by the wide publication of the facts of research.

Logic and rhetoric

Logical argument on its own is rarely sufficient to convert an opponent. We may pride ourselves on being reasonable yet we are often swayed by emotions. This fact was appreciated before Aristotle expounded on logic. The majority among Greek philosophers were not logicians but Sophists, skilled in the art of rhetoric – primordial spin-doctors and archetypal masters of the sound-bite. The experienced advocate tends to cajole a jury with rhetoric rather than convince them with logic.

It is essential when presenting a case for public consumption to realize that facts and rational argument are important but they may not be interesting or moving in themselves. They need a gloss, tuned to the audience being addressed. That is where rhetoric comes in. It should not be despised on account of intellectual snobbery. Researchers have the facts on their side – an abundance of benefits, provided both to humans and animals; ethical justification can be made out for their use of animals – cost–benefit utilitarianism; there are even ways of addressing speciesism itself – from the reality of nature, the prey–predator relationship. Such strong arguments, however, fall flat if not presented in the right fashion. The vital message of rhetoric is: 'It's the way you tell 'em'.

Later Sophists did learn something from Aristotle: the variety and nature of fallacies. These were adapted, disguised and used frequently to lead astray the unwary. In its lowest form, rhetoric can stoop to accepting the validity in practice of the preacher's marginal note: 'Argument weak, shout loud.'

The art of manipulation

In the presence of such a potent force as the modern media, the skills of persuasion have taken on more dynamic forms than was associated with rhetoric in the past. In the last section we already had a hint of how animal liberationists are prepared to manipulate public opinion. To influence people's attitudes it is now necessary to adapt to the techniques of public relations. The purpose of public relations in its best sense is to inform and to keep minds open. At its worst it misinforms and keeps minds closed. Advertising is one of the most basic forms of communication and allegedly of information. Yet obviously much of this ostensible information is not purveyed to inform but to manipulate and to achieve a result; to make somebody think something when the grounds for such a belief really don't exist.

Unfortunately, it is in this context that some of the material concerning animal experimentation is disseminated. Academic aloofness, scientific secrecy or occasional polemic forays are inadequate responses. It is imperative that those involved in the use of animals in research be prepared to explain the part they play in such areas as the progress of medical science, be ready to publicly argue the case for animal use and even to 'play the ad man'.

In an article in *New Scientist* (Morton 1992), David Morton demands more openness on the part of scientists so as to gain a better public image for animal experimentation. In his article he stresses the importance of publishing details of experiments so as to create a climate of public relations which he, a scientist himself, thinks would be more favourable to animal experimentation. He makes the following points:

> 'Researchers can no longer write scientific papers just for their colleagues. All sorts of other people, including antivivisectionists and animal welfare campaigners scrutinize published papers in an attempt to judge whether the research meets an acceptable ethical standard. The traditional format of research reports was never intended to justify the specific use of the animals in the venture.'
>
> (Morton 1992)

Morton suggests they ought to, and thinks that such an approach would constitute better science and even save animals from unnecessary, avoidable suffering.

Failing to mention adverse effects leads critics to assume the worst. The omission of such details also handicaps other scientists trying to make sense of the findings, as the result could have been influenced by the ill-effects or the steps taken to lessen them. The case that the animal cannot be replaced by an alternative and that the species chosen is the most suitable in every way should be clearly presented.

Many people are now concerned about the use of words which imply that animals are objects that lack sentience – words such as the animal 'preparation', the animal 'model' or 'harvesting' of tissues.

Details of the environment of the animals and any features of enrichment should be described. Details of special staff training and techniques beneficial to the comfort of the animal should be mentioned. The use, determination, and justification of humane end-points should be fully explained. Such reporting could illustrate the care taken by the scientist, thus allaying fears that the use of animals in research is unjustified.

Good news is no news

The dictum 'good news is no news' is obviously true, the implication being that the steady progress of the scientist is hardly newsworthy. People in the media do not see themselves as standard-bearers for medical research. The tremendous boon that animal experimentation has proved to be, does not sell papers like a blown-up or even invented story of animal suffering in laboratories. Unfortunately, initially at least, the odds are stacked against favourable publicity concerning the use of laboratory animals. This should be a greater spur to present as often as possible and in the best light not only the benefits from the use of animals but also the great concern within research for the welfare of the animal and the constant awareness of the need for alternatives to animals. If the national media are interested only in more spectacular news, then local media outlets – papers and radio – may be persuaded to give an airing to the case for using animals. Parochial though such an approach may be, it can influence a lot of people in a lot of different places.

Sir Walter Bodmer sounded a clarion call for scientists to go on to the offensive:

> 'Research organizations have a responsibility to speak up for the work they support. If they don't, they can't expect anyone else to.'
>
> (Bodmer 1989)

Sir Walter is particularly keen to dispel the idea that the scientific facts put forward by antivivisection groups are accurate. He claims that these groups often distort the science. He thinks that some of the animal rights organizations take advantage of the impressionable and the vulnerable by bombarding children with propaganda. He claims that children as young as seven have been recruited to the young defender group of the British Union of Antivivisectionists.

Neurobiologist Professor David Hubel of Harvard University told a Research Defence Society meeting in the summer of 1991 that he was shocked at the extent of animal rights groups in the UK. Professor Hubel said that those who are doing research should speak up in its favour. To remain silent is too easily interpreted as agreeing. He called on doctors to display literature in their waiting rooms which described why animals are important in research. He stressed the need for all organizations – schools, charities and pharmaceutical companies – to unite to launch big-spending promotional campaigns to counter the animal rights propaganda.

William Harvey Research Institute director and Nobel Laureate Sir John Vane told the same meeting:

> 'It is an unacceptable fact of a modern-day society that scientists who have worked all their lives to enhance the quality of life, to prevent suffering and

distress and combat disease should have to be advised to kneel at the end of the day, not to pray but to inspect the underside of their cars for terrorist bombs.'

(Vane 1991)

The Foundation for Biomedical Research (FBR) in the USA has set a lead in advertising the benefits of animal experimentation. Three advertisements are particularly striking:

(1) A child lying in a hospital bed with two stuffed animals. The caption reads: 'It's the animals you don't see that helped her recover.'
(2) Several demonstrators carrying anti-research signs in front of a barricade. The caption reads: 'Thanks to animal research, they'll be able to protest for 20.8 years longer.'
(3) A view through a microscope of cancer cells, diseased heart tissue and the AIDS virus. The caption reads: 'If we stop animal research, who will stop the real killers?'

All the advertisements carry text explaining how they relate to the use of animals in research.

The role of education

This is the most important factor in the presentation of the case for animal experimentation. At the meeting of the Research Defence Society (1991) already referred to, Sir Walter Bodmer encouraged medical researchers to go into schools to explain how their research works and the small, but crucial, part of it involving animals.

The FBR in the States runs media training workshops for spokespersons. A willingness to talk about research and a concerted effort to educate the public and legislators has become a high priority of most research institutions.

The message of those dedicated to research may be slowly and gradually making some progress in influencing public attitudes. A shift of opinion in favour of animal use in research appeared in a telephone poll associated with a Channel 5 TV Series, 'Tell the Truth', (Channel 5 1998). It was the last programme in the series. The question, 'Should we ban all medical experiments using animals?', received 48% Yes votes and 52% No votes. The total number of votes was about 7000, an average number for the series. It was a close finish but a higher percentage voted in favour of animal use than had been anticipated on the basis of previous polls.

References

Barley, J.B. (1997) This dissertation *The Ethics of Animal Experimentation*, submitted to the Middlesex University, City of Westminster College, for the degree of Master of Science by Jasmine B. Barley, traces the evolution of ethical attitudes among scientists to the use of animals in research. It is the most comprehensive mapping of the change of views on the matter for the period from 1796 to the 1990s.

Bodmer, Sir W. (1989) *Scope*, Winter.

Channel 5 (1998) *Tell the Truth* (television programme) 11 October.

Hall, M. (1831) *A Critical and Experimental Essay on the Circulation of the Blood*.

Hansard, Vol. 814, No. 116, Col. 1642 46. HMSO, London.

HMSO (1989) *Animal Procedures Committee Annual Report for 1989*. Paragraphs 3.12 and 3.13. HMSO, London.

Mason, P. (1997) A graphic account of this famous case appears in his work *The Brown Dog Affair*, Two Sevens Publishing, London.

Morton, D. (1992) *New Scientist*, 11 April.

RDS (1998) *RDS Newsletter*, July.

Rowan, A. (1992) This striking anomaly of Teutonic totalitarian jurisprudence was well written up by Anthony Rowan in the *WARDS Newsletter*, **3**, No. 2, Spring, 1–2.

Spectator (1997) Portrait of the week, 5 July.

The Times (1983) There is no implication that *The Times* condones in anyway the opinions expressed in such publications as the *Liberator*, in its article on the subject on 19 December.

Vane, W.H. (1991) Speech at RDS meeting, Summer.

Chapter 12

The Use of Alternatives – The Three Rs

Introduction

An emphasis on the importance of finding alternatives to animals in research springs naturally from a utilitarian approach to the question. The essential hedonism of utilitarianism obviously views pain as evil and thus calls for the reduction of suffering to a minimum and that includes the suffering of animals. Consequently, the meticulous weighing up of the relative worth of alternatives is not a form of casuistry to be rejected by a common-sense approach. Such attention to the details of possible alleviation of animal suffering is fully in line with the ideal of 'the greatest happiness of the greatest number'. This ideal implies allowing for a relative priority of desirability. The end-product of an application of this ethic is: first, a minimum use of animals and a minimum level of suffering of those used; and second, a greater good accompanied by the realization that worthwhile benefits accrue to animals and humans from animal experimentation.

Other, perhaps more righteous, absolute and certain forms of ethics need not be so committed to the search for alternatives. The more traditionalist deontologists tended to regard the divide between animals and humans as of such a degree that animals did not qualify for consideration in moral terms. Since animals were there for the use of the human race, a need to search for alternatives would be meaningless. Those moral philosophers and their disciples, who either on deontological or on teleological grounds oppose animal experimentation as such, cannot talk consistently in terms of alternatives because they would only tolerate *in vitro* procedures, thus effectively obviating any options.

The possibility of selecting from real options is essential to the notion of alternatives. Those who accept extreme teleology (machiavellianism) would be unconcerned with alternatives, except perhaps for economic or scientific reasons. There are few, I am sure, who would publicly espouse Machiavellism on this matter, at least not in theory. There may be those who would act privately in keeping with this approach without actually formulating their moral tenets. Finally, to avoid confusion, it must be pointed out that not all deontologists, especially modern ones including animal-loving Christians, would eschew the desirability of alternatives. They would emotively accept the goodness of alleviating suffering by research and at the same time conscientiously feel that we should try to limit as much as possible the causing of pain to animals.

The preocuppation with the three Rs (reduction, refinement and replacement) so apparent among many involved in laboratory animal science implies a recognition that the use of animals in research is undesirable. However, the reduction of the number of animals used, after many have been replaced, and the refinement of the procedures on those reduced numbers, is certainly indicative of a concern for the animals. The continued use of animals within these humane parameters does also indicate that those using the animals regard animal experimentation as acceptable. The 'reduction' is no idle boast. Remember, in 1973, in this country 5.5 million animals were used in research. This number had been reduced to 2.7 million by 1997. The striving for greater implementation of the three Rs flows naturally from the hedonism of a utilitarian approach to animal use, employing a cost–benefit assessment.

Numerous works have appeared on the need for and nature of alternatives in the last three decades, for example Smyth (1978).

Inadequacies of alternatives

In the exposition on alternatives in practice and the pursuit of the three Rs, so well outlined in a recent pamphlet (UFAW 1998), specific difficulties will be dealt with in detail. Here it is merely a matter of looking in general at the possible deficiencies of alternatives to animal use in research. In spite of the laudable progress in the development and the use of alternatives, there are factors that militate against a complete abandonment of the use of animals in research.

The reliability of results of research is paramount if they are to be accepted into medical practice or are to be regarded as guarantees of the safety in use of various suspect substances. It is essential therefore that the reliability of any suggested alternatives will need to be compared with accepted animal tests, involving of course the use of animals.

Unfortunately, once the use of alternatives becomes widespread and diverse, their relative value is liable to become a matter of opinion, as will also, their relative merit in comparison with animal experimentation. Pressure groups would be quick to force acceptance of non-animal tests without taking valid scientific arguments into account. For instance, I witnessed on television a spokesman for Greenpeace admit, but rather late in the day, the scientific inadequacy of their arguments in the Brent Spar Rig controversy in 1996.

The most telling argument in favour of at least sometimes using the whole living animal is that, in biology unlike in mathematics, the sum total of the parts do not equal the whole. Even the greatest amount of research in depth on the effects of a hazardous substance on hepatic tissue cannot give you the complete and real picture of what reactions might occur between the same substance and a liver functioning in a living organism and acted upon by the various metabolic cycles.

The three Rs and the law

The obligation to constantly seek more acceptable expressions of the three Rs in practice is not only ethical but is also solidly grounded in the Animals (Scientific Procedures) Act 1986 which states:

'The Secretary of State shall not grant a project licence unless he is satisfied that the application has given adequate consideration to the feasibility of achieving the purpose of the programme to be specified in the licence by means not involving the use of protected animals.'

(s. 5(5))

The Act also states:

'The conditions of a personal licence shall include – a condition to the effect that the holder shall take precautions to prevent or reduce to the minimum consistent with the purposes of the authorised procedures any pain, distress or discomfort to the animals to which those procedures may be applied.'

(s. 10(2)(a))

The Home Office Guidance is equally insistent on the importance of the three Rs:

'Besides weighing the benefits of a project licence against the likely adverse effects on the animal concerned, a number of other considerations are taken into account before a project licence is granted. These include:
(ii)   The consideration which has been given by the applicant to reducing the number of animals used, refining procedures to minimize suffering and replacing animals with alternatives.

(4.32)

It goes on to say:

'In applying for a licence (education and training) applicants must show that they have carefully considered alternatives, such as video material and computer simulations, and that none is suitable.'

(4.40(5))

Among the official instructions on the project licence application is the following instruction: 'Consider alternatives, particularly with reference to reduction and refinement' (s. 18). Section 21 demands a signature to this effect. The legal importance of the three Rs might be further stressed by moving this demand to consider them, to an earlier section of the application.

A Home Office communication (Home Office 1997) reiterates the significance of alternatives:

'This government will insist that applicants for licences demonstrate their efforts at finding alternatives before the use of animals is proposed.'

(Response to Animals Procedures Committee Report)

And finally:

'An experiment shall not be performed if another scientifically satisfactory method of obtaining the result sought, not entailing the use of an animal, is reasonably and practicably available.'

(Directive 86/609/EEC.Art.23)

The concept of the three Rs presented by Russell and Burch in *The Principles of Humane Experimental Technique* (Russell & Burch 1959) has been presented in various forms over the last few decades. The most recent authoritative interpretation of and outline of the application of the three Rs in practice is to be found in *Selection and Use of Replacement Methods in Animal Experimentation* (UFAW 1998). This publication was issued in 1998 under the auspices of FRAME (Fund for the Replacement of Animals in Medical Experiments) and UFAW (Universities Federation for Animal Welfare). This booklet from which much of the following material comes will be referred to as UFAW 1998.

Marshall Hall's principles

The drive to replace the use of animals in research is by no means new. Marshall Hall struck a similar humane note in his work *A Critical and Experimental Essay on the Circulation of the Blood* (Hall 1831). The principles have appeared in more than one form. They were reiterated in the *The Lancet* in 1847:

'We should never have recourse to experiments in cases in which observation can afford us the information required. No experiment should be performed without a distinct and definite object, and without the persuasion, after the maturest consideration, that, that object will be attained by that experiment, in the form of a real and uncomplicated result.

We should not needlessly repeat experiments which have already been performed by physiologists of reputation.

An experiment "should be instituted with the least possible suffering" and in all cases the subject of the experiment should be of the lowest order of animals appropriate to our purpose as the least sentient; whilst every device should be employed, compatible with the success of the experiment, for avoiding the infliction of pain.

Every physiological experiment should be performed under such circumstances as will secure due observation and attestation of its results, and so obviate, as much as possible, the necessity for its repetition.'

(*The Lancet* 1847)

The three Rs

It is usual to accept the term 'alternatives' as not only referring to replacement methods, but as including all the three Rs – reduction, refinement and replacement as defined by Russell and Burch:

(1) *Reduction*: a means of lowering the number of animals used to obtain information of a given amount and precision.
(2) *Refinement*: any development leading to a decrease in the incidence of severity of inhumane procedures applied to those animals which have to be used.
(3) *Replacement*: scientific methods employing non-sentient material which may replace methods which use conscious living vertebrates.

Russell and Burch wrote within the context of the Cruelty to Animals Act 1876.

The three Rs approach combines animal welfare with good science and best practice. Each of the three Rs is not to be taken in isolation. To be most effective they should be considered as complementary to each other – each employed in concert with the others. The use of non-animal alternatives does not only offer the possibility of reducing the number of animals which might have to be used subsequently, for example when screening candidate chemicals during the early stages of product development, but can also lead to refinement of such animal experiments, when they are necessarily used.

When considering the application of the three Rs there must always be the overriding caveat that they should only be applied when attainment of the scientific objective of the proposed, and worthwhile investigations will not be compromised.

Details of appropriate methods of replacement, reduction and refinement will be presented under their respective headings. It must be stressed that each of the three Rs may overlap somewhat. The exact interpretation of the precise scope of each of the three Rs has varied somewhat in the literature over the last few decades. Similarly, in some commentaries on the subject, the order in which the three Rs are given differs. Dr Smyth defined alternatives using the concept of the three Rs but arranged the concepts in the following order – replacement, reduction and refinement:

> 'Alternatives include any procedures which do away with animals altogether, lead to a reduction in the total number of animals used or lead to less distress to the animals employed.'
>
> (Smyth 1978)

Putting replacement as the initial 'R' seems both logically and ethically preferable. Especially in respect to ethics because many opposed to the use of animals in research seem to be more concerned about animals actually being used rather than about how they are used. It seems more desirable to try to dispense with the use of animals if possible before going on to consider the reduction of the numbers required. Attention to the care and welfare of the animals comes within the scope of refinement. The requirement for refinement follows naturally from an ethical approach to animal experimentation. On the other hand the most suitable form that refinement should take in keeping with the nature of the procedure, the level of husbandry appropriate and the biology of the animal, is a scientific and/or technical, not an ethical affair. These factors need to be adjudicated by those directly involved with the research programme and who are the most likely to be experts in the matter.

As a general introduction to the separate topics, a broad classification would be fitting. Four broad categories of alternative techniques that may replace or reduce animal experimentation are:

(1)   *in vitro* tests
(2)   life forms presumed to be less sentient
(3)   computers, models, films, videos and statistics
(4)   human and epidemiological studies.

A practical implementation of the three Rs is not simply to attempt to apply specific categories of alternatives, rather it is an atmosphere in which all the following considerations are brought into play. There should be a careful selection of the species of animal and careful attention to the manner of their use. The species chosen must always be the most appropriate, both biologically and ethologically. Species which are regarded as having the least developed nervous system are to be preferred. The design of the experiment must ensure that the objective is achieved with as few animals as possible and the least interference as possible. Always the ultimate aim is to replace the animal by an alternative wherever possible.

Although not given a great amount of publicity there has been an accelerating rate of scientific and pharmaceutical breakthroughs which have helped to reduce the number of animals required for research.

The Animals, Byelaws and Coroners Unit on the advice of the Animal Procedures Committee, in support of alternative methods sponsors 3Rs research on the scale of a quarter of a million pounds per annum.

Unless the demands set by regulatory bodies for safety testing, etc. are accordingly reduced or amended in keeping with these ideals, it is difficult to see how even moderate reductions can be achieved.

Replacement

Russell and Burch's definition of 'replacement' – 'Any scientific method employing non-sentient material which may, in the history of animal experimentation replace methods which use conscious living vertebrates' – is expanded somewhat in this subsection. Among the three Rs 'replacement' is the term most closely aligned with the concept of 'alternatives'. Consequently, it appears more fitting to include within this topic of replacement the requirement to select for use in experiments the least sentient creature which is adequate to the particular line of research. This is not strictly speaking a replacement of animal use but it is an attempt to reduce animal suffering. For this reason some would regard this choosing of a lower (the term is used with caution) species as reduction.

A salient feature of any comment on or discussion of replacement must contain an acknowledgement of the complexity and fluidity of the subject matter. As animal procedures are used in such a wide range of scientific areas, it is impossible to describe all available replacement methods in all the various areas of research. New possibilities of replacement will continue to be developed. It is the responsibility of those carrying out animal experiments to remain up to date in their field of research on this matter. Any serious discussion of the value of any specific alternative method can only be validly conducted by experts in that line of research. It will necessarily be conducted in the relevant technical language.

Types of replacement

Relative replacement is, for example, the humane killing of a vertebrate animal to provide cells, tissues and/or organs for *in vitro* studies.

Absolute replacement means that animals would not need to be used at all. Examples are the permanent culture of human and invertebrate cells and tissue. There is a presumption here that the work is being done within the context of the 1986 Act and that neither cells nor tissue of the *Octopus vulgaris* are being used.

Direct replacement occurs, for example, when the human skin or guinea-pig skin is used *in vitro* to provide information that would have been obtained from tests on the skin of live guinea-pigs.

Indirect replacement is said to occur in cases such as the replacement of the pyrogen test in rabbits by the limulus amoebocyte lysate (LAL) test or a test based on whole human blood.

Total replacement – the ideal form – is taking a decision not to use any animals because of a lack of justification for such use, or because, in the circumstances, there is no doubt about the reliability of using either a human volunteer or an *in vitro* method.

Partial replacement is, for example, the use of non-animal methods as pre-screens in toxicity testing strategies.

Replacement methods in detail

In vitro *methods and tissue culture*

In vitro (literally, 'in glass') appears to be a generic term not always clearly defined, but generally applied to systems of research using subcellular fractions, short-term maintenance of tissue slices, cell suspensions and perfused organs and tissue culture proper (cell and organotypic culture), including human tissue culture. Similarly, the phrase 'tissue culture' seems to be used in a generic manner, covering the *in vitro* cultivation of organs, tissues, cells and embryos.

Cells, tissues and whole organs, as well as parts of organs, can now be kept alive outside the body. The cells are kept in buffered solution with nutrients under conditions which closely resemble their normal physiological situation. Consequently, physiologists and pharmacologists make wide use of animal and human tissues. In toxicology, *in vitro* methods act as pre-screens, so that the most toxic compounds can be screened out before less toxic compounds are tested on animals. This process not only complements animal studies but allows for the accomplishment of subsequent improved and more detailed *in vitro* work.

The advantages of *in vitro* systems are as follows:

(1) Once validated, *in vitro* systems can provide information in a cost-effective and time-saving manner.
(2) *In vitro* systems can sometimes be used to produce data which are more reliable and more reproducible than data from animal studies. In other cases, they can be used to increase the efficiency of whole-animal studies and decrease the number of animals required.
(3) *In vitro* systems are ideal for mechanistic investigations at the molecular level, as well as for target organ and target species toxicity studies.
(4) Human tissues can be used in *in vitro* systems. The use of human cells obviates the need for cross-species extrapolation, and thus is more relevant to the human situation.
(5) The use of *in vitro* methods can be done in the absence of complex body systems which might introduce confusing factors. This allows studies to be done which could not be conducted in animals.

The disadvantages of *in vitro* methods are as follows:

(1) *In vitro* methods lack the complex interaction of the numerous factors within a living organism, for example immune responses, the endocrine system, the nervous system, the circulation of the blood.
(2) Models are not yet available for all tissues and organs, or for all toxicity end-points.
(3) It can be difficult to relate concentrations of drugs and test chemicals *in vitro* with those occurring in body fluids.

Cell culture

(1) Primary cell culture
A primary cell culture involves the isolation of cells by the disruption of the tissue, often with proteolytic enzymes. The major advantages of primary cultures are the retention of the capacity for biotransformation and tissue-specific functions. One limitation of primary cultures is the necessity to isolate cells for each experiment. This may result in the loss or damage to the integrity of the membrane and loss of cellular products. During the interval necessary to establish monolayer cultures, damage is often repaired (see Table 12.1).

Primary cultures have a limited life span and changes in metabolism and tissue-specific functions will occur with time.

Cell culture techniques are commonly used for monoclonal antibody production, virus vaccine production, vaccine potency testing, screening for cytotoxic effects and studying the function and make-up of cells.

(2) Cell lines
The use of cell lines provides a number of advantages for the study of many biological phenomena, including toxicity. A wide variety of cell types can be used, including human cells and those from specific tissues for investigations of target organ specificity.

Table 12.1 Examples of advantages and limitations of tissue culture systems (from Table 1 of FRAME and UFAW (1998), Table 1).

Systems	Advantages	Limitations
Organ culture	Retention of structural integrity. Maintenance of cell–cell interrelationships.	Large degree of experimental variation. Short-term viability. Statistical sampling problems.
Primary cell	Retention of several differentiated functions.	Loss of tissue architecture. Requires recovery period owing to damage from isolation.
Continuous cell culture	Increased cell viability period. Easier to maintain than primary cultures. Can assume characteristics of transformed cells. Can differentiate *in vitro* to assume new phenotypes.	Loss of tissue architecture. Loss of differentiated organ functions. Can assume characteristics of transformed cells. Significant loss of metabolizing capacity.

Most cell lines can be stored at ultra-low temperatures and they either have a finite life span, or they are capable of an unlimited number of population doublings (continuous cell line). However, the differentiated functions may be altered in cell lines depending on the culture conditions, The metabolic capacity of the cells may also decrease depending on the culture conditions (see Table 12.1).

Isolated and cultured cells offer many advantages both in the study of mechanisms of cellular toxicity by chemical agents and for *in vitro* bioassays.

Established animal cell lines, such as Chinese hamster ovary (CHO) and mouse lymphoma L5178Y, suffer from inter-laboratory variation, especially in basic properties like chromosome number. This is because they have been maintained for many years in culture collections. One attempt to minimize the problems of differentiation, senescence and instability has been to generate immortalized cell lines by introducing viral oncogenes into primary cells. Examples of cells which have been immortalized include rabbit kidney, mouse macrophages, rat liver and human lymphocytes.

(3) Subcellular fractions
Fractionated organelles and membranes prepared from defined cell types can be used for specific cell-free investigations. These *in vitro* systems which are usually prepared by differential centrifugation, include nuclei, mitochandria, lysosomes and membrane vesicles.

Organ culture
Organ culture refers to a three-dimensional culture of tissue, retaining some or all of the biological features of the tissue and preservation of its architecture, usually by culturing the tissue at the liquid–gas interface on a grid or gel. Organ cultures cannot

be propagated and experiments in organ cultures generally involve a large degree of experimental variation between replicates, making organ cultures less suitable than cell cultures for quantitative determinations. The production of organ cultures requires fresh tissue from the relevant organ, although one organ can provide material for several cultures. Table 12.1 refers.

Organ cultures can be used to study pharmacodynamics. The functions studied include oxygen consumption, glucose uptake and release, pyruvate release, lactate release, nitrogenous excretion and cell proliferation. Complex human skin models have been developed and some are available commercially. Test protocols have been developed for use with these human skin models, which enable topically applied aqueous and non-aqueous test materials to be screened for their skin irritancy potentials.

Use of early developmental stages of vertebrates
There is a presumption in this context that there is less likelihood of the occurrence of animal suffering if we accept that the nervous systems of the organisms are not sufficiently well-developed to arouse an awareness of pain. This method of research has special legal significance in the UK. The Animals (Scientific Procedures) Act 1986 does not protect mammals, birds or reptiles before they reach a stage halfway through gestation, nor other vertebrates or the *Octopus vulgaris* before the larvae become capable of independent feeding.

Tests based on mammalian whole-embryo culture systems are well-developed for *in vitro* methods for the detection of reproductive toxicity and teratogenicity, and for elucidating mechanisms of teratogenesis. Chick embryos and frog tadpoles are also being used for these purposes. Chicken eggs have been used for identifying irritants, for example the CAM (chorioallantoic membrane) irritancy test.

Use of lower organisms
This method of research is acceptable on the basis that less suffering is being experienced by the organisms used because they are presumed to be less sentient than the more common experimental animal. Even more preferable is the use of organisms that are presumed to be completely non-sentient, for example bacteria and algae. Examples of this sort of replacement are the following:

(1) The AMES (Bruce) Test is well-established for screening large numbers of chemicals for potential toxic effects. This assay utilizes *Salmonella* bacteria to detect chemical mutagenesis. The AMES test has been validated for regulatory toxicology purposes as a screen for genotoxic chemicals.
(2) Certain species of light-emitting bacteria are being used in toxicity tests. The energy for their light production comes from respiration. As the biochemical processes of respiration are very similar in all organisms, then any chemical which disrupts respiration in bacteria may possibly do the same in humans and would therefore be toxic to humans.
(3) Since yeasts are eukaryotes their cells are more like mammalian cells than bacteria cells. As their chromosome structure resembles that of mammals, yeasts

are more suitable for revealing certain kinds of genetic damage. Yeasts are also used to detect substances that might cause skin damage in the presence of light.

(4)   The coelenterate, *Hydra attenuata*, is used in pre-screening techniques for teratogenicity. This technique is commercially available. It is based on the ability of the hydra to rapidly regenerate from dissociated polyps, which are used as artificial embryos.

(5)   The nematode, *Caenorhabditis elegans*, is widely used in genetic research and in fundamental studies in biology. Substantial progress has been made in complete sequencing of the genome of *C. elegans*. It is becoming clear that many of its genes are conserved in humans. Its use in research has made contributions to fundamental studies in neurophysiology and behaviour, developmental biology, including mechanisms of programmed cell death (apoptosis), and genetics.

(6)   The fruit fly has proved invaluable in genetic research and in fundamental studies in cell biology. Studies with *Drosophila* spp. provided the first evidence that X-rays are mutagenic. *Drosophila* spp. are being used for pre-screening to test for chemical mutagens and carcinogens.

(7)   One unusual piece of research had been designed to test the effects of narcotic drugs. Spiders were given controlled doses of a drug and the extent of their consequent deviant behaviour in web-spinning was then carefully observed and recorded.

(8)   The LAL pyrogen test, already referred to as replacing the traditional test which used rabbits, is more sensitive, economical, convenient and reliable. Blood is taken from the horseshoe crab (*Limulus polyphemus*) and the *Limulus* amoebocyte lysate is extracted from the blood cells for the detection of endotoxins. Unfortunately, this particular alternative method has had an impact on the population of horseshoe crabs. Perhaps, in cases of this nature, attention needs to be paid to overall environmental considerations.

Assays using the organisms referred to can only give limited information. They are, however, useful as pre-screen systems for agrochemicals and environment pollutants.

Physico-chemical methods

Assessment of the chemical properties of a substance will provide some information about its possible toxic effects. For example, compounds with high or low pH values and low buffering capacities are likely to be irritant to the skin, so testing on animals is not necessary. Physical and chemical techniques can be used to study enzyme structures and the mechanisms of their action. In pharmacology and toxicology, physico-chemical analysis can be used in predicting both the likely beneficial and harmful biological effects of chemical substances.

Progress has already been made in developing alternatives to the Draize eye (rabbit) test, for example EYTEX whereby a protein matrix is exposed to the suspected eye irritant. However, recent (1998) validation studies have shown that more *in vitro* test development is required if the Draize eye test is to be replaced by a non-animal testing strategy. HET–CAM (hen's egg test–chorioallantoic membrane) assay, isolated rabbit eye and bovine cornea have been proposed to replace the original undesirable test.

Mice were once used to check the purity of each new batch of insulin. HPLC (high performance liquid chromatography) is now used to analyse insulin for impurities.

Mathematical and computer models

Molecular modelling
In molecular modelling, the three-dimensional structural and electronic properties of a biological site are used to predict whether a novel molecule would interact with it, producing a biological effect. In some cases the detailed structures of such biological sites are known (for example, from X-ray crystallography or other studies). In other cases, the nature of the site of action is inferred from the structures of the molecules known to interact with it, compared with similar structures that do not. This technique is known as pseudoreceptor modelling. Molecular modelling is restricted to making predictions about biological sites whose structures are reasonably well understood.

CADD
Computer assisted drug design (CADD) uses interactive graphics in the early stages of development of new compounds. Receptor sites of cells are explored. Once the shapes of receptor sites are known, attempts can be made to design molecules to fit them. The compatability of the potential molecule to a particular receptor can be observed.

QSAR
Quantitative structure–activity relationships (QSAR) in the form of equations attempt to define relationships between the structure of chemicals – the shape, size and reactivity of the particular groups of atoms present – and their biological activities. QSAR can be used to predict the possible biological effects of new compounds. The information collected may indicate ways of changing the structure of a molecule to alter its therapeutic or toxic properties.

DEREK
Deductive estimation of risk from existing knowledge (DEREK) interfaces on-screen structural information with a toxicity database so that qualitative predictions about novel structures, drawn by the toxicologist, can be made and toxicophores identified.

PBPK
Physiologically based pharmacokinetic (PBPK) modelling predicts the disposition of xenobiotics and their metabolites by integrating three types of information: species-specific physiological parameters, partition coefficients for the chemical parameters, and partition coefficients for the metabolic parameters. PBPK can provide information to predict tissue exposure to xenobiotics and their metabolites for various doses and species. PBPK presents a clear potential for refining ADME (absorption, distribution, metabolism and excretion) studies.

Final comments on computer models

As previously indicated, the variety of possible alternatives is immense and new methods are constantly coming on line. A new laser/computer model has been developed to simulate orthodontic tooth movement.

So significant is mathematical and computer modelling to replacement that as far back as 1993 the RSPCA sponsored a research programme at the University of Surrey. Its object was to develop a computer modelling approach for the testing of chemicals. Such methods, however, are even now in an early stage of development. The computers' ability to predict beneficial or toxic effects of chemicals depends on the amount and quality of the information available for use in their programming. In the future it may be possible to assess the biologically useful and toxic effects of untested substances simply from a knowledge of their three-dimensional structure.

The use of models, films and videos

Some very realistic models of experimental animals have been developed for the replacement of live animals in teaching and training. The Japanese silicone rat model has proved useful as a teaching aid. A further advance has been an artificial rabbit with all the necessary characterisitics of the live animal. This model is an accurate simulation of a female New Zealand White rabbit weighing 2.4 kg. It has lifelike fur and body plasticity. The abdominal wall can be simply opened to show the position of the stomach, while the abdominal cavity conceals small tubes which conduct and drain fluids during practice injections.

The usefulness of films and videos of animal handling and procedures made by experts, for use in teaching and training as a replacement of live animals, is self-evident.

Human beings

The use of humans for replacement of animals includes the use of human tissues and human volunteers as well as post-marketing surveillance and epidemiology.

Human tissues have been used to establish organotype culture models such as skin equivalents. Immortalized human cells have been established to overcome problems of the supply of fresh tissue. This has been done mainly by DNA virus oncogene transfection.

There are problems with obtaining human tissue samples. Logistics problems include safety issues associated with the necessity to screen for HIV, hepatitis and other infections. Furthermore there will be a need to obtain detailed histories of donors relating to genetic background, drug intake and details of any other exposures, as well as a need for a system to keep track of tissues obtained from each donor, in case of future problems. In the UK, statutory regulations require informed consent from donors/relatives and from local research ethics committees. Morally there are potential ownership problems and many commercial and legal implications. Reflecting on the course of events in the USA, consideration should be given to the possibility of future patenting of genetic material. The use of fetal tissue brings its own complex legal and moral aspects.

Human beings would seem to be ideal subjects for biological, physiological or medical research concerning humans. There need be no dependence on the weak argument from analogy. The discrepancies which are bound to occur even with the best method of extrapolation are obviated. Unfortunately, the human being is not always the ideal model for studying some aspects of human biology and there are circumstances when an animal model is a better choice. We are certainly not gnotobiotic animals; in fact, we are far from specified pathogen-free (SPF), so that in any tests involving humans, varying health status will tend to introduce unacceptable variables into the procedure.

Moreover, the life of the human subject may prove to be longer than that of any member of the research team, so it is much easier to assess long-term effects (relative to a life span) in animals which reach old age in a much shorter period. The length of human generations militates against any meaningful research within the working life of the average scientist whereas there is a rapid turnover of mice generations in a matter of a few years. This means that in some areas the animal model is much more likely to provide testable results, valid for human beings, than could be ascertained by using human beings, either law-abiding or criminal (the more commonly suggested subjects).

The use of human subjects obviously has its place and must ultimately be a vital part of clinical trials. This, of course, evokes a different ethical scenario because informed consent must always be a main feature. And there are those who would say that consent is not always an entity in these procedures because full information is not always made available to the people involved (*Guardian* 1992).

Validation

Apart from the time it takes to develop alternative techniques, the factor that has emerged as causing the most delay in the acceptance of various proposed methods of replacement has been validation. Validation refers to the process whereby the reliability and relevance of an assay are established for a particular purpose. The time-consuming aspect of the whole process of achieving validation is due to the need to:

- establish the accuracy of the new technique or approach, for example in the case of epidemiology;
- establish the repeatability of the method;
- perform trials using genuine products in real situations;
- obtain acceptability by official bodies who use the result to issue safety certificates. This is probably the most time-consuming part of the venture, impeding rapid progress. This delay is exacerbated by a variety of national attitudes and a mosaic of bureaucratic practices of Byzantine complexity.

The nature and the scale of the validation is dictated by the purpose of the assay. If an assay is designed to replace an animal method and to be used widely for regulatory purposes then validation trials are often conducted at several different laboratories according to specific internationally harmonized criteria which are intended to facilitate regulatory acceptance of the alternative method.

ECVAM (European Centre for the Validation of Alternative Methods) is specifically concerned with the drive to replace animals in research (ECVAM 1998).

Reduction

The ideal method of reducing the number of animals used in research is of course by replacement. In the more restricted sense in which the word 'reduction' is used in this context the term has a more specific connotation. The term 'reduction' here denotes strategies for obtaining comparable levels of information from the use of fewer animals in scientific procedures or for obtaining more information from a given number of animals. There are areas of overlap between reduction as such and replacement.

There is evidence that although fewer animals are being used, neither scientific progress nor medical research are being curtailed. The call for such reduction has come from within the scientific community. ICLAS (International Council of Laboratory Animal Science) has in the past called upon regulatory authorities to help reduction still further by revising the number of animals used in toxicity testing and to avoid duplications from one country to another.

The 1986 European Convention on animal use in research reflected this spirit in Article 29:

> 'In order to avoid unnecessary repetition of procedures for the purposes of satisfying national legislation on health and safety, each Contracting Party shall, where practicable, recognize the results of procedures carried out in the territory of another party.'

The drive for reduction may sometimes have to be balanced against the comparative severity of proposed procedures. It would appear to be preferable, if the choice needs to be made between using a larger amount of animals in milder procedures or fewer animals in more severe procedures, to select the former option. This decision, of course, presumes that other factors are equal and that the principles of good science are observed.

Reduction methods in detail

Communication of information

Proper use of all available data can obviate unnecessary repetition of research using animals and can ensure that the best use of the least animals for a particular purpose can be achieved. In these days of the 'global village' and rapid extension of electronic means of communication, the dissemination of relevant information is not only possible but should be given priority by those responsible for using experimental animals. Research establishments should provide adequate information and a centralized efficient retrieval system of useful data. Laboratories ought to publish results of animal studies to avoid unnecessary repetition of animal procedures. Furthermore, researchers may be made aware when animals are to be killed so that any spare tissue, etc. can be shared among researchers thus reducing the overall numbers of animals used.

Individual researchers now have access to on-line databases which give up-to-date lists of published research in all areas of science. Before planning an experimental procedure, a scientist should be aware of any similar work which has already taken place, with either animal or non-animal procedures, so that unnecessary repetition is avoided. There is no lack of informative literature in this field. FRAME (Fund for the Replacement of Animals in Medical Experiments) publishes abstracts giving information about methods of reducing the number of animals used in experiments.

The ideal model

The significance of using a specialized animal model for a specific type of research has already been mentioned. The direct result of this good practice is a reduction in the numbers of animals used because the animals that are used are more suitable for providing the required data in smaller numbers. An example is the use of nude mice which, being athymic, are immunologically incompetent. Consequently, fewer individuals are needed than those of other mice strains for the passaging of tumours.

In-breeding

This topic has been alluded to, so it will be apparent that by the use of an inbred strain, strain variation will be eliminated from the data. Some inbred strains may have a characteristic that is significant in a particular area of research, rendering that strain the ideal model in the work being done.

Transgenic and chimeral animals

In this area of research we have the possibility of producing the ideal model animal rather than trying to select the best from those available. In the case of inbred strains, time is a major factor because at least 20 generations are needed to develop a desired strain, if at all possible. Genetic manipulation can certainly contribute directly to the reduction of the number of animals required for research. In the wider aspect of genetic engineering, cloning could lead to the production of groups of animals which lacked even individual variations, at least as regards the genotype – a further opportunity of reducing animal numbers in research.

Unfortunately, from experience, I realize that the number of animals needed for initiating a transgenic programme, starting with superovulation, can be very high. Since the early days in this research, methods have been duly refined and this particular difficulty is now less problematical.

Among the many examples of how genetic manipulation can produce the ideal model animal for research and thus reduce the number of animals needed in a procedure, is the case of the Duchenne muscular dystrophy mouse. This mouse, ideal as a model for the effects of Duchenne on both the skeletal muscle and the heart, was produced by the Washington School of Medicine in St Louis. The new mouse strain develops muscle wasting and heart disease, dying before adulthood, thus mirroring the effect of the disease in humans. The disorder results from a defect in the gene for an enormous protein called dystrophin which forms on the scaffold in muscle fibres.

Known health status
The use of animals protected from infection and maintained in a healthy condition obviates a potent source of variations between individuals; this ensures that a smaller number of animals will be sufficient for producing valid results in research. Disease in animals masks and distorts reaction, producing a greater demand for experimental animals to offset these defects. A further reason why reduction can result from using barrier-maintained or isolator animals is that there will not usually be a loss of animals due to death or disease during a research programme. Such an unfortunate occurrence would necessitate the use of even more animals if the programme is to be successfully completed. It was not unknown in the past for research programmes to be 'rubbed out' and done again because the regular supply of rodents had suddenly dried up due to an outbreak, say, of tyzzers, a virulent murine infection.

In gnotobiotic animals, the complete micro-organic burden is known. If it is known that in fact there is no micro-organic burden whatsoever, then these gnotobiotic animals are referred to as germ-free or axenic. In the use of gnotobiotic animals, variations between individuals is minimized and data are not affected by pathogenic conditions which are often not fully accounted for or understood. Consequently, fewer animals will be needed to achieve the level of statistical precision or the use of the same number of animals will lead to better experiments with fewer incorrect results. This could obviate the need for repetition which might otherwise be required for confirmation purposes.

Interest in gnotobiotes seems to have waned somewhat since the enthusiasm of the 1980s, perhaps because of high costs and a certain dislike of isolators on the part of some workers. There might be an increased demand for gnotobiotes as the interest in and the real need for germ-free animals, for example pigs, grows in order to advance progress in xenotransplants.

Experimental design
It is a prime principle of research that any animals used, are used economically. 'Economically' is meant to apply to the minimizing of the discomfort of the animal, not to the cost of the project in monetary terms.

By judicial planning, superfluous experiments can be discarded and effective experimental projects using the minimum number of animals can be designed. The number of products going forward for conventional tests using animals have been reduced by trying to predict potential carcinogenic or other hazardous qualities in groups of chemicals. By this type of early investigative work, many suspect substances can be screened out at an early stage.

Expert care and thoughtful management of animals is conducive to the accuracy and validity of experimental results. The application of such expertise on the part of researchers can effectively reduce animal use.

Critical appraisal of the worthiness of the proposed project can lead to reduction in the number of animals required for an experiment. It may be possible to carry out small pilot studies using only a few animals, which can be reviewed before committing larger numbers of animals to a major research programme.

Statistics

So important are statistics to the proper implementation of the three Rs that the mandatory study module for obtaining a project licence must have a statistical content. Proper statistical design, prior to undertaking the study, and appropriate analysis of the resulting data, can make it possible to obtain results of comparable or greater precision while using fewer animals.

There is evidence that poor experimental design, together with inappropriate statistical analysis of experimental results, is leading to inefficient use of animals and of scientific resources in toxicological research and testing, and in other areas of biomedical research. A study of papers in *Index Medicus* carried out on behalf of the Humane Society of the USA in 1961, showed that a saving of 23–40% of the animals used could have been achieved if better statistical methods had been employed. The statistician, rather than the moral philosopher, has probably been more directly responsible for the greatest amount of reduction in animal use.

Refinement

In keeping with what has been said about reduction, an apt comment on refinement is that more effective refinement of procedures on animals has been accomplished by competent anaesthetists than by anything learned in ethics. Refinement encompasses those methods which alleviate or minimize potential pain and distress, and which enhance animal well-being. The details of refinement are so varied and numerous that it is only possible in this text to indicate the general areas in which animal suffering can be alleviated and the care of laboratory animals improved. Attention must be payed to:

(1) The expertise employed in experimental work, for example as regards surgery and all other relevant skills.
(2) The proper use of anaesthetics and a readiness to use them on all appropriate occasions, as would be done in the case of humans undergoing similar procedures.
(3) The use of analgesics.
(4) The provision of sedation to obviate stress or eliminate discomfort.
(5) Post-operative care in all cases in which it would effect the alleviation of animal suffering.
(6) Meticulous observance of humane end-points which ought to be set so as to prevent as much animal suffering as possible. The demand for the fixing of appropriate end-points is the most significant legal requirement for refinement. In practice, the actual end-point will vary greatly according to the

procedures involved; in some cases it may be tumour size (UKCCCR 1988). I have known cases involving primates where it was fixed as the geriatric state.

(7)   There must be strict adherence to the permitted level of severity which preferably should be set as low as is feasible in the circumstances.

(8)   The most suitable form of euthanasia, usually in keeping with Schedule 1 of the Animals (Scientific Procedures) Act, must always be available without delay at all times.

(9)   In order that projects are properly planned, procedures are correctly performed and the animals are properly cared for, it is essential that all those involved in animal experimentation are fully trained. The mandatory Home Office modules are designed to provide a modicum of instruction on these matters to all concerned. However, more extensive and intensive in-house training should be provided so that refinement of animal use in research can be fully accomplished.

(10) There must always be sustained efforts to replace severe procedures by more refined and less severe ones. An obvious case in point is the various attempts to obviate the need for the undesirable LD_{50} by milder forms of assessment of the toxicological nature of substances, for example the FDP (fixed dose procedure) or the HID_{50} (hypothermic inducing dose).

Good husbandry as the ongoing expression of refinement

Husbandry of the highest order must be the accepted practice throughout every animal unit. The animal welfare should not only be in keeping with the relevant Codes of Practice but also the specific biology and behavioural patterns of the experimental animal must be considered so that suitable environmental enrichment can be provided. The choice of the form of environmental enrichment will be influenced, if not sometimes restricted, by the type of research being practised.

A base line of the provision of refinement in the area of animal welfare must be those principles of good stockmanship – the five freedoms as formulated by Professor Brambell in 1979 with the Farm Animal Welfare Council. These tenets on the care of animals have been dealt with under the heading of the nature of rights in respect to animals. Their significance in the practice of animal technology cannot be over-stressed.

A multiplicity of Rs

So popular has the whole concept of the three Rs been in laboratory animal science that various usages of 'R' have proliferated. A suggestion of the 'right animal for the right reason' was put forward by Dr H.C. Rowsell. Other letters were not to be ignored: Dr Carol Newton posited three Ss – 'good science, good sense and good sensibility'. A favoured contender for significant initials was the four Rs, adding 'respect' to the three Rs. There is no denying the importance of respect when it comes to dealing with experimental animals. This respect is not inspired by mere anthropomorphism or emotive sentiment. Unless respect is paid to the animal within the context of its specific nature, those dealing with that animal are going to run into many difficulties. We need to treat a dog in the context of its canine nature, or a goat within the context of its caprine nature, etc. or we will fail to achieve anything of worth in our work with the animal. Respect for the animal as an individual and in keeping with its species must be the main plank of any effective welfare. Figure 12.1 illustrates the UFAW strategy for implementation of the three Rs into a research protocol.

Other relevant 'Rs' that come to mind are as follows:

(1) *Responsibility.* This concept is an integral part of the managerial role of a project licence holder. Responsibility for an experimental animal springs directly from the fact that, being captive, it depends completely for its needs on those responsible for it. Responsibility for an animal under a procedure is an important duty of the personal licensee.

(2) *Reason.* This concept is relevant to justifying the use of an animal in research. There must be a good reason for subjecting any animal to a regulated procedure which by definition may involve pain, suffering, distress or lasting harm.

(3) *Recognition.* This concept implies that not only the need for alternatives should be recognized but also the most appropriate form of alternative be recognized and adopted.

(4) *Reflection.* This concept refers to the need to seriously reflect on all relevant literature in a search for suitable methods to implement the three Rs.

(5) *Reconsideration.* This concept demands a readiness to be prepared to keep an open mind, even after the initiation of a programme, so that if the feasibility of a new validated alternative appears, it will be seriously considered.

(6) *Relief.* This is an essential feature of the approach to the use of experimental animals. Every means will be used to relieve the suffering of the animal.

The list, I suppose, could go on to include 'Rs' with a negative connotation, such as Repetition and Reuse. I recall one harassed scientist who quite rightly pointed out, after being presented with an even longer list, that the most striking relevant 'R' was omitted – Regulations (not forgetting that some of those Regulations demand the use of animals in tests).

No doubt it was in this spirit that a rather irreverent article appeared on this topic (Landsell 1993).

In the animal room among the animals there is one 'R' of special significance – rapport. This term expresses the ideal interface with the animal. It is a result of gentling the animal. This is a method of caring for the animal that puts it at its ease. Its proper performance depends on an understanding of not only the particular species but if possible the individual animal and its needs. The establishing of a rapport with an animal is not just a matter of good husbandry but it is also a requisite of good science. An effective rapport with the animal will obviate panic and create the circumstances in which an animal will react normally and give normal reactions to tests being carried out. The overall importance of this caring attitude to the achieving of animal welfare and good science can not be overemphasized.

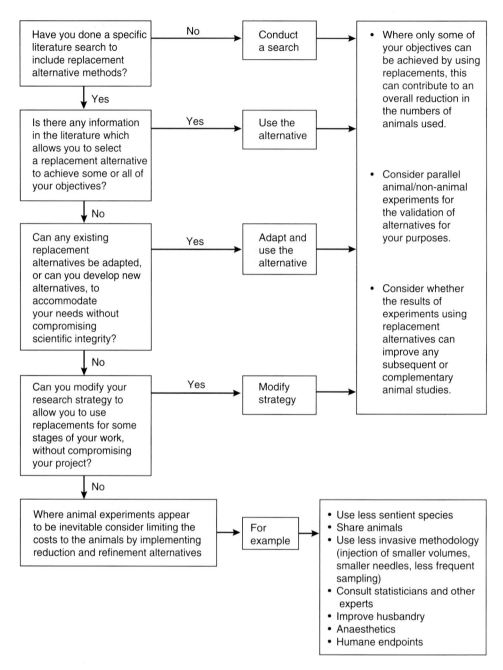

Fig. 12.1 A strategy for the assessment of the potential for implementation of the three Rs into a research protocol (UFAW 1998).

The scientific basis for such a claim was provided by Russell and Burch. They indicated that besides the genotype and phenotype of which we are all aware, we should take into account another deciding factor which can influence the animal's reactions – the dramatype. By the dramatype they meant the pattern of performance in a single physiological response of short duration. The response elicited will be influenced by the proximate and immediate environment (see Figure 12.2).

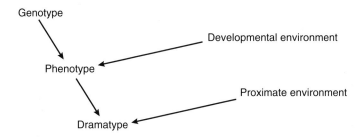

Fig. 12.2   The determination of the dramatype (Russell & Burch 1959).

Relevant data resulting from any animal experimentation will be affected by the conditions of the proximate and immediate environment; that is, whether the environment tends to induce panic or, because a rapport with the animal has been built up, the animal does not anticipate distress nor experience fear. In the latter case there is a relationship of trust between animal and handler. A calm animal is the ideal subject for research.

In practice the degree of rapport which can be achieved will vary greatly from species to species and even in respect to individual animals. Even the same animal will vary from time to time in amenability. From decades of close encounters with rodents, I am of the opinion that in the matter of attaining a successful rapport with animals, the watershed comes between rats and mice. Rats are readily reactive with humans. Whereas mice seem to be usually indifferent to human attention.

Indubitably, the drive to validate alternatives to animals and the ethical imperative to implement as much as possible the three Rs, is paramount in research. This is a praiseworthy function of ethics in animal experimentation. The fulfilment of this ideal in practice is a matter of expert technology, not ethics. Reading through some laboratory animal science literature, one could get the impression that ethics is spelt only with three Rs.

References

ECVAM (1998) ECVAM is ready to supply any relevant information on the three Rs. Contact: JRC Environment Institute, 21020 Ispra (Va), Italy. E-mail address, julia.fentem@JRC.it.

Guardian (1992) An article entitled 'Trafficking begins in human flesh', 10 April, made apt and valid comments on this topic.

Hall, M. (1831) *A Critical and Experimental Essay on the Circulation of the Blood.*

Home Office (1997) *HO Communication HO/PCD-H*, November. This was a response to an Animals Procedures Committee Report.

Landsell, H. (1993) This unusual and somewhat adversatorial approach was presented with skill in an article by Landsell entitled *The 3Rs: A Restrictive and Refutable Rigmarole*'. It appeared in *Ethics and Behaviour*, **3**(2) 177–185.

Russell, W. & Burch, R. (1959) This diagram appeared in their work *The Principles of Humane Experimental Technique*, Methuen, London. The diagram shows the relationship between variables. The arrows represent causal relations. Variation in the system at the back end of an arrow contributes to the variance of the system at the front end.

Smyth, D.H. (1978) Smyth's book was an important milestone in the drive towards awareness of alternatives to experimental animals, producing the arguments and explaining the methods. *Alternatives to Animal Experimentation* by D.H. Smyth, Emeritus Professor of Physiology at the University of Sheffield, a Scolar paperback, London.

The Lancet (1847) *The Lancet*, **i**, 58–60, 135–161.

UFAW (1998) *Selection and Use of Replacement Methods in Animal Experimentation*. UFAW, Wheathampstead. (Compiled by FRAME and UFAW.)

UKCCCR (1988) Details of this valuable pamphlet have already been given in the reference section at the end of Chapter 10.

Chapter 13

Cost–Benefit – the Balancing Act

'... through clouds of "Ers" and "Ums"
Obliquely and by inference, illumination comes.'

The Puzzler, Rudyard Kipling

Introduction

Dr Robert Watt, a past Chief Inspector at the Home Office, pointed out rightly that the big ethical decision, i.e. that animal experimentation should be allowed under specified conditions, had already been taken at a national level by the passing of the Animals (Scientific Procedures) Act. Dr Watt went on to indicate the role of the Secretary of State, acting through, and using the experience and expertise of, the Inspectorate:

'To weigh the likely adverse effects on the animals concerned against the benefit likely to accrue as a result of the programme to be specified in the licence.'

In difficult cases requiring specialized knowledge, external assessors and the Animal Procedures Committee are consulted. Work is considered to be justified if the likely benefit exceeds the likely cost to animals in suffering (LASA 1994).

A model of the cost–benefit process was published in the Animal Procedures Committee Report (1993: p. 27) and is reproduced in Figure 13.1.

The representation of the Animal Procedures Committee shown in Figure 13.1 has the appearance of an algebraic equation – something quite different from the obtuse notions of ethics that this work commenced with. Yet on one side of the

$$\text{Justification} = \frac{\text{Benefit}}{\text{Cost}}$$

$$\text{Justification} = \frac{\text{Importance of objectives} \times \text{Probability of achievement}}{\text{Cost to animals in suffering}}$$

$$\text{Justification} = \frac{\text{Background/objectives potential benefits} \times \text{Scientific quality}}{\text{Adverse effects and coping strategies}}$$

Fig. 13.1 Model of the cost–benefit process.

equation is 'justification', certainly a term with an ethical tone. Since the process mapped out here is intended to portray the crucial issue of establishing the accept-ability of using individual animals in research, it is imperative that it be considered seriously; not only seriously but item by item – 'justification', 'cost' and 'benefit'.★

Justification

There is no doubt that if you are issued a licence to perform a particular action then you have justification in law for what you do. That is what a licence is – a permission to do something, which if you did not have that permission, it would be unlawful for you to do. The above formula, however, is prior to any granting of a licence. It seems to be concerned with whether there is justification for issuing a licence. If the desired balance is present, if the assessment produces a positive answer, it is implied that there is a reason for granting such a licence. We are back into the realms of *why* it is morally right to go ahead. We have investigated the morality of the proposed deed. We have strayed into an indulgence in ethics. It must be stressed that much of the detail used to make the case will be scientific and technical. It is only the weighing-up of the relative worth, the persuasion value of the testimony of relevant experts such as the researcher and the animal carer, which pertains to the final moral judgement on the intended experiment. Once the credibility of the science in the case is established then others, who are regarded as being able to contribute constructively to a moral judgement on the matter, can cooperate with those involved in arriving at a decision. An ethics committee might prove to be an ideal crucible in which to discuss and explore the elements of this assessment so as to arrive at an acceptable solution. This ethical exercise – looking at the 'why' – will argue on the basis that any pain an animal experiences in research must be directly related to the value of the experiment.

In the context of the cost–benefit assessment we move into casuistry – the useful moral art of weighing up the ethical worth of an action on a case-by-case basis. As a practical application of ethics, this exercise will stem from some basic ethical theory. An ideal ethical theory for this pursuit would appear to be utilitarianism. It homes in on consequences and particularly on benefits, in keeping with its principle of 'The greatest happiness of the greatest number'. A special feature of utilitarianism which is particularly relevant in this endeavour to find a proportionality between pain and beneficial concequences is that, of all forms of moral philosophy, as a hedonistic theory, it pays particular attention to pain. Bentham, himself, points out that as pleasure is good, so of course pain is evil. It is to be avoided as much as possible. There is a serious intent within utilitarianism to avoid suffering, an attitude undetectable in many other moral philosophies. The Stoics seem to have delighted in suffering. The Puritans appeared to glory in it. Schopenhauer wrote of it in glowing terms.

Neither utilitarianism, nor indeed any other ethical theory, is able to settle each and every problem occurring in the making of a decision on the rightness or

---

★A more sophisticated exposition was published in the APC 1997 Report (p. 44) along with com-mentary on the concept of 'disbenefit'.

wrongness of any intended project. Utilitarianism provides an ethical justification for deciding on the goodness or badness of an act by reference to the consequences in the context of given circumstances such as pain. The final decision will depend on the expertise in presenting all germane facts, experience, study and casuistry. Unfortunately, arguments in casuistry tend to depend on the history of previous decisions; in short, on precedent. Authoritative published precedents have not been a feature in the practical application of the cost–benefit assessment. Such useful points of reference may be built up by busy, well-informed and consistent ethics committees.

The crux of the ethical problem being considered is the 'permission to hurt'. Can that ever be permissible, particularly in the context of hedonistic utilitarianism? Other moralists, as already indicated, did not have such difficulty as regards suffering; indeed, some religions, abundant sources of morality, seemed to revel in it. Nature itself is awash with pain but within modern culture and accepted mores the infliction of suffering is undesirable, if not unacceptable. Is there any way in which a case can be made out for the justification of causing suffering?

A salient feature of modern humanity is an all-pervading indulgence in sport. This is undoubtedly a hedonistic pursuit. Yet one of its acclaimed axioms is 'There's no gain without pain'. Perhaps then, pain is not all bad, even for the hedonist. On the positive side, pain plays a crucial part in the preservation of health, both of humans and animals. A rather extreme and indeed untrue statement, in the light of medical progress, makes the following point. A French surgeon, Alfred Velpeau, wrote in 1832:

> 'The abolition of pain in surgery is a chimera. It is absurd to go on seeking it today. "Knife" and "pain" are two words that must forever be associated in the consciousness of the patient.'
>
> (Harris 1994)

Given that pain is of the very warp and weft of life, can we feel justified in 'hurting a little to help a lot'? Indeed the carnivores amongst us may have already made the ethical quantum leap of accepting as justified a lot of hurt for a preferred cuisine. We may be willing to accept discomfort, even pain for an advantage to ourselves. We are even prepared to accept proxy permission from parents, guardians, etc., for painful but beneficial treatment of others. In these cases the benefit is to the sufferer. It is a different matter in the case of animals in research, no consent is forthcoming and the benefit is for others, not for the experimental animal being used.

We need to look further than a mere playing-down of suffering or a dependence on the raw consequentialism associated with the name of Machiavelli – the end justifies the means. That can and has justified the worst atrocities.

The application of the subtle moral principle of double effect is not relevant in this setting. While there is obviously no desire to hurt the experimental animal, such hurt is an immediate effect of any painful experiment. Any desired benefit is not an integral result of the action being performed and so cannot be presented as a double effect of the operation. To claim otherwise would be unacceptable sophistry. The single apparent effect of feeding a test substance to a rat may be distress. The consequent knowledge gained is not an essential effect of the administration of the suspect diet.

To turn to another moral principle of much wider application, can we consider as relevant the classical moral dilemma of the choice between two evils? What could those two evils be? It is here taken for granted that suffering, in this case the suffering of animals, is an evil. It is to be avoided and it is undesirable to cause it. It must be stated that in many case of animal experimentation, speaking from experience, the suffering is not severe and always as minimal as possible.

Set against this evil of animal suffering we have the ever-present evil of universal suffering of animals and humans alike. There is no doubt that, as intelligent creatures, we can do something about reducing that evil. In fact, of course, long lines of scientists have progressed knowledge so that some of that suffering has been alleviated; sometimes, of course, by the use of animals.

Is the choice then between the acknowledged evil of causing pain to animals and what some would see as an evil, ignoring suffering, not using the gifts we have to reduce that suffering of animals and humans alike?

Animals may have rights but do all creatures have rights to safe medicines etc?

We by no means claim that the use of experimental animals is desirable but is there a case for saying it may be acceptable? This may be so if we choose to regard restricted animal suffering in research as a lesser evil than allowing a continuation of suffering which could be prevented by science.

Such a decision is not a comfortable one. It has none of the self-satisfaction of high moral righteousness. It is following a line we do not particularly like. We realize that for us it is an acceptable compromise. Is not this often the case in the real world, i.e. the least worst option is the best? Our attitude may be confusing but so are facts. Reality is not black and white, rather it is an infinity of greys. Because this ethical approach is far from absolute, there is certainly lacking the solid ring of confidence of deontology. Consequently, caution is inherent in making decisions in the context of the teleological approach. Judgements are formed on a case-by-case basis. It is necessary to pay attention to details and circumstances. It is all-important to ask the right questions. It could be argued that the suggested formula of the Animal Procedures Committee is an appropriate framework for working out the justification of a project in research involving experiments on animals. The formula deals with the essential features of the polemic – pain and benefit.

The cost in animal suffering

This factor in the assessment has been dealt with at length, in respect to the nature of pain, its measurement and gradation, in Chapter 10. Suffice it to stress that it is this factor that calls for the greatest amount of monitoring and control.

Benefits

There is no hesitation in using the plural since the benefits accruing over the centuries from animal experimentation have been numerous.

Before considering those benefits in general and in particular, it is important to stress that the level of probability of achievement of the desired benefits must be seriously considered. Another essential feature of the process should be the assessment of the scientific quality of the proposed project. The questions which ought to be asked in this context should include:

(1) Is the use of animals necessary?
(2) Is it the right choice of species and at the lowest level?
(3) Is the number of animals to be used as small as possible?
(4) What is the scale of the project and are the various procedures properly staged?
(5) Is there an appropriately statistical design, maximum efficiency and minimum group size?
(6) What is the track record of the research team?

The fundamental nature of the demand for defined benefits is illustrated by the fact that within the scope of both the European Convention and UK legislation, animal experimentation will only be permitted if proposed work can claim to be orientated to one of seven categories of benefits. In brief these seven 'whys' are:

(1) targeted medical research
(2) blue-sky physiological research
(3) environmental monitoring
(4) advancement of biological and behavioural knowledge
(5) education and training
(6) forensic enquiries
(7) specialized breeding of experimental animals.

Progress through the ages

Medical skill and the living sciences progressed through the use of animals in research probably before the time of Arasistratus (*c.* 300 BCE). In Alexandria he used animals in his study of nerves and anatomy, He explored and named the trachea as well as developing the catheter. About the same time in Athens, Aristotle, the founder of biology, was extending his knowledge by a hands–on use of animals. The use of animals in research had advanced far enough to justify the publication of a book on veterinary surgery in AD 65 (Pascoe *et al.* 1968). Galen (AD 129–200), the great Greek physician in Rome, through his studies using apes and pigs, was able to increase the knowledge of medicine enormously, publishing 500 medical treatises.

As time passed, each century increased our knowledge in the living sciences by the use of animals in research. The effective use of animals produced the advances by Harvey (1578–1657) in haematology. He first described the circulation of the blood in animals *De Motu Cordis et Sanguinis in Animalibus (On the Motion of the Heart and Blood)*. The title indicates how he achieved the great progress in medical science. He stated categorically the need to use animals in research. It is said that he used more than 40 species of animals in his experiments. By the next century, similar research using animals established a basis for measuring blood pressure. In the nineteenth century, the use of experimental animals brought us vaccination through the work of such scientists as Pasteur and Jenner.

Charles Darwin, who deplored some forms of animal experimentation, testified to the Royal Commission (1875) that he thought that a ban on animal experimentation would be 'a great evil'. The implication of this remark was that he appreciated the many advantages which had accrued from the use of animals in research. He regarded refraining from animal experimentation as a greater evil than ignoring and tolerating suffering that could be alleviated by research using animals.

In this century each decade has brought more and more useful discoveries through the use of animals. In the first decade of the century antibodies were discovered. By the 1920s vitamins had been recognized in detail and insulin had been discovered.

In the 1930s the mechanism of the nervous system was being fully explored and modern surgery was being developed. The 1940s brought an understanding of embryonic development and antibiotics were established as efficient remedies. Transplants were proving their worth through animal experimentation in the 1950s. A start was made on methods of treatment of mental illness by animal use in the 1960s. A whole spectrum of tested drugs were brought into use during the 1970s. At this time, also, there was the discovery of prostaglandins and monoclonal antibodies. In the 1980s great advances were made in understanding immune reactions, and, with the development of transgenic animals, research could become more precise and there was the opportunity to reduce the number of animals needed in research. Drugs to treat viral diseases were also developed. In the 1990s, progress in medical research through the use of animals is indeed accelerating. New knowledge concerning the brain and the causes of inherited diseases is continually being published.

All these benefits have, of course, where possible, been spread to animals and adopted by veterinary medicine. In fact, some research establishments are solely concerned with the therapeutic needs of animals.

This is not the place to produce long lists of achievements. Suffice it to point out that had there been a mandatory moratorium on the use of animals in research at any time in the past, there could have been dire consequences for the progress of medicine and the living sciences. Such a moratorium in 1910, for example, could have deprived humankind, in the years immediately following, of extensive knowledge regarding vitamins. In the same vein, such a moratorium in 1950 could have deprived that particular generation of polio vaccine.

The valuable contribution to the well-being of animals and humans alike continues. A single injection that will protect against the dominant form of meningitis could soon be available thanks to genetically engineered vaccines (IAT 1997).

Benefits in the cost–benefit assessment

Recording past benefits of animal experimentation which are apparent and speak for themselves is a comparatively easy task. Estimating specific future benefits is quite another matter. Any future programme is liable to be afflicted by the operation of the law of unintended consequences. In fact, suggested benefits may be what the Scholastics called 'futurabilia', things or events that are possible but might never actually come into existence. There is no doubt that assessing animal suffering precisely is extremely difficult. Estimating actual benefits clearly would call for all the foresight of a Hebrew prophet. However, if the cost–benefit process is to have any validity, whenever the use of animals in research is proposed, an attempt must be made to evaluate the specific benefit which is suggested.

The Institute of Medical Ethics suggests the categories of considerations which appear the most worthy of evaluation in the weighing-up of the benefits of research.

> 'To judge the probable benefits of research, policy-makers must weigh up the proposed project's likely contribution to:
>
> (1) the improvement of health and welfare in humans or other animals;
> (2) science, in terms of its originality, timelessness and likely effect on understanding;
> (3) education and training;
> (4) employment and economy;
> (5) the conservation of natural resources or to the reduction of the impact of humans on the environment.'
>
> (IME 1991)

Application in detail of this general approach to investigating the comparative worth of benefits *vis-à-vis* animal suffering will be dealt with in the following section.

Trying to strike the balance

Although the above title appropriately sets the scene for considering the all-important cost–benefit assessment, balance is perhaps the wrong term to use in this context. If we use the term 'balance' in this setting we must stress that it has to be a balance with a definite bias. The scales must be weighted in favour of the animal. The expected accruing benefit from the project must outweigh the suffering of the animal. The burden of proof, to justify the use of animals in a regulated procedure, by definition involving pain, suffering, distress or lasting harm, rests on the prospective licensee. No regulated procedure may be performed unless initially a reason can be given for performing it. Neither the law nor any other authority nor ethical speculation produces a clear definition of the border between acceptable interference with an animal such as slight restraint for visual inspection in the pursuit of knowledge and minimal distress for the same purpose. There is no doubt that the simplest of injections within the scope of a scientific procedure counts as a regulated procedure.

To avoid possible confusion and to anticipate censure for inaccuracy, it is necessary to deviate into legal matters. Specifically within our legislation as expounded in the Home Office Guidance (paragraph 1.6–9) an injection of a microchip for purposes of identification would not be regarded as a regulated procedure. Why not if it is being done for scientific purposes? Because the law says it is not a regulated procedure.

Similar provisions, which to some people may have the appearances of anomalies, occur regarding clinical trials of veterinary medicines; veterinary, agricultural and animal husbandry practices; and killing animals under Schedule 1 of the Animals (Scientific Procedures) Act 1986.

Various approaches to solving cost–benefit evaluation

Squares, cubes, trees, diagrams, questionnaires and algorithms of varying complexity and restricted relevancy to particular forms of research have beeen called into play to discover the touchstone of justification in respect to specific projects.

Optimistic speculation by Professor Bateson that there could be an end to controversy by the use of a square of estimation (Figure 13.2), spurred on moves to find more sophisticated means to resolve cost–benefit dilemmas. Professor Bateson himself went on to better things.

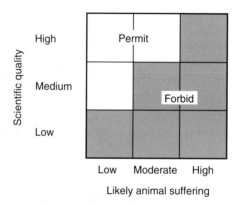

Fig. 13.2 An end to controversy? A first attempt to decide whether a research project should be carried out on animals.

Professor Bateson went on to develop the Decision Cube as a way of bringing together the various judgments that should be made about research on animals (Figures 13.3 and 13.4). He denies that it is a cost–benefit exercise since it does not depend on a common currency or on the balancing of incommensurable properties. He presents the cube rather as a set of rules that could be helpful in determining whether or not a particular piece of research should be done. Professor Bateson described the application of his cube in the *New Scientist*:

'The cube had three separate dimensions: the scientific quality of the research, the probability of human benefit and the likelihood of animal suffering. I argued that animal suffering should be tolerated only when both research quality and probability of benefit were high. Moreover, certain levels of animal suffering would be unacceptable regardless of the quality of the research or its probable benefit. The decision rules used in this model would permit research of high

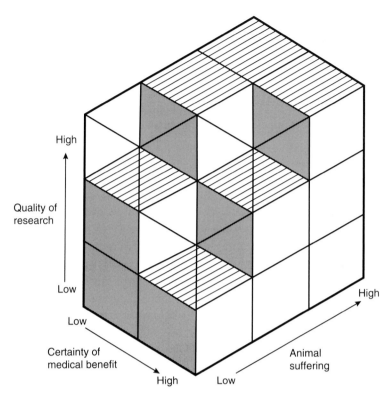

Fig. 13.3 Professor Bateson's Decision Cube. When a research proposal falls into the opaque part of the cube, the experimental work should not be done.

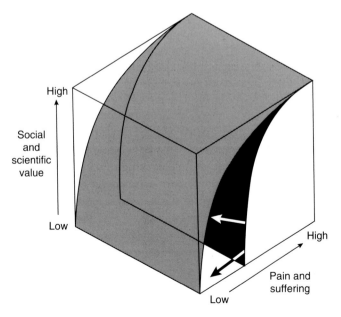

Fig. 13.4 Experiment, yes or no? A 'decision cube' spells out the trade-offs (left). Now, less suffering is acceptable at a given level of 'benefit' (right).

quality involving little or no animal suffering even if the work had no obvious potential benefits to humans. This would enable scientists to work to understand phenomena even where they foresaw no immediate and obvious practical benefit.'

(Bateson 1992: p. 33)

The professor expounds on the elements cognate to the possible suffering of the animals:

'Plausible assessments of the suffering that animals may experience can be based on how the animals were obtained, housed and treated experimentally and how likely they are to experience in a human-like way changes to their environment and damage to their bodies. Understanding the animals requires projections from the behaviour and nervous system of humans combined with good knowledge of the natural history and behaviour of the animals in question.'

(Bateson 1992: p. 33)

Ethical scores for animal experiments

David G. Porter, the holder of the Chair of the Department of Biomedical Sciences, University of Guelph, Ontario, Canada, proposed a scoring system as valuable in what he regarded as the polarized debate concerning the ethics of animal experiments. His proposal has been criticized as not having an acceptable level of discrimination and for not providing the researcher with any pragmatic tools to optimize the research design. He does however attempt to deal with speciesism by proposing a scale of 1 to 5, ranging from apparently relatively insensitive creatures to highly sensitive and intelligent mammals. He suggests the desirability of a unit of ethical concern (an ethicon?). The mollusc might score 1 and a chimpanzee 1 000 000. To complete the mathematical flavour of the cost–benefit ethic, one might propound a unit of pain (a dol)? Just the slightest intensity of sensation above an itch.)

Porter admits that any scoring system must have its limitations. He writes:

'The premise of my scoring system is that every experiment on a sentient animal represents a departure, however small, from the Schweitzerian ideal. The more points scored, the further the departure. The ideal should generate constant pressure to avoid experiments on animals wherever possible, to seek alternatives, and to reduce the cut-off for unacceptable experiments.'

(Porter 1992)

Proposed scoring system to minimize suffering in animal experiments

(A) Aim of experiment
(1)   Alleviation of substantial human or non-human pain.
(2)   Alleviation of moderate human or non-human pain or suffering.
(3)   Clear benefit to human or non-human health or welfare.
(4)   Some benefit to human or non-human health or welfare.
(5)   Fundamental research for the advancement of knowledge (no clear alleviation of pain or benefit to human or non-human or animal health).

Note   For item (5), such 'curiosity-driven research' has often led to unexpected, valuable discoveries, but given the fairly high probability that it will not do so, it is difficult to quantify the inflicting of suffering in such inquiry. Its weighing therefore requires experiments to have low costs in the remaining categories, in keeping with the ideal.

(B) Realistic potential of experiment to achieve objective
(1)   Excellent.
(2)   Very good.
(3)   Average/fair.
(4)   Limited.
(5)   Very limited or impossible to assess.

(C) Species of animal
(1)   Low sensibility/consciousness.
(2)   Some sensibility.
(3)   Sentient but possibly limited consciousness.
(4)   Sentient and conscious.
(5)   Sentient, highly intelligent and precognitive.

Note   Examples of animals are as follows: group 1, molluscs; group 2, cephalopods, fish, amphibia; group 3, reptiles; group 4, mammals (except group 5), birds; group 5, primates (some lower primates in this group because endangered), carnivores, cetaceans.

(D) Pain likely to be involved
(1)   None.
(2)   Minimal/slight.
(3)   Moderate.
(4)   Considerable.
(5)   Severe.

Note   The use and effectiveness of analgesics should be taken into consideration, as well as such factors as post-operative pain and the skill of the experimenter.

(E) Duration of discomfort or distress
(1)   None or very short.
(2)   Short.
(3)   Moderate.
(4)   Long.
(5)   Very long.

Note   All aspects of the procedure must be considered, for example, restraint, deprivation of social contact, and environmental conditions.

(F) Duration of experiment
(1)   Extremely short 10^{-5} LS.
(2)   Short 2×10^{-4} LS.
(3)   Moderate 2×10^{-2} LS.
(4)   Long 2×10^{-1} LS.
(5)   Very long, above 2×10^{-1} LS.

Note   LS stands for lifespan. An eight-hour experiment with mice (assumed lifespan one year) will score 10^{-3} LS and will be considered moderate (3 points). The same experiment with chimpanzees (assumed lifespan 50 years) will score 2×10^{-5} LS, which will be regarded as extremely short (1 point). Perhaps small animals with a high metabolic rate, which live shorter lives, live more intensively.

(G) Number of animals
(1)   1–5.
(2)   5–10.
(3)   10–20.
(4)   20–100.
(5)   Above 100.

Note   Whether death *per se* is an 'evil' is debatable, but to kill 100 animals in an experiment represents a greater departure from the ideal than to kill five (category G). It is not always easy to score category G appropriately, because using more animals for a shorter period (category F) could generate lower scores than fewer animals used for longer. This is a dilemma that no scoring system can resolve, for there is no ethically acceptable number. Experiments should be statistically designed so that excessive numbers of animals are not used and that unnecessary repetition does not occur.

(H) Quality of animal care
(1)   Excellent.
(2)   Very good.
(3)   Average.
(4)   Good.
(5)   Poor.

Note   In this category, attention is focused on the animal's environment when not under an experiment; for example, the suitability of the environment for specific animals – caging, skill of attendants, quality of post-operative care, lighting, temperature, humidity, etc.

Porter goes on to state:

'The next step is to arrive at a total score out of a maximum of 40. The minimum unavoidable score of 8 reflects the tension between ideal and practice and is a reminder that every experiment on a sentient animal represents a departure, in at least some measure, from the ideal.

The cut-off score should be as low as possible. Because the animal categories account for up to 30 points, their contribution should be no worse than 15. Categories A and B should contribute no more than 7 together, giving a working cut-off of about 21. If experiments are carried out *in vitro*, without previous procedures on the animal *in vivo*, only categories A, B, C, G and H would be scored and a cut-off point of around 16 could be used. Under the imperative of the ideal, the cut-off score should be revised downwards as time goes on. Additional categories could be made, for example, for endangered species.'

(Porter 1992)

The Dutch system

In the Dutch system the estimation of pain and distress experienced by the animal is scored at three levels (minor, moderate and severe) in combination with four durations (under 1 day, 1–7 days, 8–30 days, and over 30 days). According to recent advice from a special working group of the National Committee on Animal Experimentation (an independent committee which advises the Minister of Public Health) the three levels of pain and distress should be based on physiological and behavioural signs rather than on a (black)list of scientific procedures. The philosophy underlying this advice is, among other considerations, that skilful investigators might be able to perform experiments which are labelled as severe without inflicting more than moderate distress on the animals. It would be incorrect to treat these investigators as if they were no better than a moderate investigator (and vice versa), who would probably inflict severe harm on the animals.

Once the level of discomfort has been established, it can be aligned with the significance of the project for assessment for a designation of approval or rejection. Table 13.1 illustrates this process, where balancing three levels of discomfort (minor, moderate, severe) against three levels of significance (minor, moderate, great) results in nine combinations.

Table 13.1 Designation of approval and rejection at nine combinations of discomfort and significance.

	Discomfort		
Significance	Minor	Moderate	Severe
Minor	Reject	Reject	Reject
Moderate	Approve	Approve	Reject
Great	Approve	Approve	Approve

The designation of approval and rejection on the discomfort/significance balance is decided upon after due consultation with the National Inspectors of the Animal Experimentation Department of the Veterinary Public Health Chief Inspectorate. This weighing matrix is slightly more restrictive than most researchers are inclined to formulate. Researchers usually prefer to approve a combination of minor discomfort and minor significance. Pressure groups, however, prefer a ban on experiments of moderate significance and a moderate level of discomfort (de Cock *et al.* 1994).

The Dutch tree

A feature of the Dutch approach, known as the Dutch tree, moves on the process of ethical evaluation into a further stage (see Figure 13.5)

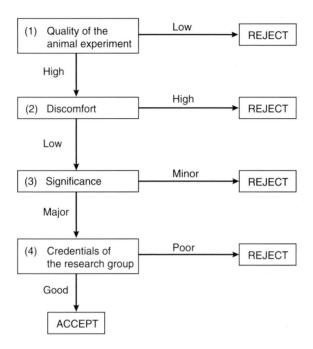

Fig. 13.5 Decision tree used in the Dutch model in deciding whether to accept or reject an animal experiment proposal (de Cock *et al.* 1994).

The fuller diagram shown in Figure 13.6 presents the four parts of the Dutch model. Each branch of the tree is backed up by detailed questions to help committee members trace morally significant aspects of a proposal. The questionnaire is designed in such a way that by circling the chosen answers one obtains a visual impression of the overall score: positive (right side) or negative (left side). In order to avoid visual overestimation, the design is such that all questions are necessary and are independent of each other. In this way each part will lead to a qualitative conclusion (minor/moderate/great; sufficient/insufficient).

A detailed checklist helps the making of clear decisions. It broadens and deepens discussion in animal experimentation committees. A properly completed checklist can serve as a 'document of argumentation' for anyone who wants to question an animal care committee's decision. The checklist might also serve as a discussion paper in the public debate on animal experiments: on the basis of it one could argue for or against proposed aspects of the decision-making. Note: The earlier an aspect is evaluated in the decision tree the more it can work as a limiting factor. The basic questionnaire is shown at Figure 13.7 and the following boxed checklists and commentaries.

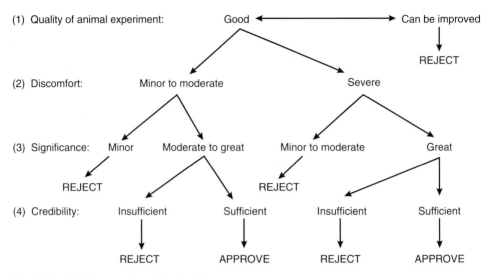

Fig. 13.6   The four parts of the Dutch model.

(A) Quality of animal experimentation
(1)   How good are the statistics?
      Was there a pilot scheme? Is there reuse?
(2)   Have alternatives been researched?
(3)   Can less animals be used? Is there repetition?
(4)   What are the refinements?
      Is there maximum reduction of pain and discomfort?

(B) Discomfort for the animal
(1)   What is the extent and duration of the discomfort?
(2)   How comfortable and beneficial is the accommodation?

(C) Significance of the animal experiment
(1)   How necessary is this particular form of research? For example, is there interest in
      the substance's toxicity?
(2)   How important is the substance under investigation? For example, a new
      cosmetic?
(3)   How useful is a diagnostic identification to health?
(4)   How necessary is a demonstration for education?
(5)   What is the danger of the disease under review?
      How does this research contribute to therapy?
(6)   What are the chances of success?
(7)   How valid is the extrapolation?
(8)   What is the worth of the knowledge and insight to be gained?

(D) Credibility of the group/researchers
(1)   How extensive is the group's experience and how wide are their contacts with
      regard to alternatives?

Fig. 13.7   Ethical assessment questionnaire: Dutch model.

The Checklist and commentary

(A) *Quality of animal experiments*	Circle the answer of your choice	
1 General		
1.1 Has the scientific quality already been judged elsewhere as being 'good'?	No	Yes
If not, did a statistician approve the research proposal?	No	Yes
1.2 Has a statistical account been given?	No	Yes
1.3 Is it a pilot study?	No	Yes
If not, has a pilot study been done?	No	Yes
1.4 Are animals used again after an experiment which causes severe discomfort?	Yes	No
2 Replacement		
2.1 Have adequate sources (journals, databases) been consulted for alternatives?	No	Yes
2.2 Do alternatives exist?	Yes	No
If so, what is your opinion about the reason for not using them?	Insufficient	Sufficient
3 Reduction of the number of animals		
3.1 Is it possible to perform the animal experiment with a smaller number of animals?	Yes	No
3.2 Is it a case of repeating research?	Yes	No
If so, what is your opinion about the arguments in favour of repetition?	Insufficient	Sufficient
3.3 Does closely related research occur elsewhere?	Yes	No
If so, does collaboration exist?	No	Yes
3.4 Are organs/animals shared with others?	No	Yes
4 Refinement (in consultation with animal welfare officer)		
4.1 Are pain and discomfort avoided as much as possible?	No	Yes
4.2 How is the prevention of pain and other discomforts dealt with?	Insufficient	Sufficient
4.3 Are the animals killed at a well-considered time and in a well-considered way?	No	Yes
4.4 Is the discomfort per animal reduced by increasing the number of animals?	No	N/A/Yes
4.5 Does the accommodation provide sufficient 'relief' for animals who emerge ill or in pain from an experiment?	No	Yes
5 Judgement		
Quality of animal experiment? Arguments in favour of dismissal	Could be improved Good	

Commentary

A.1.1   A statistician ought to be consulted.

A.1.2   A statistical account must be given for the number of animals used.

A.2.2   For example, models, cell and tissue culture, organs, lower species, and research with humans (epidemiological research).

A.3.1   Not a question of statistics; rather, is a different experiment-planning possible?

A.4.5   Possible withdrawal from experiment, good accommodation, social contact and environmental enrichment.

(B)	*Discomfort for the animal*				
1	Discomfort caused by experiments Experimental group 1				
1.1	What is the extent of the discomfort during the experiment?	Severe	Moderate	Minor	N/A
1.2	What is the duration of the discomfort in days?	>30	8–30	1–7	<1
	Experimental group 2 (control group)				
1.3	What is the extent of the discomfort during the experiment?	Severe	Moderate	Minor	N/A
1.4	What is the duration of the discomfort in days?	>30	8–30	1–7	<1
	Experimental group 3 (if applicable)				
1.5	What is the extent of the discomfort during the experiment?	Severe	Moderate	Minor	N/A
1.6	What is the duration of the discomfort in days?	>30	8–30	1–7	<1
	Experimental group 4 (if applicable)				
1.7	What is the extent of the discomfort during the experiment?	Severe	Moderate	Minor	N/A
1.8	What is the duration of the discomfort in days?	>30	8–30	1–7	<1
2	Discomfort caused by housing conditions				
2.1	Does the accommodation guarantee good physical health at the outset of the experiment?	No		Moderate	Yes
2.2	Does the accommodation impede species-specific behaviour?	Severe		Moderate	No
2.3	Does the animal display abnormal behaviour caused by the accommodation?	Yes			No
3	Judgement				
	Discomfort for the experimental animal	Severe		Moderate	Minor

Commentary

When answering, it is advisable to make a distinction between more or less 'sensitive' animal species, and between more or less social animal species. The discomfort of a specific operation will differ widely for different animal species (e.g. guppy or anthropoid). As a general rule, one must assume that, when animals are exposed to certain procedures, they experience a comparable discomfort to humans, unless the opposite is proven. One must also take into account that the extent of the discomfort of an experiment can be determined by the frequency of the operation, as well as, of course, the duration of the discomfort.

(C)	*Significance of the animal experiment*	Please answer one cluster of questions only		
(Cr)	*Routine research*			
	• production, control or biological standardization of sera, vaccines, diagnostica or other biological products			
	• production, control, or biological standardization of medicines			
	• production or control of other medical or veterinary expedients or applications			
	• other biological standardizations			
	• testing of alternatives for animal experiments			
	• toxicity (routine) testing			
1	Necessity of animal experiment			
1.1	Is the animal experiment a liability?	No	N/A	Yes
1.2	If not, what is the extent of the (safety) interest regarding health and nutrition of man or animal?	Minor	Moderate	Great
2	Assessment of the necessity of the product			
2.1	How important is the product with regard to the health or nutrition of man or animal?	Minor	Moderate	Great
3	Judgement			
	Significance of the animal experiment	Minor	Moderate	Great

Commentary

The Dutch law permits an experiment either in the case of a direct or indirect significance regarding health or nutrition of man or animal, or in the case of answering a scientific question. Other reasons for animal experiments are only allowed after explicit governmental exemption.

Cr: This question makes a distinction between the importance of the animal experiment and the significance of a product. This implies a distinction between the production, quality or safety of a substance and the significance of the substance itself; for example, the importance of testing the safety of a new cleaning product and the significance of the cleaning product itself.

(Cd)	*Diagnostics (identification and detection of diseases or other physical symptoms)*			
1	Necessity of animal experiment			
1.1	How important is the identification or detection for the health of man?	Minor	Moderate	Great
1.2	How important is the identification or detection for the health of animals?	Minor	Moderate	Great
2	Judgement			
	Significance of animal experiment	Minor	Moderate	Great
(Ce)	*Education (transfer of knowledge and proficiency training)*			
1	Necessity of animal experiment			
1.1	What is the importance with regard to the future health of man or animal?	Minor	Moderate	Great
1.2	What is the importance with regard to future handling of animals?	Minor	Moderate	Great
2	Judgement			
	Significance of animal experiment	Minor	Moderate	Great

Commentary

Cd: More and more alternatives are available for diagnostic purposes. However, there is an increase of animal use for the production of monoclonal antibodies, and in transgenic work.

Ce: For education the standard must be that an animal experiment must be of direct or indirect significance for the health or nutrition of humans or animals. This means that an experiment can only be permitted to students, who will certainly perform similar actions with animals in their future profession.

(Cp)	*Problem-oriented research*			
	• research into the course of a disease, pathophysiology, prevention, nutrition and housing			
	• development of biological, pharmaceutical and biopharmaceutical products			
	• development of toxicological and pharmacological methods			
	• development of alternatives for animal experiments			
	• development of transgene animals			
	Either answer questions listed under 1 *or* 2			
1	Medical or veterinary significance			
1.1	How severe is the disease?	Minor	Moderate	Great
1.2	How often does the disease occur?	Seldom	To some extent	Often
1.3	Can a high-risk group be indicated?	Yes		No
	If so, is it a large group?	No	To some extent	Yes
	If so, is the risk avoidable?	Yes	To some extent	No

Contd

		Minor	Moderate	Great
1.4	What is the extent of the health benefit expected from the new or improved therapy/product/method?	Minor	Moderate	Great
1.5	What is the extent of the contribution to improvement of the therapy/product/method from this concrete experiment?	Minor	Moderate	Great
1.6	What is your estimation of chance of success?	Minor	Moderate	Great
1.7	Is the animal model extrapolatable?	Insufficient		Sufficient
2	Broader social significance (short or medium term)			
2.1	Is the research directed at replacement, reduction or refinement of animal experiments?	Not much		Substantial
2.2	What contribution to the improvement of health or nutrition of man or animal do you expect?	Minor	Moderate	Great
2.3	What is your estimation of the chance of success?	Minor	Moderate	Great
2.4	Is the animal model extrapolatable?	Insufficient		Sufficient
3	Judgement			
	Significance of animal experiment	Minor	Moderate	Great

Commentary

Cp.1.1. and 1.2: For estimation of urgency.

Cp.1.3: Some diseases, e.g. influenza, are not serious as a rule, but for specific groups of people they are a potential fatal disease.

Some diseases are avoidable, because with humans they are caused by their own behaviour or by poor working conditions.

Cp.1.7. and 2.4: The extrapolatability of the animal experiment depends on the question to what extent the disease develops in the same way in animals as in humans and/or to what extent the animal functions in a comparable way to the human, on the grounds of build, metabolism or behaviour.

(Cf)	*Basic scientific research (research into biological functions, biological processes and behaviour)*			
1	Scientific significance			
1.1	How great is the scientific significance of the knowledge or the insight?	Minor	Moderate	Great
1.2	What is the estimation of the scientific quality?	Minor	Moderate	Great
1.3	How great is the scientific context of the research project?	Insufficient		Sufficient
1.4	What is your estimation of the chance of success?	Minor	Moderate	Great
1.5	Does the concrete research fit in with the research project?	No	N/A	Yes
2	Judgement			
	Significance of the animal experiment	Minor	Moderate	Great

(D)	*Credibility (of the group/researchers)*			
1	Group/researchers			
1.1	Is the subject new to the group?	Yes		No
1.2	Does the group often conduct pilot studies only?	Yes	N/A	No
1.3	Is this type of animal experiment new to the group?	Yes		No
1.4	Do all members have sufficient experience with these animal experiments?	No		Yes
1.5	Does the group develop alternatives on its own or does the group participate in validity research?			Yes
1.6	Do the researchers have/create sufficient opportunities to look for alternatives?	No		Yes
2	Judgement			
	Credibility of the group/researchers Arguments in favour of rejection	Insufficient		Good

(E)	*Assessment*	
1	Model (please circle the chosen answer)	

Commentary

Cf.1.1: What does the research produce with regard to breaking new ground in knowledge or insight?

Cf.1.2: What estimation of the scientific quality has been made by a research committee or an official?

Cf.1.4: Is it a realistic project with a well-founded research hypothesis?

Cf.1.5: Does the concrete research fit in with the research project or is it just an interesting but not very relevant sideline?

D: Answer these questions in consultation with the authority on experimental animals. She or he will have insight regarding the activities of the group. All the questions together form a picture of the care exercised by the group and the researchers in handling the animal experiments and, consequently, the animals.

A British ethical approach

The lists associated with the Institute of Medical Ethics approach to the ethical evaluation of animal experimentation appeared in *Lives in the Balance* (Smith & Boyd 1991). Questions from schemes for the assessment of potential and likely benefit in research involving animal subjects and of the likely cost to those animals are summarized here.

(1) Assessment of the potential benefits	N/A	L	M	H
1.1 Value – social				
1.2 – scientific				
1.3 – economic				
1.4 – educational				
1.5 – other				
1.6 Originality				
1.7 Timeliness				
1.8 Persuasiveness				
1.9 Applicability				

N/A = not applicable; L = low; M = medium; H = high.

Commentary   Part 1 is an evaluation of the project's potential benefits; an assessment of the value of its hoped-for outcome.

1.1   The potential contribution towards the improvement of human and/or animal health and welfare (including safeguarding or improving the general environment).

1.2   The potential contribution to the total fund of scientific knowledge.

1.3   The potential contribution to employment and profitability in industry and/or conservation of national resources.

1.4   The contribution towards education and training.

1.5   Such values would need to be specified in detail.

1.6   The relation to other projects in progress.

1.7   Its necessity in relation to the range of problems which might be addressed.

1.8   Its links to and implications for other areas of research.

1.9   Its potential to lead to further benefits.

(2) Assessment of the proposed approach	N/A	L	M	H
2.1.1 Relevance of approach to potential benefits				
2.1.2 Quality of hypothesis				
2.1.3 Quality of experimental design				
2.1.4 Background research				
2.2.1 Applicability of scientific procedures				
2.2.2(i) Necessity of animals				
(ii) Necessity of species				
2.2.3(i) Necessity of procedure in relation to severity				
(ii) Necessity of procedure in relation to number				
2.2.4 Maximization of information				
2.3.1(i) Training of staff				
(ii) Experience of staff				
(iii) Competence of staff				
2.3.2 Quality of equipment and facilities				
2.3.3 Adequacy of funding				

Commentary   Part 2 is an assessment of the quality, validity and necessity of the methods it is proposed to use in achieving the potential benefits.

2.1   Assessment of the scientific merit of the project's general approach.

2.1.1   Relevance of approach to the stated potential benefits.

2.1.2   Quality of the working hypothesis.

2.1.3   Quality of experimental design and statistical aspects.

2.1.4   Appreciation of the relevant background literature and other relevant research in progress.

2.2   Assessment of the necessity and validity of the scientific procedures to be used in the project.

2.2.1   Applicability of the procedures to the proposed approach.

2.2.2   What about possibilities of replacement and must it be the species suggested?

2.2.3   Can severity and the number of animals be reduced further?

2.2.4   The best statistical use must be made of each animal used.

2.3   Assessment of the quality of the project workers and facilities.

2.3.1   What training have the project workers received? What is their experience and competence? Are there opportunities for supervision and consultation?

2.3.2   Are all the necessary equipment and facilities available?

2.3.3   What is the financial basis of the project? Is it adequate?

(3) Overall assessment of the project; assessment of likely benefit	N/A	L	M	H
3.1 Overall potential benefits 3.2(i) Likelihood of realization (ii) – in time 3.3 Necessity of approach (three Rs)				

Commentary   Part 3 is an overall assessment of the project, to judge the likelihood that the potential benefits will be realized, given the proposed scientific approach.
3.2   Are the benefits likely to be actually realized and, indeed, in the time available?
3.3   Have all aspects of the three Rs been explored? Is there further possibility of the use of replacement, reduction and refinement?

(A) Quality of facilities and project workers	N/A	L	M	H
A1.1 Quality – housing A1.2 – equipment A2.1 – assisting staff A2.2 – performing staff A2.3 – responsible staff				

Commentary   Part A examines the quality of the facilities and personnel involved in caring for and carrying out the proposed procedures on animals.
A1.1   What are the facilities for feeding, watering, hygiene, bedding and environmental enrichment? What are the cage sizes?
A1.2   What is the quality and reliability of the technical equipment? Is it appropriate? What is the standard of operating theatres? Is there adequate recording facilities?
A2.1   What is the training, experience and competence of the animal technicians?
A2.2   Are the personal licence holders trained, experienced and competent? Is appropriate supervision available and are there senior staff who can be consulted for advice?
A2.3   Can all the project workers recognize adverse effects, such as pain, distress and anxiety in the animals? Are they capable of taking appropriate action when and if animals are found to be suffering adverse effects?

(B) Severity of effects of husbandry and procedures on animals set in the context of the assessment in Part A	N/A	L	M	H
B3.1 Severity of distress for the species				
B3.2.1 – during capture and transport				
B3.2.2 Threat to wild population				
B3.2.3 Adaptation to laboratory				
B3.3 Genetic defect				
B4.1 Housing				
B5.1 Scientific procedures				
B6.1 After analgesia				
B7.1 Number of animals				

Commentary   Part B examines the likely effects of the specific husbandry and scientific procedures to be used on the chosen species of animal. It is suggested that since more than one animal will be involved in the project, the effects on all the animals should be considered but special attention must be paid to those that will suffer the most. Consequently, it is proposed that the assessment should be based on the worst cases. B3 is concerned with the types of animals to be used.

B3.1   Deals with the animal's capacity for experiencing adverse effects including anxiety, and its ability to appreciate what is being done to it during the experiment.

B3.2   Deals with animals taken from the wild.

B3.2.1   What may be the special adverse effects arising from method of capture, mode of transport or quarantine conditions?

B3.2.2   Is the species being used endangered in any way?

B3.2.3   Will the novelty of laboratory surroundings (given a suitable period of acclimatization) cause hardship?

B3.3   How severe is any adverse effect associated with a genetic defect (naturally occurring or induced)?

B4.1   What increase of suffering might accrue from adverse effects, including anxiety and boredom, caused by housing and husbandry conditions? This assessment should take into account the length of time the animals will be maintained in such conditions.

B5.1   What is the severity of adverse effects directly due to the scientific procedure? End-points must be fixed and clearly defined. Appropriate anaesthetics must be expertly administered and the most suitable forms of euthanasia must be readily at hand with the availability of competent operators.

B6.1   Any adverse effects must always be ameliorated, especially pain for which analgesics should be administered.

B7.1   The estimate of the number of animals needed for the efficient performance of the project should be carefully appraised.

(C) Overall costs	N/A	L	M	H

Commentary   Part C demands a definitive assessment of the overall costs likely to be imposed on the animals used in the proposed project.

A further, more detailed, questionnaire is associated with this scheme of assessment proposed by the Institute of Medical Ethics. It evokes fuller responses within the categories already outlined. These supplementary schemes for the Assessment of Potential and Likely Benefit in Research Involving Animal Subjects and for the Assessment of Likely Costs to Animals in Research Involving Animal Subjects are useful methods of evaluating a proposed project. They can certainly be recommended to anyone who wishes to go further into this topic.

A selection of other approaches to the ethical assessment of experiments on animals

Three further approaches to the ethical assessment of experiments on animals now follow. They are as follows:

(1)   the Swiss ethical guidelines (Figure 13.8)
(2)   an algorithm to determine ethical acceptability (Figures 13.9 and 13.10)
(3)   the Utrecht University decision system (Figure 13.11).

References

Animal Procedures Committee (1993) *Report of the Animal Procedures Committee.* HMSO, London.
Bateson (1992) *New Scientist,* 25 April, 33.
de Cock Buning, T.J. & Theune, E.P. (1994) An article entitled 'A comparison of three models for ethical evaluation of proposed animal experiments' which produced an account in detail of the Dutch approach to cost–benefit evaluation, as well as a comparison of this system with others, appeared in *Animal Welfare,* **3**, 107–128.
Harris, M. (1994) This interesting snippet from the history of medicine occurs on p. 285 of *ITN Book of Firsts.* Michael O'Mara Books Ltd, London.
IAT (1997) *IAT Bulletin,* November. IAT, Oxford.
IME (1991) An abundance of material on evaluating the cost–benefit assessment is provided in the book *Lives in the Balance* edited by J. Smith and K. Boyd, Oxford University Press. This work has been widely accepted as authoritative on this subject.
LASA (1994) A workshop organized by the Laboratory Animal Science Association on the topic of ethics and animal experimentation was reported in LASA Newsletter September, pp. 14–16.
Pascoe, L.C., Lee, A.J. & Jenkins, E.S. (1968) *Encyclopaedia of Dates and Events.* English Universities Press, London.
Porter D.G. (1992) Porter's suggestions for assessing animal suffering was published in *Nature,* **356**, 12 March, 101–102.
Smith, J.A. & Boyd, K.M. (eds) (1991) *Lives in the Balance: The Ethics of Using Animals in Biomedical Research.* Oxford University Press, Oxford.

**Swiss Academy
of Medical Sciences
(SAMW)**

**Swiss Academy
of Natural Sciences
(SANW)**

Ethical Requirements for the Conduct of Experiments on Animals

1. It is the duty of all persons participating in experiments on animals to be heedful of the well-being and ensure the least possible suffering of the experimental animal. The decisive criterion on which the fulfilment of this duty depends is their professional competence and express acceptance of their responsibility towards the animal.
2. If pain, suffering, or fear are inevitable accompaniments of an experiment, all possible measures must be taken to limit their duration and intensity to the essential minimum. The animals should therefore be kept under observation by trained personnel and all necessary and appropriate measures taken to minimize their suffering.
3. In all experiments which lead to chronic suffering or necessitate repeated interventions, every possible measure must be taken to mitigate suffering and dispel anxiety. It is particularly important in such cases that the animals should be cared for in the proper fashion by trained personnel before, during, and after the experiment.
4. Experiments apt to cause the animal severe suffering must be avoided by modifying the hypothesis to be tested in such a way as to allow the choice of alternative experimental procedures, or by forgoing the anticipated gain of knowledge.
5. Continued physical restraint must only be resorted to after other procedures have been considered and found wanting. All possible measures must be taken to alleviate anxiety, including, in particular, careful and gentle accustoming of the animal to the experimental conditions.
6. Whenever distressing measures such as restriction of the supply of food and drinking water, or the application of painful stimuli are essential for the purposes of an experiment, they must be precisely documented in the experimental protocol. The effects of such measures on the animals must be checked by determining relevant parameters, to ensure that the discomfort caused does not exceed an acceptable degree.
7. The accommodation and care of the experimental animals should be in keeping with the recommended standard practices appropriate for the species in question. Every effort must be made to ensure that the animals are not deprived of social contacts and can engage in an adequate range of activities.
8. Animals experiencing grave suffering must be killed humanely and as rapidly as possible by a method appropriate to the species in question.

10 October 1996

Extract from *Ethical Principles and Guidelines for Scientific Experiments on Animals* (1995). The full document in English, French or German may be obtained free of costs from:
- Schweizerische Akademie der Medizinischen Wissenschaften, Petersplatz 13, 4051 Basel
- Schweizerische Akademie der Naturwissenschaften, Barenplatz 2, 3011 Bern

Fig. 13.8 Extract from the SAMW and SANW ethical principles and guidelines for scientific experiments on animals.

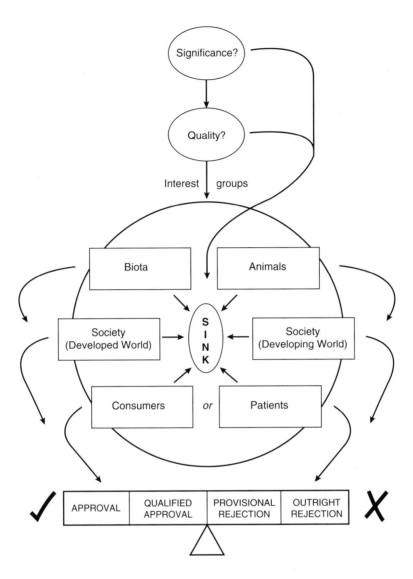

Fig. 13.9   Decision model (associated with the algorithm devised by Crilly & Mepham.

Introduction

The aim is to design a tool to facilitate assessment and evaluation of ethical issues relating to the use of transgenic farm animals, viz:

- Agricultural applications – e.g. productivity promotion.
- Xenotransplantation – 'humanized' organs for use in human transplant surgery.
- Bioreactors – production of human therapeutic proteins.

Existing assessment schemes were devised before the current explosion in genetic technology and so fail to take into account questions specific to transgenesis, e.g. issues of species integrity. These schemes are also limited to a comparison of reduced welfare of the experimental animals with potential benefits, usually to humans.

Genetic engineering, with the power to radically alter the world we live in, demands a fuller examination. The proposed algorithm presented here extends the assessment process to include wider societal, global and ecological impacts.

Question 1

Does the research proposal address a significant concern for which no viable alternatives exist?

The basis of this scheme is the precautionary principle, namely the sceptical position that animal transgenesis should not be undertaken without good cause. Only projects which demonstrate a certain degree of necessity, rejection of which would infringe some fundamental human concern, are allowed to progress.

This stance broadly accords with existing animal welfare regulations and public opinion. For example, Dutch law promotes a 'No, unless' approach to animal experimentation. Thus, research is not permitted except where a clear need, usually human nutrition or health, can be shown.[5] Public opinion, measured by the Eurobarometer surveys in the EU, is also more supportive of certain applications of biotechnology than others. Thus, genetic engineering receives higher approval when applied in medicine than in agricultural research.[6]

Question 2

Is the quality of research capable of meeting the objective?

Once the overall objective has been assessed, the likelihood of actually achieving that goal needs to be established. This is an essential part of a decision process which assigns significant weight to the stated aim in advance of any experimentation.

Factors to consider will include:

- Existence and results of pilot studies.
- Efficacy and suitability of techniques.
- Validity of any hypotheses.
- Quality of research workers and facilities.
- Suitability of the chosen species.

Several of these points have been included in other schemes.[7]

The sink

The sink exists to add a further level of discrimination to what would otherwise be a straightforward cost–benefit analysis (CBA). CBAs have the disadvantage of allowing major costs to be outweighed by a number of relatively minor benefits acting together. Question 1 of this algorithm ensures that transgenic technologies are only employed in return for potentially substantial gains. The sink complements this action, ensuring that a single significant cost can be enough to reject a project, regardless of potential benefits.

This principle is derived from the UK Banner Report which highlights the issue of intrinsic objections, that 'harms of a certain degree and kind ought under no circumstances be inflicted on an animal'.[1] Thus, in the scoring system presented here, values for animal welfare of −3 lead to automatic rejection.

The principle of intrinsic objection is further extended to all interest groups so that 'harms of a certain degree and kind' cannot be inflicted on the environment, consumers, patients and the wider local and global society.

Ethical acceptability: the options

According to this scheme, the seven individual scores are summed to produce an aggregate score which can be allocated to one of four outcomes:

- APPROVAL – though subject to monitoring for adverse impacts.
- QUALIFIED APPROVAL – the proposal is approved provided that a number of recommendations are acted upon.
- PROVISIONAL REJECTION – rejection, although the proposal may be resubmitted once a number of specified improvements have been made.
- OUTRIGHT REJECTION.

These categories are comparable to, but distinct from, the 'YES, YES BUT, NO UNLESS, NO' used elsewhere.[2] This balancing process may need to be refined in the light of experience.

Further work

The aid to decision-making presented here is a speculative attempt to provide the foundation for a more comprehensive evaluation process than is currently available. To develop this approach, a number of tasks need to be undertaken:

- Performance of ethical analyses – which highlight those questions that need to be addressed by the decision process and collate the raw data by which to score the prospective transgenic animal project.
- Compilation of checklists – a questionnaire is currently being devised to aid the assessment of each category within the flow diagram.
- Application to specific examples.

Scoring

The first level of the flow diagram [see Figure 13.9], consisting of Questions 1 and 2, uses a scale of 0–3. Use of only four categories allows a consensus to be reached, while still retaining a degree of discrimination.

The rest of the model comprises six interest groups which are rated for three ethical principles based on those of Beauchamp and Childress[3]:

- Respect for well-being.
- Respect for autonomy.
- Respect for justice.

Each principle is converted to a term relevant to the interest group being considered, e.g. animal well-being becomes animal welfare, and is shown in the matrix below.

Specification of the three principles[4]

	WELL-BEING	AUTONOMY	JUSTICE
TREATED ANIMALS	Animal welfare	Behavioural freedom	Telos
CONSUMERS	Food safety	Consumer education and choice (labelling)	Universal affordability of food
PATIENTS	Quality of life	Informed choice of treatment	Universal availability of treatment
SOCIETY	Standard of living	Public consultation	Fair distribution
BIOTA	Conservation	Maintenance of biodiversity	Sustainability of biotic populations

Scores are then assigned on a scale of –3, representing a gross infringement of the principle and diversion to the sink, to a maximum of +3. The score of 0 is the neutral point at which the principles are neither respected nor infringed significantly.

This results in a maximum possible score of +51 and a minimum of –45.

References

1. Ministry of Agriculture, Fisheries and Food, UK (1995) *Report of the Committee on the Ethical Implications of Emerging Technologies in the Breeding of Farm Animals*. HMSO, London.
2. Ministry of Agriculture, Nature Management and Fisheries, Netherlands (1993) *Ethical Aspects of Plant Biotechnology*.
3. Beauchamp, T.L. & Childress, J.F. (1994) *Principles of Biomedical Ethics*, 4th ed. Oxford University Press, New York.
4. Mepham, B. (1996) Ethical analysis of food biotechnologies: an evaluative framework. In: *Food Ethics* (ed. B. Mepham). Routledge, London, pp. 101–119.
5. Brom, F.W.A. & Schroten, E. (1993) Ethical questions around animal biotechnology – the Dutch approach. *Livestock Production Science* **36**, 99–107.
6. Commission of the European Community (1993) Biotechnology and genetic engineering: what Europeans think about it in 1993. *Eurobarometer* **39.1**.
7. de Cock Buning, T.J. & Theune, E. (1994) A comparison of three models for ethical evaluation of proposed animal experiments. *Animal Welfare* **3**, 107–128.

Fig. 13.10 An algorithm to determine the ethical acceptability of transgenic farm animal applications (R.E. Crilly and T.B. Mepham, Centre for Applied Bioethics, The University of Nottingham).

Functions of the system

1	2	3
Checklist function: the system provides a checklist containing the morally relevant factors which should be assessed.	A heuristic function: the system helps to find the basic decision points by asking for explicit justification of choices and by showing the consequences of each choice.	A normative function: the system poses a moral stance by making basic assumptions and by assigning a numeral weight to relevant factors.

1. Formulate the ultimate goal of the experiment

2. Assess and score the human interest involved in the ultimate goal

Score gains in health interest

Item	Possible score
Lowering?	H
Mortality?	
Morbidity?	(0–10)

Score gains in knowledge interest

Item	Possible score
Hypothesis?	K
Originality?	
Problem worth solving?	(0–5)

Score gains in economical interest

Item	Possible score
Affect industry?	E
Affect national economy?	
Economic losses due to disease?	(0–5)

3. Compute the total interest of the ultimate goal (IG). Use the formula which produces the highest score

$$H \;[\;\;] = UG \;[\;\;] \quad (0–10)$$

$$K \;[\;\;] + E \;[\;\;] = UG \;[\;\;] \quad (0–10)$$

$$H \;[\;\;] + \frac{(\,K \;[\;\;]\; \text{or}\; E \;[\;\;]\,) \times 2}{2} = IG \;[\;\;] \quad (0–10)$$

$$H \;[\;\;] + \frac{K \;[\;\;] + E \;[\;\;]}{2} = UG \;[\;\;] \quad (0–10)$$

4. Assess and score the relevance of the proposed experiment

Replacement possible?	Yes: score 0	No: score 10
Methodological quality (general)?	Score 7–10;	score <7 = score 0
Methodological quality (laboratory animal science)?	Score 7–10;	score <7 = score 0
Necessity?	Score 5–10;	score <5 = score 0
Reliability	Score 0, 5 or 10	
Quality research group?	Score 1–10,	score <5 = score 0

Total relevance

One or more '0' leads to relevance 0 => experiment unacceptable.

$$\frac{[\;\;]}{6} + [\;\;] = R \;[\;\;] \quad (0.65–1)$$

5. Compute human interest (HI) involved in experiment

[IG] × [R] = [HI] (0–10)

6. Assess and score the harm to animal interest

Actual discomfort	
0 or positive	0
Light	1
Medium	2
Severe	3
Very severe	4
	[A]

Duration of discomfort	
Short and/or once	0
Medium and/or frequently	1
Long lasting and/or very frequently	2
	[D]

Numbers of animals involved	
<10	0
10–100	1
>100	2
	[N]

Total Discomfort

[A] + ([D] + [N]) / 2 = [T] (0–6)

Intrinsic value

(fixed score) [2 1]

Psychological complexity	
Non-human primates	2
Cold blooded	–2
Other vertebrates	0
	[P]

7. Compute the harmed interest of the involved animals (AI)

[T] + [2 1] + [P] = [AI] (0–10)

8. Assess acceptability of the experiment

If [HI] ⩾ [AI] Experiment acceptable

If [HI] < [AI] Experiment unacceptable

Lay out: Hanneke de Waal, Utrecht University, Faculty of Veterinary Medicine

Fig. 13.11 A decisional system for the ethical evaluation of animal experiments (F.R. Stalleu, R. Tramper, J. Vorstenbosch, Centre for Bio-ethics and Health Law, Utrecht University, Heidelberglaan 2, 3584 CS Utrecht; J.A. Joles, Department of Nephrology, Medical Faculty, Utrecht University, The Netherlands).

Chapter 14

Ethics Committees

> The committee came to a decision:
> it was 5.00 PM.

Introduction

In relevant literature and more so in casual conversation at meetings, the bodies being discussed seem to be referred to indiscriminately as ethical or ethics committees. Since the application of the adjective 'ethical' to a committee in this field might imply the possible existence of an unethical committee, I prefer to use the expression 'ethics committee' though the phrase 'a committee on the ethics of animal use' might be more grammatically correct.

One perhaps could regard the Animal Procedures Committee, asssociated with the Home Office, as the supreme example or a prototype, within the UK system, of the formation of an ethics committee and, maybe, as an indication of the desirable *modus operandi* of lesser bodies. It does, of course, have quite different functions in some areas, for example monitoring the administration of the 1986 Act, and is in a unique legal position – a sort of quasi-autonomous non-governmental organization (QUANGO).

In other countries with a different legislative structure, greater importance may be ascribed to the impact of ethics committees on cost–benefit assessment and protocol adjustment. A more fundamental question may arise about low-level institutional ethics committees. In their case the main ethical discussion on whether it is right to use animals in research is already presumed to be settled. Discussion turns on details of method, the amount of suffering involved and the relative merit of benefits. In some countries, ethics committees arose as a public relations exercise to allay anxiety but like many bureaucratic structures they took on a life of their own. They can become an obstacle to much that is worth while in research by promoting the trivial and inhibiting the original. Difficulties arise if the committee fails to reach a consensus. This may reflect either legitimate questioning of the study or the personal dynamics of the group, where, for example, one of the group routinely opposes the rest.

Early drafts of the European Convention on the Use of Animals in Experiments (1986) suggested the formation of ethical committees but this recommendation did not appear in later editions.

The Swedish experience

Swedish Animal Ethics Committees (AECs) became statutory in 1979 with the duty to review researchers' applications to carry out experiments likely to cause pain or other suffering to animals. There are seven regional AECs each consisting of 12 members – six representing the 'research interests' (i.e. research workers and animal technicians) and six representing the 'general interest' (i.e. lay persons). Since 1982 the lay persons may include official representatives of the Swedish Antivivisectionist Society. Since 1988, all planned experiments, including those which involve killing animals for *in vitro* tests must be reviewed in advance by an AEC. The AEC issues advisory decisions.

How can an advisory body have influence? The government authority responsible for animal protection is the National Board of Agriculture. Its regional veterinary officers supervize the local public health inspectorate which inspects animal quarters and has the duty to take action against animal abuse in conjunction with the regional officer or the police. The authorities respect the opinions of the AECs.

If an AEC advises a researcher to refrain from an experiment, he can still perform it and the committee will not inform on him. The authorities, however, have access to the protocols of the AEC.

The researcher submits his project with a short description of the experiments, emphasizing what happens to the animals, together with the number of animals of different species which are being used. He has to describe briefly what kind of post-operative care the animals will have and what he plans to do to alleviate and diminish their suffering. He sends the form to the selected research worker on the AEC. He may ask for clarification but will, anyway, consult with one of the lay persons and one of the technicians on the committee. They will all read the application and then discuss it with the applicant, perhaps suggesting alterations. If the members of this subcommittee agree with the proposals of the applicant, they sign the form. The form is then sent to the Central Veterinary Bureau and the applicant can start work immediately.

This scheme has not been without difficulty. In the early years there were many conflicts between radical lay members and researchers. The collision between diverse conceptions of the world entailed cultural shock. No one side seemed to be able to understand how the opposite side could look upon the problem in the way they did. Some of the radical lay members eventually resigned or became passive. The majority adapted, shifting from an ideological to a technical perspective and have begun to have an effect on the conduct of animal research. They now talk of refinement of animal experiments. In public, abolitionist protests seem to have declined, to be replaced by talk of reduction and limitation of the use of animals. The other members of the committee appeared to become more ready to discuss questions concerning procedures.

The AECs have promoted discussion of animal research ethics, leading to a heightened awareness of the issues and an enforced self-policing by researchers. A convergence of opinions has come about. The frequent meetings between lay persons and laboratories have increased mutual understanding and sympathy for the views of the opposite side. The antivivisectionists have gained experience of the reality of animal experimentation and had the opportunity of having their concerns discussed and treated with a certain respect.

Of the 6786 applications considered between 1979 and 1989, 6512 were approved, 13 disapproved and 261 returned for reconsideration. A total of 621 of the studies approved were the subject of written objections, mainly from lay members (Forsman 1993).

The Canadian system

The Canadian Council of Animal Care is the national authority responsible for monitoring the use of animals in research in Canada. The whole approach is ethical with a legal flavour.

The official principles laid down for the guidance of those using animals in research is surprisingly like the tenets of practice within our own legislation and goes under the Canadian Ethics of Animal Investigation. Starting with the statement of the fundamental requisites for ethically permissible use of animals in research, to the restrictions on for example neuromuscular blocking agents, the Canadian Ethics of Animal Investigation includes many of the details of the administration of the Animal (Scientific Procedures) Act 1986.

The Ethics of Animal Investigation illustrates an attempt to bring ethical principles to bear even on the technical details of animal experimentation and how such an ethical approach can mirror a legal framework. The following is an extract from its guidlines:

> 'The use of animals in research, teaching and testing is acceptable only if it promises to contribute to understanding of fundamental biological principles, or to the development of knowledge that can reasonably be expected to benefit humans or animals.
>
> Animals should be used only if the researcher's best efforts to find an alternative have failed. A continuing sharing of knowledge, review of the literature, and adherence to the Russell-Burch "3R" tenet of "Replacement, Reduction and Refinement" are also requisites. Those using animals should employ the most humane method on the smallest number of appropriate animals required to obtain valid information.
>
> The following principles incorporate suggestions from members of both the scientific and animal welfare communities, as well as the organizations represented on Council. They should be applied in conjunction with CCAC's *Guide to the Care and Use of Experimental Animals*.
>
> (1)   If animals must be used, they should be maintained in a manner that provides for their physical comfort and psychological well-being, according to CCAC's *Policy Statement on Social and Behavioural Requirements of Experimental Animals*.

(2) Animals must not be subjected to unnecessary pain or distress. The experimental design must offer them every practicable safeguard, whether in research, in teaching or in testing procedures; cost and convenience must not take precedence over the animal's physical and mental well-being.

(3) Expert opinion must attest to the potential value of studies with animals. The following procedures, which are restricted, require independent, external evaluation to justify their use:

(a) burns, freezing injuries, fractures, and other types of trauma investigation in anaesthetized animals, concomitant to which must be acceptable veterinary practices for the relief of pain, including adequate analgesia during the recovery period;

(b) staged encounters between predators and prey or between conspecifics where prolonged fighting and injury are probable.

(4) If pain or distress are necessary concomitants to the study, these must be minimized both in intensity and duration. Investigators, animal care committees, grant review committees and referees must be especially cautious in evaluating the proposed use of the following procedures:

(a) experiments involving withholding pre- and post-operative pain-relieving medication;

(b) paralysing and immobilizing experiments where there is no reduction in the sensation of pain;

(c) electric shock as negative reinforcement;

(d) extreme environmental conditions such as low or high temperatures, high humidity, modified atmospheres, etc., or sudden changes therein;

(e) experiments studying stress and pain;

(f) experiments requiring withholding of food and water for periods incompatible with the species' specific physiological needs; such experiments should have no detrimental effect on the health of the animal;

(g) injection of Freund's Complete Adjuvant (FCA). This must be carried out in accordance with *CCAC Guidelines on Immunization Procedure*'.

(5) An animal observed to be experiencing severe, unrelievable pain or discomfort should immediately be humanely killed, using a method providing initial rapid unconsciousness.

(6) While non-recovery procedures involving anaesthetized animals, and studies involving no pain or distress are considered acceptable, the following experimental procedures inflict excessive pain and are thus unacceptable:

(a) utilization of muscle relaxants or paralytics (curare and curare-like) alone, without anaesthetics, during surgical procedures;

(b) traumatizing procedures involving crushing, burning, striking or beating in unanaesthetized animals.

(7)   Studies such as toxicological and biological testing, cancer research and infectious diseases investigation may, in the past, have required continuation until the death of the animal. However, in the face of distinct signs that such processes are causing irreversible pain or distress, alternative endpoints should be sought to satisfy both the requirements of the study and the needs of the animal.

(8)   Physical restraint should only be used after alternative procedures have been fully considered and found inadequate. Animals so restrained must receive exceptional care and attention, in compliance with species-specific and general requirements as set forth in the Guide.

(9)   Painful experiments or multiple invasive procedures on an individual animal, conducted solely for the instruction of students in the classroom, or for the demonstration of established scientific knowledge, cannot be justified. Audiovisual or other alternative techniques should be employed to convey such information.'

(CCAC 1989)

The making of an ethics committee

Those who set up an ethics committee should be clear about the function of such a committee, its remit and how it slots into the chain of command within the establishment. All these factors will vary greatly between different designated establishments according to the nature of work being done which will differ in, for example, universities, hospitals, research institutes, pharmaceutical companies and contract establishments. Ethics committees will accordingly have a different format in keeping with the needs and circumstances of the place in which they operate. In spite of this necessary flexibility as regards constitution, a paramount concern for any such committee must be an assessment of the cost–benefit balance. All ethics committees will provide the mechanism for serious discussion and provide a setting for any concerns for animal welfare to be constructively debated.

The *modus operandi* of an ethics committee

The *modus operandi* of an ethics committee should conform to the following format:

- regular meetings convenient to all members, if possible;
- relevant reports available to all interested parties;
- advice to the authorities of the establishment on ways of improving the impact of the committee;
- provision of training in ethics for its members;
- issuing of guidelines with special emphasis on the need for promptness of replies and consistency of decisions;
- maintenance of an efficient secretarial service.

The disadvantages of ethics committees

Most of the disadvantages associated with ethics committees have surfaced abroad where many ethics committees have been given official status, have been compelled to include representatives of animal rights groups and have been given wide powers.

An often recurring complaint about ethics committees is delay. This follows from the very nature of the venture. Frequently, the members are fully committed in the pursuit of their own careers and because of their expertise and high profile have few free slots in any week. To collect such a galaxy of stars in one place, at one time is never easy. Often the opinion of some members will need to be sought by correspondence and that inevitably entails delay in arriving at a decision.

An important possible disadvantage of ethics committees, is the possible lack of confidentiality and consequent danger of disclosure of trade secrets.

It would not be desirable to either completely exclude or ignore the views of those unfavourable to the use of animals in research in the deliberations of an ethics committee. On the other hand, however, some animal activists could continually frustrate the operations of a committee. In spite of the favourable reports of the 'Swedish experience', even there, difficulties can arise. An antivivisectionist lady in Gothenburg caused trouble by prolonging the meetings until people had to leave (a Viking filibusterer). This caused clinical members of the committee, who had other work to do, to refuse to take on an appointment for a second period. It is difficult to recruit worthwhile members in the face of sabotage (RDS 1983).

A shift of legislation in respect of animal experimentation could have a catastrophic effect on research in Germany. According to Rainer Klinke, professor of zoology at the University of Frankfurt, the present delay in the granting of applications to use animals in research, of four to six months, could become much longer. In some of the state committees there may be a high proportion of members from animal rights movements. The original constitution of these state ethical committees had been balanced – two university researchers, two industrial scientists and two from animal rights organizations. Unfortunately, the new law specifies 'animals' rather than just 'vertebrates' as being protected in research. Discussions within ethics committees as to whether the term 'animal' included drosophila could prove not interesting but alarming to workers in research. The opportunities for filibustering on this topic are unlimited (NS 1993).

A Parthian shot

Draft legislation (1994) on animal use in research drawn up for the government of Brazil by the lawyers' association, could threaten the future of biomedical research in that country. The proposed Superior Committee for Scientific Ethics with Animals (COSETICA), an autonomous body, would have the power to close down laboratories in the case of perceived cruelty, and to license researchers to use animals. The sting is in the tail. Any scientist who has recently been involved in animal experiments would be excluded from membership. Decisions could be arrived at by uninformed ignorance. The law's authors say that the draft is based on British and

Swedish legislation – an initial misconception based on a misunderstanding of their source material. The law's authors, lawyers (perhaps, they know the law but do they know about research?) deny it would hinder research (LASA 1993).

The hidden agenda is a hazard in any committee. Politics, with a small 'p' is bound to play its part even in such idealistic gatherings as ethics committees.

It is not always predictable who, within a committee, will eventually be primarily responsible for 'drawing the line in the sand'. In theory, of course, the majority will be responsible for the decision but the individual who will by persuasion mould that majority will vary. Among those deciding the opinion for the majority might be:

- the person of authority within the establishment;
- the person who can interrupt most loudly;
- the known worthy from the local community;
- the one regarded as the most knowledgeable, the honorary professor;
- the accepted moralist, perhaps a cleric;
- the committed fanatic;
- the sceptre of the Inspector. What will be allowed? How far can we go?

One advantage of the UK's present legal system is a clear provision for appeal against any decision regarded as unacceptable by an applicant. The first Statutory Instrument under the 1986 Act, in December 1986, granted this concession in no uncertain terms. This type of consideration for possible aggrieved parties does not appear to be a defined feature of ethics committees. Some have suggested that such a precaution against possible questionable decisions by a committtee is hardly necessary. Deliberations of such bodies may be above suspicion but even the vaunted 'trial by peers' has never been regarded as infallible.

The advantages of ethics committees

These advantages are similar whether we are dealing with a high-level ethics committee, an ethical committee (if that is what you wish to call it), or an animal care and use committee. Obviously the impact of the committee will vary with the level at which it operates within the institution. Among the benefits accruing from these bodies the following seem most important:

- Responsibilities for serious decisions on animal experimentation and welfare are shared. Unfortunately, shared responsibility can sometimes mean that no individual need feel responsible and so will more readily align with their peers. It is not only mariners who don't want to rock the boat.
- Decisions are shared but this may be the result of a trade-off or a compromise which may partly evade a crucial issue.
- Mutual support for all involved in the research.
- Increased awareness of the problems involved, due to open discussion and the expression of various views.
- An imperative to continually consider the three Rs.

- Production of a specific ethos on animal work within the establishment as a guide to the certificate holder and management on the running of the animal facility.
- Provision of material on ethics which might lead scientists and other interested parties to pursue a further study of the subject.
- Fruitful involvement in public relations, particularly in defence of research work.
- Improvement of staff morale by providing an outlet for their moral concern and making both counselling and appropriate training available.
- Liaison between various departments, particularly in large institutions, to achieve the most economic use of animals.
- Dissemination of all relevant material to workers who should be aware of such information.
- Finally, a serious appraisal of proposed benefits, the most unforeseeable factor in the cost–benefit equation. The Home Office Guidance (4.4.) bears witness to the difficulty of assessing future possible consequences which may never come to fruition and are liable to be subjectively overestimated by an interested individual.

The ethical review process

Impetus was given to the development of ethics committees on the use of animals in research by a letter (25/4/96) from the Animals Byelaws and Coroners Unit of the Home Office sent on the advice of the Animals Procedures Committee (APC) to all holders of Certificates of Designation. The letter was couched in a moderate tone, but stressing that the missive was advisory and not mandatory. The gist of the guidance was a suggestion regarding the adoption of some form of 'local ethical review', a more amorphous phrase than 'ethics committee'.

   The recommended options were as follows:

(1)   Ethics committees. This option seemed to lack whole-hearted support.
(2)   Care and use committees which could consider animal experimentation and welfare.
(3)   The named veterinary surgeon as a one-person ethics committee. Although feasible in law (in *re Opera Photographic Ltd* (1989) I W.L.R. 634), a quorum of one was not highly commended.
(4)   Project refinement reviews having retrospective features.
(5)   Awareness-raising activities. This final option illustrated well the wise and tolerant approach of the Home Office.

   Once the concept of another layer of arbitration prior to the granting of a project licence as a universal factor, had been launched, it gathered its own momentum. It was driven by imperatives from various quarters. One of the first casualties of this reforming zeal was liberal expression of intent:

   '6. The Home Secretary does not intend that any process over and above what is already required by the 1986 Act should be mandatory. He invites you to consider, however, whether or not your own establishment would benefit from one or other of the local ethical review processes described above. The aim would be to maintain the awareness of all involved in laboratory animal care and use of their responsibilities towards their animal charges. Any of the ways described above would encourage this. Some of the processes will be more suitable for some institutions than others.'

Change of emphasis did not come rapidly. The APC were silent on the matter in their interim report in July 1997. However, on 6 November, Lord Williams (Under Secretary of State) announced that every designated establishment must set up and maintain an ethical review process.

In the Home Office letter of 1 April 1998, we read:

'6.2. This condition will require that an appropriate form of ethical review process is in place which demonstrably meets the needs of the establishment and the aims of the policy. The ultimate sanction for not complying with this condition will be revocation of the certificate, subject to the right to make representations.'

An excellent and comprehensive presentation of the case for an ethical review process appeared in the form of a report on a workshop *Progressing the Ethical Review Process* (Boyd Group 1991).

The growth of the project can be traced from the suggestion by the Working Party of the Institute of Medical Ethics in 1991 which concluded that there was a place for a local research review process in this field. Then in 1994 the RSPCA published a document by M. Jennings (Jennings 1994), putting forward ideas for the composition and function of ethics committees in the UK, in the light of both UK and international experience.

Having had the privilege of interviewing on a weekly basis and at close quarters would-be licence holders from as far afield as Slovenia and Finland to Japan and Ecuador, and having gathered through industrious graduates animal law from Ghana to Thailand and from Catalonia to Los Angeles, I am aware that the sometimes complex but often scant data can be read many ways. This is particularly true when we realize that, in spite of the European Convention, few countries have legislation on the matter which is in the same league as that of the UK. In many cases a committee is the sole form of control. The Laboratory Animal Science Association convened a workshop on the ethical review process in 1995. The Boyd Group, a laudable addition to the animals in research controversy, since it represents the consensus view of a group of individuals spanning a wide range of perspectives on the use of animal research, produced a discussion paper on the topic. Its conclusion was that institutional ethics committees 'could enhance the ethical review process by widening consultation and providing a clear institutional focus for consideration of relevant ethical issues.'

The 1997 workshop, produced a precise workable definition of the ethical review process:

'A local framework acting as an adjunct to the Home Office Inspectorate to ensure that all animal use in an establishment is carefully considered and justified, and that proper account is taken of all possibilities for reduction, refinement and replacement.'

This clarity and efficiency of approach to the subject was due to the business-like efforts of the organizers of the workshop under the leadershp of M. Jennings. She has given a lot of time and worked hard in the pursuit of this ideal.

The report of the workshop summed up well the thinking behind the ethical review and the envisaged format. It was concluded that every establishment in which animals are used should have a well-documented effective ethical review process to help create a 'culture of care' and complement the work of the Home Office in ensuring implementation of the law. Necessary to the fulfilling of this aim is the commitment to it of senior management, particularly the certificate holder.

Guidance on the implementation of the ethical review process (ERP) stressed the importance of flexibility and the tailoring of the process to individual establishments:

'The first stage in setting up a local process should be to decide on the most suitable model, taking into account the existing framework, including the management structure, relationship between those with statutory responsibilities, the nature and number of project licences, the species of animals and training arrangements. Consideration of what works well in the existing system and the kinds of problems encountered is also important. It would be useful to consult people outside the establishment to provide an objective perspective.'

The desirable functions of the ERP are listed as:

'(1) assisting the certificate holder and other named persons in discharging their duties effectively;
(2) promoting awareness of animal welfare issues and developing initiatives leading to greater applications of the three Rs, thus minimizing suffering and optimizing animal welfare;
(3) considering wider ethical issues and assisting in communication within the establishment and with the public.
Ensuring good communication throughout the establishment, providing a forum for members of the establishment to raise concerns and facilitate early detection and solution of problems, promoting training (particularly in order to enhance competence and sensitivity towards animals), and encouraging critical scrutiny of the utilitarian harm versus benefit justification for animal use, all come within the overall remit.'

Authoritative source material

The material on the ERP already presented covers the topic of authoritative source material and is in tune with what is being required by the Government. It will, however, be useful to look at the source documents to clarify some important details.

In the first instance, in the Home Office letter of 25/4/96, the flexibility of any ERP was stressed. This theme of adaptability to local circumstances is a recurring refrain throughout the proposals on this subject:

'44. We (that is the APC) believe that the Home Secretary should encourage the local considerations of ethical issues, aimed at a continual improvement in the awareness of what it means to use animals in laboratories and the consequences for the animals. ... We have therefore recommended that the Home Secretary should provide advice to certificate holders and project licence holders on the ethical review process, but neither specify the form that these review processes should take nor add to the regulatory requirements.'

The broadening out of the remit of an ERP is indicated in the Home Office letter of 23/2/98:

'2.3. These processes need to be informed by a wider ethical consideration. There should be a continual and improving awareness of what it means to use animals in laboratories and the consequences for animals. This extends to current work as well as to work in prospect. It goes beyond the regulated procedures to the 3Rs and the welfare of all animals in the establishment.'

The individuality of the ERPs is not only allowed for but indeed encouraged:

'3.2. It is critically important to devise and adopt a system appropriate to the individual establishment. The outcome of the ERP is more important than how it is done. Proportionality should be observed: the ERP should be appropriate to the size and complexity of the establishment.'

The Home Office letter of 25/2/98 deals with a special issue in respect to membership of the ERP:

'3.5. One potentially contentious area contained in the Annex (official directives on the ERP) is the suggestion that people outside the establishment should be involved. This should be considered seriously by all establishments. The main payoff of their involvement comes from the input of relevant expertise or morality, concern for animal welfare, and the perspective of the ordinary person that those independent and outside the establishment and its hierarchy can bring. There may also be dividends in terms of public relations and improved communications.

3.6. At the same time, there may be concerns that the establishment's security and the commercial or intellectual features of the work proposed or under way will be compromised. Experience shows that these can be met with goodwill and appropriate systems and that the consequences are worth while when the concerns can be surmounted. Establishments are therefore urged to consider the widest forms of ERPs, and if necessary, to broaden the base of existing systems.'

After consultation on the Annex in February 1996, a further missive was sent to all holders of Certificates of Designation (Reference 3.–4.98) reporting the consultation. The reaction was indicative of the level and source of interest in this matter:

'2.3. Over 50 responses were received, only one arguing against establishment of local ethical review processes. Comments were received from a range of organizations and individuals, including professional and scientific associations, medical and veterinary research centres, universities and colleges, commercial establishments, breeders, interest groups and animal protection societies, and an accredited trainer. Some were very detailed, suggesting changes in the particulars of the requirement; others raised more general concern. These points are addressed below and in the Annex to this letter.'

The text of the Annex was amended in keeping with the results of the consultation. In the same letter, encouragement was given to use existing structures:

'3.4 Thus, where helpful structures already exist, where project refinement processes are in place, where there are suitable fora, or where responsibility and advisory systems are already working, these need not be duplicated but should be drawn creatively into the wider process. Consideration of what already works well in existing systems and of the kinds of problems encountered is to be encouraged. By the same token, there is no requirement to collapse all existing systems into one set of structures.'

The relationship of the Inspector to the ERP was spelt out by the Home Office (PCD holders Reference 3.–4.98):

'4.2. First, it is our intention that an Inspector be allowed occasionally to join meetings and to see the records associated with the ethical review process. It is to be hoped that the Inspector will not limit openness of discussion, nor be regarded as a formal member of any committee. His or her involvement should not be used to bypass the need for local ethical review. We intend that the Inspector will need to assess occasionally how effectively the process is operating. This puts the new requirement on the same basis as other aspects of the establishment's operation under the 1986 Act – open to inspection and advice. 5.2. Inspectors will be pleased to discuss initial ideas and, as at present, be available to advise on the continuing refinement of project plans. But, when the plan is getting to a stage when application to the Home Office is likely, or even before this, it will need to be considered within the local ERP. 5.6. In this, and in all other features of the ERP, it will be the responsibility of the Certificate Holder to present to the Inspectorate, in the first instance, a description of an ERP suitable for the establishment. The Inspector will give a view on whether the features of the system appear to meet the requirements set out in the Annex and are as extensive as the situation allows. A sustained dialogue may be required in some cases to ensure the process has evolved locally as far as possible during the year. The Inspectorate will be setting up procedures to ensure internal consistency.'

A controversial issue in the past, the system of dealing with amendments to licences, is referred to in this letter from the Home Office:

'5.5. Equally, it is not possible to set out generalised rules about the handling of amendments or secondary availabilities. These must be evolved locally, again because establishments differ and projects certainly differ. Every application should, at some stage, be reviewed in the process but not every amendment need be. Each establishment will need to set a threshold for scale and type of amendment which makes sense in that setting and to the project in hand. It would be ideal if the spirit of ethical review were applied, not a minimal requirement of the Home Office.'

The text of the revised Annex (1/4/98)

The Policy

'1. The Secretary of State requires that an ERP be established and maintained in each establishment designated under s. 6 or 7 of the Animals (Scientific Procedures) Act 1986. Every establishment should explain to and test with the Animals (Scientific Procedures) Inspectorate a viable process, appropriate to that establishment, before 1 April 1999. From that date, the requirement for a local ERP will be a standard condition for every designated user and breeding/supplying establishment.'

Ethical review process

'2. The Certificate holder should ensure as wide an involvement of establishment staff as possible in a local framework acting to ensure that all use of animals in the establishment, as regulated by the Animals (Scientific Procedures) Act 1986, is carefully considered and justified; that proper account is taken of all possibilities for reduction, refinement and replacement (the 3Rs); and that high standards of accommodation and care are achieved.'

Aims

'3.1. To provide independent ethical advice to the Certificate holder, particularly with respect to project licence applications and standards of animal care and welfare.

3.2. To provide support to named people and advice to licensees regarding animal welfare and ethical issues arising from their work.

3.3. To promote the use of ethical analysis to increase awareness of animal welfare issues and develop initiatives leading to the widest possible applications of the 3Rs.'

Responsibility of the certificate holder

'4. The Certificate holder will be responsible to the Home Office for the operation of the local ethical review process and for the appointment of people to implement its procedures.'

Personnel

'5. A named Veterinary Surgeon and representatives from among the Named Animal Care and Welfare Officers should be involved. In user establishments, project licensees and personal licensees should also be represented. As many people as possible should be involved in the ethical review process. Where possible, the views of those who do not have responsibilities under the Act should be taken into account. One or more lay persons, independent of the establishments, should also be considered. Home Office inspectors should have the right to attend any meetings and have access to the records of the ERP.'

Operation

'6. These people should deliberate regularly and keep records of discussions and advice. All licensees and Named Animal Care and Welfare Officers must be informed of the ERP and should be encouraged to bring matters to its attention. An operating description should allow for input by colleagues and other people from outside the establishment. It should be clear how submissions can be made. The people involved should be regarded as approachable, dealing in confidence with complaints and processing all suggestions for improvement.

7. Specifically, the process should allow (where appropriate) the following:

7.1 promoting the development and uptake of reduction, replacement and refinement alternatives in animal use, where they exist, and ensuring the availability of relevant sources of information;

7.2 examining proposed applications for new project licences and amendments to existing licences, with reference to the likely costs to the animals, the expected benefits of the work and how these considerations balance;

7.3 providing a forum for discussion of issues relating to the use of animals and considering how staff can be kept up to date with relevant ethical advice, best practice and relevant legislation;

7.4 undertaking retrospective project reviews and continuing to apply the 3Rs to all projects, throughout their duration;

7.5 considering the care and accommodation standards applied to all animals in the establishment, including breeding stock, and the humane killing of protected animals;

7.6 regularly reviewing the establishment's managerial systems, procedures and protocols where these bear on the proper use of animals;

7.7 advising on how all staff involved with the animals can be appropriately trained and how competence can be assured.

8. Commonly, there should be a promotional role, seeking to educate users (in applying the 3Rs) and non-users (by explaining why and how animals are used), as appropriate. There should be some formal output from the ERP for staff and colleagues in the establishment, made as widely available as security and commercial/intellectual confidentiality allow.

9. Receipt of a project licence application signed by the Certificate holder will be taken by the Home Office to mean that the application has been through the ERP for that establishment.

10. Once the system is established, Inspectors will still be happy to discuss early ideas with prospective project licence holders and will be available for advice and clarification at any point. But an application will not be considered for formal authorization by the Home Office until the prospective project has been considered appropriately within the ERP. The Inspector will not negotiate with any advisory group. Local arrangements and the individual case will dictate whether amended applications must re-enter the ERP. It would be a matter of judgement in the particular case how best to balance the inputs of the ERP and the Inspectorate without duplicating effort or creating undue delay.'

A working model – human research ethics committees (HRECs)

There are obvious similarities between ERPs and HRECs. Both are operated at a local level and review scientific quality of proposed research.

The remit of HRECs includes consideration of the science involved since it would be unethical to subject individuals to poor science. Judgement on the quality of the science implies evaluating the worth of the research, the design of the programme, the competence of the research workers and the statistical analysis. As in the case of the ERP, the possible discomfort of the subject from the project is of vital importance.

HRECs, like the ERPS, have an official standing. The Department of Health requires each district health authority to 'appoint a properly constituted HREC which meets regularly to review and approve (or not approve) the research conducted by its staff or using its premises and facilities.' Standing operating procedures have been issued by the Department of Health and various professional bodies have published relevant guidelines.

The cost–benefit assessment so vital in the justfication for a project licence has its counterpart in the risk–benefit analysis called for in the HREC.

The issue of consent

On this issue there is bound to be a marked difference between HRECs and ERPs due to the nature of the subject matter of each one. A major concern of members of HRECs will be the nature of the consent given by the patient. They need to be sure that any consent received is fully informed. If patients lack the mental capacity to give or withhold consent, research with them is unlawful, unless it is therapeutic research of potential benefit to the patient. Non-therapeutic research may be allowed in the case of young children but rarely and only if it is non-invasive, entails no suffering, carries no more than minimal risk, has parental approval and the child does not appear to object.

The significant difference and ethical difficulty in the case of animals is that there is no practical accepted way of establishing that an animal would be a consenting participant in a project. There are no provable bases for a presumption of consent.

Membership

Two lay members are accepted as a proper feature of any HRECs. Purely professional committees settling their own problems within their élite circle could hardly, nowadays, command public confidence. Credibility gaps have sprung up where once there was nothing but unquestioning trust. Lay involvement enhances public confidence. It contributes valid comment on issues from the point of view of 'the woman or man in the street'.

As in the case of ERPs, so in the case of HRECs there is always a certain amount of concern about the choice of lay members. Lay persons will by definition be lacking in the expertise required to make a fully informed judgement on the value of the scientific material crucial to the decision-making process. Should such lay persons then have their own form of expertise, in ethics perhaps? Are there such experts, and if so are they wanted? In frequent enquiries over many years from both students and scientists, I ascertained that few would welcome a moral philosopher on to these types of committees. Some obviously do get on by stealth. In Australia it is mandatory to have one versed in moral philosophy on animal use committees. There is no evidence that ethicians are more abundant there than elsewhere.

Even in the case of HRECs there may be people who would be undesirable as members of a committee. The guidance issued by the Royal College of Physicians comments:

> 'Those who are totally opposed to research investigations or experiments on humans should be left to attack the system from outside and should not be invited onto the Committee. Likewise, individuals who are acquiescent and may be thought likely to give automatic approval are also not suitable.'

This smacks a little of 'loading the dice'. In the case of ERPs, that 'attack' may not be merely verbal but may take the form of the brick or the letter-bomb. The 'man on the Clapham omnibus' will not usually be opposed to the practice of human medicine but on a full bus there would be at least a few ready to oppose outright the use of animals in research. Screening out – an unfortunate process – if seeking unbiased decisions, will be more necessary in the case of ERPs than in the case of HRECs. There is one forceful argument, often put in a homely fashion, against excluding even opponents from committees. It is preferable to have a contentious person within the group causing a nuisance to those outside, rather than disconcerting those within from outside.

Another difficulty associated with lay members on ERPs is the hazard which may arise to the institution's security and confidentiality of scientific work. This particular difficulty is of special significance to commercial enterprises, for example in the pharmaceutical industry. A further minor difficulty which may arise is that lay people may feel overawed by professional members of the committee but 'lay' is an ambivalent term and the so-called lay person may be a highly skilled professional in her or his own right, articulate to a high degree, a lawyer for example. In its original use 'lay' simply meant non-clerical. In fact, in this context, the lay person *could* be a local cleric.

Some examples of emerging ERPs (from the 1997 workshop)

In one research company it would appear that a well-developed ERP is up and running. It is, as has been suggested the ERP should be, tailored to the company. It efficiently and effectively provides animal welfare and maintains the awareness of the 'culture of care' promoted throughout the establishment by several different structures and committees with minimal bureaucracy. Several mechanisms have been devised to raise concern.

The example of an ERP within a contract-testing environment was moulded to meet different needs from other research establishments. Safety asessment rather than evaluation, of the benefit of the product is the purpose of the operation. The firm involved in the report aimed to build ethical considerations into all procedures. Rather than a formal ERP there is the intention to create a corporate ethical environment beginning with staff selection and concentrating on staff training to instil an awareness of care and welfare. The ethical dimension is brought to the fore in written documentation, such as codes of practice, quality manuals, mission statements and project licences. Study directors are aware of the need to consider adverse effects on animals at pre-study meetings.

Monitoring and enforcement predominate. Animal welfare may be subject to detailed consideration by *ad hoc* committees or task forces and consequently disciplinary procedures may be used in this area. The named veterinary surgeon has an ethical veto on any animal work.

Outlines on embryonic ERPs within academic institutes also appear in the report (RSPCA 1997) and three of these are now discussed.

Example 1

In one academic institution the NVS (named veterinary surgeon) appears to play a pivotal role in the operation of the ERP. There are, however, two formal committees.

(1) *A Management Committee.*   This committee meets three times a year and decides general policy on animal use. Important decisions have been: not to permit primate work, to give financial support for implementation of the three Rs and to reject both the proposal to set up a formal ethics committee and the involvement of laity in the decision-making process. The committee consists of:
   - the Vice-Principal
   - the certificate holder
   - the Director of BMSU (Biomedical Service Unit) this person is also the NVS and Professor of Biomedical Ethics
   - a representative from the Faculty of Medicine
   - a representative from the Faculty of Science
   - representatives from the staffing, finance and estates departments.
(2) *A Research Advisory Committee.*   This committee seems to function as an informal ethics committee. It meets three times a year and its members are:
   - representatives of animal users on a departmental basis
   - the Director of BMSU
   - the Deputy NVS
   - the NACWO (Named Animal Care and Welfare Officer).

Example 2

In a second academic institute, the ERP is akin to editorial refereeing. A Project Review Committee has the power to withdraw facilities from those who do not conform and the certificate holder will request the withdrawal of licences from those who do not comply with direction. The particular functions of the Committee are to provide:

- an assurance that scientific work involving animals is making progress and that animals are only being used when scientific objectives are being met;
- opportunity to debate the 'benefit side' of the utilitarian weighing required by law;
- a shared understanding of the science within the institute.

Example 3

The final example of an ERP discussed in the report is more in the nature of a full-blown ethics committee and I can write about it more fully from personal experience than about the other examples.

This committee, associated with a charitable research institute, includes lay membership. It meets four times a year to review all project licence applications and important amendments. It has been active since 1990 and has dealt with more than 200 licence applications. Membership comprises the following:

- a member of Council;
- a member of senior management;
- Chairman of the animal executive committee;
- two animal-using scientists;
- a scientist who does not use animals;
- two scientific officers (the NACWO and a non-animal user);
- two lay members with an expertise and interest in ethics, currently both theologians;
- the Chairman of this committee who is one of the members who does not use animals;
- one senior person responsible for animal welfare (the NVS or head of Biological Resources) is also in attendance.

Project licence applications and amendments are circulated among the membership. Applicants are also required to submit 'lay persons summaries'. When the application has been considered, the Chairman collates members, responses and any new applications and contentious amendments are considered carefully by the committee.

The committee has refined procedures by reducing maximim permitted tumour size, discontinued the use of ascites for monoclonal antibody production and improved the provision of analgesics for mice.

The tenor of the report, when discussing this final example, lacks the heady idealism of the Groves of Academe and the strict discipline of commerce that discourages 'marching to another drum'. There is a realism here presented by one who knows the animal room from the inside. Possible disadvantges of an ERP are presented; and there is a cost awareness expressed, important to those who depend on charity and so the expense involved in the running of such reviews is spelt out both in respect of time and money.

A final note on the 1997 report

Two practical questions, apart from the matter of an appeal structure, which readily come to mind on ERPs, have not been fully addressed in the report. If it is desirable to have qualified lay persons on a committee, shouldn't they be paid? The corollary to that is, are they then in the pocket of the establishment? Should the lay members be trained? The corollary to that is, would that involve insidious programming? These are highly pertinent questions to which there is no easy answer.

References

Boyd Group (1991) *Ethical Review of Research Involving Animals*. A discussion paper. Boyd Group, Edinburgh.

CCAC (1989) *Guide to the Care and Use of Experimental Animals*. Canadian Council of Animal Care.

Forsman, B. (1993) This revealing account of the Swedish experience is entitled *Research Ethics in Practice: The Animal Ethics Committees in Sweden*, Centre for Research Ethics, Göteborg, ISBN 91–97 1672–311.

Jennings, M. (1994) *Ethics Committees for Laboratory Animals*. RSPCA, Horsham.

LASA (1993) More details on the Brazilian approach can be found in *Laboratory Animals*, **28**, 93–96.

New Scientist (1993) This information was gleaned from the *New Scientist* 17 April.

RDS (1983) This fair comment on committees appeared in *Conquest*, the Research Defence Society's periodical, March, 14.

RSPCA (1997) Report of a workshop on *Progressing the Ethical Review Process*. Covered by M. Jennings (RSPCA), B. Howard (University of Sheffield) and Graham Moore (Pfizer Central Research).

Chapter 15

Always There is a Matter of Degree

It is not easy to define exactly when push comes to shove, but you are usually aware when it happens.

Introduction

There is a tendency to concentrate on the hostile reaction to the use of animals in research. We have already considered the numerous forms of criticism that are levelled against painful experiments on animals but that is by no means the full picture. Societies such as PETA (People for the Ethical Treatment of Animals) go further with their opposition. We have already referred to the views of one of their leading members, Ingrid Newkirk, who regards even painless research as fascism, as supremacism, because it is her opinion that the very state of confinement is traumatizing in itself. Other, one-time respectable users of animals such as butchers and furriers have of late become targets of abuse and violence from self-appointed animal champions. Activists of this persuasion sometimes rely only on publicity and draw a certain amount of support from the public, particularly where there is blatant animal abuse, and rightly so. It is difficult, however, to accept the arguments of extremists who would ban even the keeping of pets on the grounds that such a practice is a challenge to the animal's individuality.

Rather than accept the stance of the extreme attitudes which would either deprive both animals and humans of mutual companionship and many other worthwhile benefits of animal–human relations, or on the other hand condone any use or abuse of animals as justified by the culture in which it may occur, it behoves us to look more closely at this matter. It is already obvious that there is a difference between the *use* and *abuse* of animals by humans. By going a little deeper into the topic we might be able to indicate where the distinction might lie between what is acceptable and what is unacceptable, or in what special circumstances some uses of animals pass from being acceptable to being unacceptable. This latter distinction may sometimes be easy to detect as in the case of a permitted load for a beast of burden.

In making a cost–benefit analysis of a regulated procedure, a precise and definitive judgement may be extremely difficult to arrive at. It might prove therefore a fruitful exercise to look at various categories of animal use and attempt to compare the relative moral worth of the activities involved. Few would regard the keeping of a cosseted pet dog to do a little barking on the side as an indication of the presence of intruders, as in any way exploiting Fido; however, the sacrificing of an animal in an alarm system, as happened with canaries in mines, while once generally accepted might now be frowned upon by some. Any attempt to reach even a consensus of opinion on the rightness or wrongness of more controversial uses of animals would be extremely difficult.

Degrees of acceptability of the use of animals

The following list (see Figure 15.1) is merely an attempt to present, on a very rough basis, the main categories of animal use, starting with the most acceptable and progressing to those uses which many would now condemn. It must be stressed that the more pronounced moral differences may occur within categories rather than between them. The gradation of the list is arranged according to a personal point of view. It is a list to be amended, added to and even, perhaps, reorganized. It may prove to be merely an interesting exercise in ethical grading of activities with animals.

USE

FULLY ACCEPTABLE

- Interest
- Concern
- Help
- Protecting
- Interfering
- Companionship
- Exhibition
- Entertainment
- Production (e.g. dairy farming)
- Work (e.g. arable farming)
- Research
- Sport
- Fighting

COMPLETELY UNACCEPTABLE

- Abuse

A NOTE ON KILLING:

Can a culture make a difference?

Fig. 15.1   The main categories of animal use (an adjustable list).

The following attempt to grade the acceptability of different forms of animal use can hardly be expected to elicit full agreement from more than a few like-minded souls. People naturally would approach such an exercise from very different stances. There is no doubt that there may be more tolerable types of use within a category lower down the scale than some more undesirable types of use within generally more acceptable categories. Always, in spite of the nature of a particular category, there will be perhaps mitigating circumstances, and always there will be the important significance of justifying reasons and approved benefits. The categories do, of course, overlap. Furthermore, killing, a crucial factor in the treatment of animals, is associated directly with more than one of the categories; that is why it is considered separately.

There is no intention in this commentary on the list given in Figure 15.1 to present answers even tentatively. It is merely an indulgence in speculation on attitudes on the topic and the provision of material for those so inclined to contemplate and probably improve upon it.

Interest

Surely no one could in any way censure a healthy interest in animal behaviour. Even if the pursuit is being done purely for human pleasure, as in the case of bird-watching, it would always be regarded as acceptable. On the other hand, interest in animals has instigated the creation of zoos and that implies captivity. In some cases poor conditions in badly run zoos could be called into question.

Concern

Ecology is now of great importance, and rightly so. It has taken on a very marked ethical dimension. It can hardly be regarded as undesirable but it must be ecology with knowledge and concern – concern with forethought. In October 1998 we witnessed the first attempt to prosecute a farmer for farming mink. Leaving aside the details of the court case, it is relevant to refer to the difficulties experienced by the mink which the animal activists released; not to mention the consequent suffering of prey animals in the vicinity.

Help

Helping animals in need, for example making veterinary treatment available to injured wild animals, is undoubtedly laudable. Some purists in this field may question the feeding of, for example, wild birds. Does it make them dependent so that they suffer accordingly when their benefactor moves elswhere? Does it make them lazy which could mean that, if they are young, they may never acquire the essential skills needed for later survival?

Protecting

Few would wish to fault those who devote time and energy to protecting animals, for example rescuing those in danger of sudden flood. Does, however, the protecting of animals from their natural predator upset the natural balance of things? Could it vitiate the principle of the survival of the fittest?

Interfering

Interfering with animals in their habitat can be done for the best of motives as already indicated. Indeed, these four categories – concern, help, protecting and interfering –

have a lot in common and overlap. In this subsection the emphasis is on special care directed towards individual animals. The possibility of even well-intentioned interference being counter-productive was made by an entomologist who was studying the metamorphosis of moths. He learnt from experience that if he assisted a struggling emerging chrysalis, that individual died soon after, whereas others which appeared to be in much more difficulty but emerged after great struggle, survived for a long period. It seemed as if the struggling process had survival value and any outside assistance, even if it mitigated apparent suffering, jeopardized the future of the individual.

Companionship

Here we are moving into more positive use of animals, into the rich and varied world of pets. In this country 50% of the the population have at least one pet each. Pet-keeping seems to be a most innocuous pursuit, especially if we think in terms of the independent lodger, the cat. There are good psychological arguments for the therapeutic value of pets, particularly for the aged and lonely. The birdman of Alcatraz was a classic example.

There are some questions which may be usefully posed. Can pets be overindulged to their disadvantage, for example the fat cat? Is the unrestricted ownership of exotic pets acceptable, knowing that many would-be owners may be completely ignorant of the specialized welfare needs of their strange companions? Do fanatical pet owners need to be looked at? Does the statement 'The more I know my fellow man, the more I love my dog', tell us more about the inadequacy of the speaker than about human nature or canine attractiveness?

Exhibition

This topic follows easily from the last. In some instances the pet is regarded as an extension of the owner's personality. The owner can shine in the afterglow of the brilliance of the prize-winner.

Surely this is harmless fun in the most serious sense. The dog obediently at heel at Crufts does not in any way seem distressed. The strutting peacock in ornate grounds can hardly be regarded as suffering any inconvenience.

However, the misshapen dog, bred to conform to a fashion, may arouse a certain amount of adverse comment. The production of what could be regarded as almost artificial animals to cater to unusual tastes goes beyond the acceptable. Exhibition of animals either for pleasure or in competitions usually causes little, if any, distress to an animal. There are, however, differences in degrees of activity having an ethical connotation. There is a variation of effort between the gentle art of dressage and strenuous circus tricks. Both of these pursuits may be better classed as entertainment or sport but the comparison makes the point of the grounds on which divergence of opinions are founded.

Entertainment

When considering the use of animals for entertainment, perhaps the first objection which springs to mind is that it exposes animals to ridicule. We have discussed animal consciousness and their capacity for suffering. It is a little late now to embark on involved polemics about whether animals are sensitive or not. The more serious discussion here is whether performing animals are properly treated and if some tricks are instilled by unsuitable methods. Few in the past even dreamt of censuring the use of Lassie, Trigger or the like, for the delight of both old and young in the cinema. The most bizarre involvement of animals, to my mind, in entertainment, although only tangential and I suspect unwillingly, occurred in Italy. In 1974, an extremely pious group demonstrated against a production of *Jesus Christ Superstar* in Rome's Opera House. The enraged devotees rodent-bombed the audience from a gallery by showering white mice upon them.

Production

In the sphere of animal use for production we enter the region of serious use of animals for the benefit of humankind. Here there is indeed a wide spectrum of acceptability, from the shearing of sheep for wool (benefiting the animal in the warmer weather) to intensive calf production of tender veal.

In many cases valuable materials taken from animals may be gained without any intrusion, for example dung for fertilization of the land. In some countries this product is the most important form of domestic fuel. Many animal products are obtained without any distress to the animals. Genetically manipulated material for medicinal purposes, for example in the milk of sheep, is available with little inconvenience being experienced by the ewe. An ample milk supply is usually given by cows without any difficulty. Some may question the attitude of those who seem to regard the cow as a milk machine and they may object to breeding programmes and dietary regimes geared only to enhance milk output.

From an ethical point of view, sight must never be lost of the importance of animal welfare. The five freedoms mentioned previously are most important. Eggs are another dairy product freely given by resident poultry. The praiseworthy free-range farming of poultry is acceptable by most people but the intensive farming methods such as battery systems for hens is to be, if not deplored, at least carefully monitored. I suppose it depends on knowing how much honey and wax is plundered from the beehive if we are to make a value judgement on such an activity. A certain amount of restraint may sometimes be necessary to obtain desired products from a particular animal, for example in the taking of venom from snakes.

Unfortunately, some important animal products can only be obtained after the death of the animal. Such use of animals entails killing the animal. The principal produce of this type is of course food in the form of meat. It is at this point that the use of animals begins to be called into question by such groups as vegetarians. Even among carnivores there is ethical concern regarding methods used in farming and methods of slaughter. Probably there is more objection on moral grounds to the killing of animals for their pelt than to hunting them for food. Fashion or adornment does not strike many as a sufficient benefit to justify the killing of an animal.

Work

Some of the topics we have already listed, for example entertainment, overlap the category of work and could be included within it. In this category of animal use there is great variation in the amount of work demanded from the animal and the amount of energy the beast of burden must expend to do that work. It is no coincidence that we have measured resulting work in terms of horse-power. The ethical dialectic in this area is bound to be influenced by the method which is used to obtain the cooperation of the animal, by beating perhaps? Would this really happen? Our first full-blown animal protection Act, back in 1822 – Martin's Act – was intended '. . . to prevent the cruel and improper Treatment of Cattle'. This enactment goes on to threaten penalties on '. . . any Person or Persons (who) shall wantonly and cruelly beat, abuse or ill-treat any Horse, Mare, Gelding, Mule, Ass, Ox, Cow, Heifer, Steer, Sheep or other cattle . . .'.

The acceptability of employing animals is bound to vary according to what service is expected. The remedy provided by the leech for the sick, hardly called for any compulsion whereas the mule under the yoke may have been spurred on by threat of violence, if not in fact by harsh treatment. The following categories vary in acceptability and may also be judged according to intensity or other factors.

Helping
I am filled with admiration when I see the gentle labrador guiding with care a blind person on to an underground escalator.

Rescuing
I accept the word of those who claim that the Newfoundland dog jumping into the waves to save a man is doing what comes naturally. The hardship imposed on the St Bernard dog seems justified. The dog seems to show little reluctance in its task.

Warning
This willingly given service is akin to rescuing. It is forestalling danger. Animals had readily performed this task long before 390 BCE when the gaggle of geese saved the Capitol of Rome from the Gauls. Ganders are still supplying this foolproof system for a famous distillery near Glasgow.

Protection
Dogs particularly seem to enjoy protecting their territory. If that includes your property and whatever is yours, they seem to equally enjoy the commitment. If you want evidence, ask a postman.

Detection
Ever since the legendary use of bloodhounds in old detective stories, animals have played their part in unmasking criminals. The readiness with which trained drug-

sniffer dogs jump on to cross–channel lorries hardly indicates exploitation of our canine associates.

Advertising

Some censure may creep in here. Unfounded suspicion rather than proof may be used as an argument that the polished performance is gained by oppression or abuse. One premise for condemnation may be that it is bringing into ridicule higher (if that word is acceptable) animals such as monkeys. This type of use of animals has a long history since the time of the Egyptians with their animal-headed gods. Symbolism was all-important in societies were there was a low percentage of literacy. In religion, animal symbolism abounded, of good and bad. The pelican drawing blood from its own breast for its starving chicks signified self-sacrifice whereas a far from photogenic pig was a give-away for gluttony. In the secular world animal symbolism was just as potent. The bulldog breed meant much to my generation. This type of 'spin' has a long history. The lands where 'Caesar's eagle never flew' were obviously barbarian. We are, of course, here in the realm of the virtual rather than the real animal. The use of the kiwi as a symbol of New Zealand has no effect on any real animal. It does, however, illustrate the intimate place that animals have in the human psyche. Sometimes, however, real animals are involved. The regimental mascot is paraded with pride and the animal itself is pampered. No hint here of exploitation of lesser breeds.

Communication

Still in the area of the media, the legendary name of 'Reuter' is forever linked with pigeons. Unfortunately, homing pigeons do not always get home; some die exhausted on the way.

Delivery

It is not just the retriever that springs to mind. Way back it is alleged that one of the most joyous sights for mankind was the dove returning with the olive branch. Bonzo coming from the front door with a wagging tail at one end and the morning paper at the other end, pales into insignificance in comparison with the deluvian vision.

Transport

We now come to, not only real use of animals, but also to abuse of animals. Many horses are the proud possessions of their doting owners. Even in the coal trade, where I spent my early working days, the cart-horse was the most esteemed member of staff. In those war days they even had a ration book, and the laying-in of supplies for Dobbin was high priority. Such concern for our equestrian workmates should not mask the amount of real cruelty that was inflicted on many beasts of burden. Our own legislators found it necessary within the context of the Protection of Animals Act 1911 (1912 in Scotland) to outlaw the use of dogs as draught animals. Again, acceptability is influenced by circumstances and the methods employed. The cry of 'Mush mush' as the huskies pull away, hardly pricks the consciences of any onlookers.

Hard work

Great pride is often displayed by ploughmen with their team. I have, however, seen oxen looking far from happy, under a hot sun grinding corn. Goads and other implements of 'encouragement' were apparent. Right and wrong can be a matter of degree.

Controlling

This is a wide category of animal use and the various categories are discussed in the following subsections.

Controlling vegetation

The keeping of a donkey to thin out the thistles, a task they perform seemingly with relish, is definitely acceptable. Even the harnessing of the herbivorous nature of the guinea pig in the role of a miniature lawn mower hardly borders on exploitation of defenceless creatures.

Controlling other animals

Sheepdog trials are a joy to behold (if there's nothing else to watch). The exercise seems to bring delight to one and all, even to the sheep perhaps. However, there is a more sinister side to this type of use of animals which is ironic: the employing of animals to eradicate other species. For example, the cat may have first been welcomed in from the desert to deal with rats in the grain store. Examples of this deployment of our associated animals, particularly in hunting, are too numerous to list. Even the innocent-looking guinea hen is kept to deal effectively with rats in the farmyard. When Queen Victoria asked the Duke of Wellington what should be done about the nuisance of sparrows in the newly built Crystal Palace, he curtly replied, 'Sparrow hawks, Ma'am, Sparrow hawks.' Among the pious Victorians in attendance, I doubt if any felt the slightest moral qualms about the suggestion.

Controlling other humans

This is a more extraordinary use of animals by humankind. Most of us probably accept the use of the guard dog to protect our property in a defensive manner. However, within the category of controlling humans it is a more aggressive use – the controlling of rioters by dogs which do not seem to be disturbed by the situation. Unfortunately, horses have suffered the alarm and indignity of marbles thrown under their feet when charging recalcitrant demonstrators.

Warfare

The cavalry has a long and glorious history. Not only horses but camels, for example, were bred to die in the pursuit of military victory. Even the righteous poet, Tennyson, wrote only of the 'six hundred' who rode into the valley of death though it was twelve hundred creatures thundering headlong to their death. Didn't the horses count? Even the noble pachyderm did not escape military conscription in the past. The elephant was, for Hannibal, the primordial tank and for the Syrians it was the ultimate weapon. Jumbo was not really suitable for use in battles; he was neither delicate nor discerning with his footwork. He could also be vulnerable as was proved by Eleazar, the belly-stabber (I Maccabees 6:46). A most reprehensible use of animals in military manoeuvres has been the employment of explosive-laden dolphins to home-in on targets.

Research

Sufficient comment has already been made on this topic. Here again, views on acceptability will vary greatly according to the type of research involved. Many would accept the use of mice in cancer research; fewer could be reconciled to the use of sheep for testing armaments. It is a moot point whether the projecting of animals into space should be classified as detection or research. Unfortunately, in the past, such satellites have become coffins.

Sport

Sport is probably the most controversial area of animal use. The distress of the animal in such pursuits varies immensely from the greyhound enjoying the chase to the possible trauma of a horse attempting Beecher's Brook. There is a difference in the ethical attitude to the somnulent angler on the river bank from that to the huntsman in full cry, at least in popular perception. Hunting belongs within the topic of control of other animals but here there is usually a greater intimacy between human and animal. Blatant cruelty in this activity is not always restricted to the treatment of the quarry. Maintenance hunting for food appears to be more readily acceptable even among non-hunters.

Fighting

We now come to one category which all but the perverted would condemn. The setting of dog against dog to satisfy some sadistic yearning is totally unacceptable. Such legislation as the Badger Acts outlaw badger baiting and have universal support. Other forms of gratuitous violence inflicted on animals, apart from fighting, such as the rapid descent of goats from ecclesiastical heights initiated on the parapet of a church tower, can in no way be justified.

Killing animals

It is more often the method of killing an animal that is in dispute rather than killing *per se*. In UK law there is no prohibition of killing animals *per se* but there is a plethora of law on the topic of animal killing.

- Permitted methods of killing – slaughterhouse regulations dating back to the late eighteenth century.
- Prohibited methods of killing, for example the use of forbidden poisons, except in the case of the the mole. Nothing seems too bad for the little beast.

- Prohibition of killing certain species of animals, for example under the Wildlife and Countryside Act 1981.
- Restriction of the killing of specified animals at certain times of the year – game laws.
- Obligation to kill animals, for example after a bad road accident, when a police officer can overrule the property rights of the animal's owner or when a Home Office inspector orders an animal to be killed to obviate excessive suffering.

The above complex of legislation on the killing of animals reflects, as far as specialized law can, a general ethical attitude to killing animals. There are extreme opinions on this matter. The Jains of India will in no way countenance the killing of an animal, however old or sick it might be. I encountered a devout Orthodox Cypriot who claimed that within the tenets of Orthodoxy, euthanasia of a sick animal was just as wrong as euthanasia of a human being. At least within his version of Orthodox Christianity, life was sacred, only to be given and taken by God. Animals could only be killed for some good reason, for example for food. Most of us are ready when appropriate to put an animal out of its suffering and would probably feel guilty if we did not extend that mercy to a beast in agony. At the same time we would feel obliged to use the least painful means to attain that end. Any real commitment to never killing an animal produces the quaint sight of the devout Jain being preceded by a servant striving to brush away any insect which may be crushed under the devout foot. Other religions have not been so adverse to killing animals. Animal sacrifice loomed large in ancient faiths and is still practised today. It was not unknown for animals to suffer capital punishment under the Holy Inquisition. The great ritual role of the scapegoat ended in death.

To finish where we started the list – the acceptability of the study of animals – can we justify the killing of rare animals to be delivered to the taxidermist to enhance a museum?

Does a culture make a difference?

Even restricted travel often brings a realization that in different countries there are varying attitudes to animal use and widely divergent opinions on animal cruelty. UK legislation admits a variation in accepted methods of slaughter. Ritualistic slaughter of meat animals as practised within Judaism and Islam enjoys exemption from standard slaughter regulations. Television coverage of Chinese cuisine involving the skinning and boiling of cats rightly horrified my students but some sedate cookery books of this century describe the process of boiling lobsters alive. Blaise Pascal, a strict moralist, did talk in terms of a geography of morality. He posited how modes of accepted behaviour varied from place to place.

Culture and animals are closely associated. There have been cultures without the wheel. There have been cultures without writing. There does not seem to have been any human culture without animals.

Animals can live without humans. Can humans live without animals?

What animals matter?

The variation in attitudes of concern for and care of animals no doubt varies according to the species being considered. Few would put the same value, in ethical terms, on obligations to a housefly as they would put on obligations to their favoured pet. A scale of appreciation in this area is bound to be subjective and heavily influenced by sentiment. I hesitate even to outline such a gradation but present the following as a tentative suggestion on the subject. It is an alignment of what I consider to be the general attitude of the public to the various species of animals. It is therefore to a certain extent arbitrary. It begins with those members of the animal kingdom which seem to be regarded by many as least worthy of our consideration. The list progresses to those animals such as the great apes, whom some would rank alongside ourselves as having rights in an ethical context. As in the previous gradation there is a variation of acceptance within a category, for example among fish there may be more sympathy for a noble salmon than a slippery eel.

Insects

In general they are not particularly valued by the majority though highly prized by some afficianados in the field. They are not absolutely beyond legal jurisdiction in research. At least in Hessen, the drosophila merits listing among protected animals. I suppose most people would take more notice of the fate of a magnificent butterfly than a dull beetle.

Earthworms, slugs and snails

The very mention of creatures of this ilk seems often to be unwelcome in polite conversation. It may be grudgingly granted that they may have their uses but further interest soon evaporates.

Octopus

Still among the invertebrates but held in high regard by some. It has been referred to as the primate of the deep on account of a perception of its intelligent behaviour. The vulgar sort has made it to the ranks of protected animals under the 1986 Act. Among all the cephalopods only the *Octopus vulgaris* has made it to such exalted heights.

Amphibia and fish

Sympathy for these watery creatures tends to vary according to their appearance. There are those who unfortunately regard toads as repulsive, in some way as evil or harmful whereas prettily speckled frogs readily gain approval. Attitudes to fish also seem to depend on their appearance. The other denizens of the deep, though not of course fish, are usually privileged to attract human concern about their welfare – i.e. the dolphin, the whale and of course the seal pup. Then again, they are cute.

Reptiles

Apart from the slow tortoise and the attractive terrapin, reptiles have had a bad press ever since Eden. The majority of snakes attract little affection except from committed devotees.

Birds

Now we are coming to creatures which most people encounter and which they tend to regards as individuals: that makes a big difference in attitudes. Tastes in ornithology differ greatly.

Rodents

Unjustifiably to my mind, the reaction of many people to rats is one of abhorrence. Consequently, any abuse of rodents is rarely called into question from an ethical point of view.

Rabbits

The fluffy bunny rabbit is one of the most effective weapons in the armoury of the antivivisectionists. Culture does play a part in these evaluations. You will find that often an Australian's reaction, even to eating rabbit, may be one of disgust. Disgust is a classic example of a value judgement and of course the very basis of all these evaluations is a matter of value judgements.

Pigs

No universal or clear reaction will be forthcoming to these intelligent beguiling creatures. Perhaps views changed for some after the film *Babe*.

Sheep

Just one example among many of the domestic animals. At this level, personal relationships can build up between humans and the animal. Beliefs regarding how they should be treated become more readily expressed. Among farm animals, although found more often outside the farmyard than not, the horse holds a special place. We referred earlier to the statement that 'history talks too little about animals'. It is a true statement but the names of horses have been recorded for posterity. The name of Alexander's horse, Bucephalus, has been remembered for over 2000 years.

Cats and dogs

As the primary companionship animals, cats and dogs are held in high esteem by many. Scientists and research workers are not immune to special pleading on the part of these animals.

Pandas

Like a whole host of cuddly creatures, pandas are probably singled out for special consideration on sentimental grounds.

Tigers

As typical of the noble beasts of the wild, lions as well as tigers are usually given special respect beyond that paid to the other members of the animal kingdom.

Monkeys

In relations with our nearest relatives, many agree that we need to be more aware of a moral dimension in our dealings with them. Some research institutes rule out any use of primates. There seems to be room for a further gradation in our attitudes to these animals according to which species they belong (BBC2 1998). In fact, in February 1999 there were moves by the New Zealand Parliament to grant legal rights to chimpanzees and gorillas.

Grading right and wrong

This topic may seem somewhat simplistic, if not eccentric. The details of such an attempted grading are bound to have a personal bias. I was instigated to write the following comments by the considered remark of a highly qualified scientific delegate at a seminar. For him, ethics was the basis of professional codes, neither more nor less. There were no loud dissenting voices from amongst his learned colleagues. There seemed to be a silent consensus that the nature and limits of ethics were to be found in codes of conduct. This may be a false notion but I have no doubt that it is not unusual. Consequently 'ethical' or 'unethical' tend to be applied only to certain grades of benevolence or malevolence. Neither mere impolite nor sheer heinous behaviour would be regarded as correctly described by the term 'unethical'.

In texts on ethics there is much discussion on what might be right or what might be wrong but little comment on the degree to which certain conduct might be right or wrong. In real life we automatically grade conduct according to its acceptability. To describe an acknowledged recidivist rapist as a 'bit of a bounder' could be regarded as an unacceptable understatement bordering on the condoning of such criminal activity. In law there is a presumption of variation in villainy. Classification of offences according to their gravity is a salient feature of the administration of justice. It would not be regarded as just if it were otherwise. The old expression 'might as well be hanged for a sheep as a lamb' wisely reflected the lack of discernment in the penal system. There always had been a distinction between misdemeanours and felonies. At one extreme in the grading of illegality there is the venerable axiom *de minimis non curat lex* (the law has no concern for the smallest things). Such a tradition certainly militates against 'zero tolerance'.

Ethicians involved in defining the 'good' do not usually confine their speculation to any specific band of acceptable behaviour or misbehaviour. Yet it seems to me from my experience that even among academics 'unethical' is regarded as rightly applicable only to a lower level of wickedness than 'immoral'. The experience referred to is not of passing comments but has been acquired in formal discussions, two or three times a month, over the last four or five years.

In the higher sphere of moral philosophy no such restriction of the term 'ethics' is evident. For a Utilitarian, the ultimate good – 'greatest happiness of the greatest number' – could be influenced by a wrong decision in a moral context, however trivial. For the scholastic moral philosophers, following Thomas Aquinas, all human acts, however insignificant, had a moral dimension. 'The just man falleth seven times a day' (Proverbs 24:16). Duns Scotus, the Subtle Doctor, alone among the medieval moralists, posited the possibility of indifferent acts – neither morally good nor bad.

I contend that in common parlance, perhaps in defiance of classical definitions of ethics by moral philosphers, 'ethics', 'ethical' and 'unethical' tend to have a restricted extension of meaning in the realm of good and bad conduct. It may be going too far to suggest that 'ethical' belongs to the middle classes, applied by them to affordable forms of good behaviour. This is reminiscent of a throw-away line of Mark Twain: 'An ethical man is a Christian holding four aces.' Academic philosophers may talk in terms of meta-ethics while learned professionals may regard an ethical document as an extended job description.

Before we reach the level of what is generally regarded as unethical, we may posit forms of behaviour which are frowned upon because they are unfair. Pushing to the front of a queue springs to mind.

Unacceptable behaviour a notch higher up than unfairness in the iniquity stakes tends to merit the adjective 'unethical', particularly in professional circles. Acting contrary to a professional code, poaching a colleague's clients is for some the epitome of unethical behaviour. No doubt the expression 'an ethical foreign policy' would concern more serious affairs.

The modern shying away from the term 'immoral' in favour of 'unethical' may be due to the strong association of the term 'morality' with religion. The intrusion of a whiff of religion into real-life affairs may be a tad disturbing to the modern secular scientific man. In spite of such prejudice there are some wrongdoings which are normally referred to as immoral because the term 'unethical' would be regarded as inadequate for expressing the spontaneous disgust aroused by such grievously mischievous behaviour. Usually, deeds of this immoral calibre are roundly condemned within the mores of the particular community in which they occur. We have now moved into the area of traditional morality, based originally on moral theology rather than on moral philosophy.

The traditional moralists in the West, like the true scholastic theologians that they were, delighted in distinctions. They talked in terms of deeds hardly meriting condemnation. These were called imperfections, such as merely spontaneously uttering profane expressions under extreme provocation. A more popular word 'peccadillos', literally, 'little sins', was much less precise and was by no means a technical term. It covered any type of mischief from 'not appropriate' behaviour to an indulgent reference to the romantic exploits of a popular Lothario. Venial sin was a technical term, as was mortal sin. Distinctions were multiplied, the highest ranking deviation being termed mortal *ex toto sui generis*, loosely translated as 'out on its own', in terms of badness (Iorio 1946). At that level one was talking real perfidy. In such an ecclesiastical setting (setting is paramount in assessing the deviation from acceptable behaviour), preaching heresy evoked the loudest and gravest 'anathemas' (CIC 1917). In the area of religious morality there was little room for the relativism of the modern ethician. The only medieval moralist who had the temerity to hint at such laxity was Peter Abelard (Dolan 1992).

The absolutism of religious morality had a marked advantage for those who wanted to know where they stood. There was little room for argument or doubt. Perhaps the flock feel more secure with an aggressive dog than an indecisive shepherd, hence the attractions of fundamentalism.

As the level of deviation from accepted mores is ratcheted up we arrive at behaviour so heinous that it could be regarded as beyond immorality or criminality. Would it ever be acceptable to express a judgemental opinion that Hitler or Stalin were unethical in their treatment of those whom they considered undesirables? A more forceful term of disapproval would usually be considered more appropriate. In the realms of such evil, speculation about the relativity of ethics tends to get scant tolerance in the popular mind.

But let us return to our main theme. Some strictly controlled, and as painless as possible, use of animals in research may be justified by ethical theories such as Utilitarianism. Use of more animals than are necessary in an experiment would certainly be regarded by many as unethical, as would be a lack of appropriate welfare, whereas for others the duty to provide animal welfare would be seen as a moral obligation. The ignoring of the obligation to extend to our animals the five freedoms could be classified as definitely immoral. Few would ever refer to deliberate cruelty to animals as merely unethical.

We have been considering how words are used in practice, albeit loosely. However, the crucial distinction presented in the first chapter is still valid. Morality is really about what is right and what is wrong. Ethics traditionally dealt, as a branch of philosophy, with why actions may be considered as right or wrong. Ethics investigated morality. The preceding material may appear as merely playing with words, but the teasing out of meanings given to words is not irrelevant. Words are all we have to express our thoughts to others. The words we use are the only effective means of expressing clearly our value judgements. It is significant, therefore, which ones we choose, what meanings they have for us and what meanings they have for others. The same word does not necessarily have the same meaning for each one of us. The fact implied by this truism is the fruitful source of controversy. Frequently one hears about any debate, 'It is all a matter of semantics.' That trite phrase is not always true. People think very differently and feel very deeply on the matter of animal use.

Concluding comments

At the beginning of this book few answers were promised; there was the suggestion that the reader would find problems and questions more than ready solutions. In fact it is much more important to concentrate on the question. It is only when you have clarified and asked the right question that you can hope for a right answer. The wrong question will invariably produce the wrong answer.

Perhaps the wrong question in this subject is to persistently ask for a universally acceptable answer from ethics. A searching for absolute value judgements. This would indeed be seeking shadows in the dark because 'absolute value judgements' is a contradiction in terms.

This scepticism does not obviate completely some useful application of ethics in the forming of a consensus. This consensus can influence legislation. It can form opinions and persuade by peer pressure, thus improving both conduct and behaviour. We may not be talking in terms of high moral sense but merely pointing to the existence of enculturation or a type of 'institution' in the ethical sense previously discussed, always admitting that moral philosophy will never have the compelling force that comes from the authority of law or religion, truth well illustrated by the fact that, when older and wiser, Plato wrote his *Laws* and Dostoyevsky's character could boast 'If God is dead all is permitted.'

Perhaps the Bard expressed more clearly the truth of the matter than Hume's law – 'You can not pass logically from the "is" to the "ought" – when he wrote:

> 'There is nothing either good or bad,
> but thinking makes it so.'
>
> (*Hamlet* II, ii, 259, Shakespeare)

References

BBC2 (1998) This television programme (BBC2, 9.25 PM) presented a vivid protrayal of the use of chimpanzees in research in America. Of particular interest was the study of their possible language skills and their use of signs. It also dealt with their redundancy when funds ran out and their re-employment in the search for an AIDS vaccine.

CIC (1917) Canons 2314–16 of the *Codex Iuris Canonici* is outright in its condemnation of those involved in false doctrine. This Roman Codex of Canon Law was in force throughout most of this century and expressed the official attitude to wrong doing within the Church.

Dolan, K. (1992) An account of Abelard's views and his consequent sufferings for his opinions appears on pp. 204–209 of *The Gods that Were* by Kevin Dolan, Dorrance, Pittsburgh.

Iorio, T. (1946) For a fuller exposition of these various scholastic distinctions in evil-doing refer to *Theologia Moralis* by Thomas A. Jorio S.J., Vol. I, No. 179–81. S. Sedis Apostolica Typographus, Naples.

Bibliography

General Ethics

Ackrill, J.L. (ed.) (1973) *Aristotle; Ethics*. Faber.

Bierman, A. & Gould, J. (eds) *Philosophy for a New Generation*. Macmillan.

Bond, E.J. (1983) *Reason and Value*. Cambridge University Press, Cambridge.

Brinton, C. (1990) *A History of Western Morals*. Paragon House, New York.

Bullock, A. & Stallybrass, O. (eds) (1977) *Fontana Dictionary of Modern Thought*. Fontana/Collins.

Carritt, E.F. (1928) *Theory of Morals*. Oxford University Press, Oxford.

Cavalier, R.J. (ed.) (1989) *Ethics in the History of Western Philosophy*. Macmillan, London.

Gauthier, D. (1986) *Morals by Agreement*. Oxford University Press, Oxford.

Honderich, T. (1995) *The Oxford Companion to Philosophy*. Oxford University Press, Oxford.

Hudson, W.D. (1969) *The Is–Ought Question*. St. Martin's Press, New York.

Kardiner, A. (1939) *The Individual and His Society*. Columbia University Press, New York.

Mackie, J.L. (1977) *Ethics: (Inventing Right and Wrong)*. Penguin, London.

Mackie, J.L. (1980) *Hume's Moral Theory*. Routledge and Kegan Paul, Boston.

Martin, R. (1985) *Rawls and Rights*.' University of Kansas Press, Kansas.

Mellor, D.H. (ed.) (1980) *Science, Belief and Behaviour: Essays in Honour of R.B. Braithwaite*. Cambridge University Press, New York.

McGinn, C. (1983) *The Subjective View*. Clarendon Press, London.

Mill, J.S. (1979) *Utilitarianism*. Hackett, London.

Plato (1974) *The Republic*. Penguin Classics, London.

Rorty, R. (1982) *Consequences of Pragmatism*. University of Minnesota Press, Minneapolis.

Schick, F. (1984) *Having Reason*. Princeton University Press, Princeton.

Sidgwick, H. (1907) *Methods of Ethics*. Macmillan, London.

Singer, P. (ed.) (1992) *Applied Ethics*. Oxford University Press, Oxford.

Singer, P. (ed.) (1992) *A Companion to Ethics*. Blackwell, Cambridge, Massachusetts.

Warnock, M. (1963) *Ethics since 1900*. Oxford University Press, Oxford.

Williams, B. (1985) *Ethics and the Limits of Philosophy*. Harvard University Press, Cambridge, Massachusetts.

Ethics and animals

Broadie, A. & Pybus, E.M. (1974) Kant's treatment of animals. *Philosophy*, **49**, 375–83.

Carpenter, E. (1980) *Animals and Ethics*. Watkins, London.

Clark, S.R.L. (1977) *The Moral Status of Animals*. Oxford University Press, New York.

Evans, E.P. (1987) *The Criminal Prosecution and Capital Punishment of Animals*. Faber and Faber, London.

Fox, M.W. (1967) *Between Animal and Man*. Coward, McCann and Geohegan.

Godlovitch, S. & Harris, J. (1971) *Animals, Men and Morals*. Gollancz, London.

Gompertz, L. (1824) *Moral Enquiries: On the Situation of Man and of Brutes*. Centaur Press, Fontwell (reprinted 1992).

Halsbury, Earl of (1972) Ethics and the exploitation of animals. *Stephen Paget Memorial Lecture*, London. *Conquest*, No. 164. Research Defence Society, London.

Herzog, H.A. (1988) The moral status of mice. *American Psychologist*, **43**, 473–4.

Hume, C.W. (1962) *Man and Beast*. Universities Federation of Animal Welfare, Potters Bar.

Hume, C.W. (1980) *The Status of Animals in the Christian Religion*. Universities Federation of Animal Welfare, Potters Bar.

Linzey, A. (1987) *Christianity and the Rights of Animals*. SPCK, London.

Mallinson, J. (1975) *Earning your Living with Animals*. David and Charles, Newton Abbot.

Midgley, M. (1973) The concept of beastliness: philosophy, ethics and animal behaviour. *Philosophy*, **48**, 111–35.

Midgley, M. (1983) *Animals and Why they Matter*. University of Georgia Press, Athens.

Miller, H.B. & Williams, W.H. (eds) (1983) *Ethics and Animals*. Humana Press, Clifton, New Jersey.

Paton, W. (1993) *Man and Mouse*. Oxford University Press, Oxford.

Rodd, R. (1992) *Biology, Ethics and Animals*. Clarendon Press, Oxford.

Rowan, A.R. (1988) *Animals and People Sharing the World*. University Press, New England.

RSPCA (1994) *Ethical Concerns for Animals*. RSPCA, Horsham.

RSPCA (1995) *On the Side of Animals: Some Contemporary Philosophers' Views*. RSPCA, Horsham.

Ruse, M. (1973) Teleological explanation and the animal world. *Mind*, **82**, 433–6.

Sapontzis, S.F. (1987) *Morals, Reasons and Animals*. Temple University Press, Philadelphia.

Serpell, J. (1986) *In the Company of Animals: A Study of Human–Animal Relationships*. Blackwell, Oxford.

Animal rights

Donnellan, C. (ed.) (1993) *Animal Rights: Issues for the Nineties*. Independence, Cambridge.

Frey, R.G. (1977) Animal Rights. *Analysis*, **37**, 186–9.

Frey, R.G. (1983) *Rights, Killing and Suffering*. Blackwell, Oxford.

Hardy, D.T. (1990) *America's New Extremists: What You Need to Know About the Animal Rights Movement*. Washington Legal Foundation, Washington DC.

Jamieson, D. & Regan, T. (1978) Animal rights: a reply to Frey. *Analysis*, **38**, 32–6.

Linzey, W. (1984) *Animal Rights*. SCM Press, London.

Paterson, D. & Ryder, R. (eds) (1979) *Animal Rights*. Centaur Press, London.

Regan, T. (1983) *The Case for Animal Rights*. University of California Press, Berkeley.

Regan, T. & Singer, P. (1989) *Animal Rights and Human Obligations*. Prentice Hall, New Jersey.

Rickaby, J. (1908) Of the so-called rights of animals. In: *Moral Philosophy, or Ethics and the Natural Law*. Longmans, London.

Rollin, B.E. (1993) *Animal Rights and Human Morality*. Promotheus Books, Buffalo.

Animal welfare and behaviour

Duncan, I.J.H. (1993) Welfare is to do with what animals feel. *Journal of Agricultural and Environmental Ethics*, **6** (Special Supplement 2), 8–14.

Duncan, I.J.H. & Petherick, J.C. (1991) The implications of cognitive processes for animal welfare. *Journal of Animal Science*, **69**, 5017–22.

Harrison, R. (1964) *Animal Machines*. Stuart, London.

Lawrence, A.B. & Rushen, J. (eds) (1993) *Stereotypic Animal Behaviour: Fundamentals and Applications to Welfare*. CAB International, Wallingford.

Mason, G.J. (1991) Stereotypes: a critical review. *Animal Behaviour*, **41**, 1015–37.

Mason, G.J. (1991) Stereotypes and suffering. *Behavioural Processes*, **25**, 103–115.

Mason, G. & Mendl, M. (1993) Why is there no simple way of measuring animal welfare? *Animal Welfare*, **2**, 301–319.

Mench, J.A. (1993) Assessing animal welfare: an overview. *Journal of Agricultural and Environmental Ethics*, **6** (Special Supplement 2), 68–75.

McGlone, J.J. (1993) What is animal welfare? *Journal of Agricultural and Environmental Ethics*, **6** (Special Supplement 2), 26–36.

O'Donoghue, P.N. (ed.) (1996) Harmonization of laboratory animal husbandry. *Proceedings of the Sixth Symposium of the Federation of European Laboratory Animal Science Associations*, FELASA, BCM Box 2989, London WC1N 3XX.

Sainsbury, D.W.B. (1986) *Farm Animal Welfare, Cattle, Pigs and Poultry*. Collins, 1986.

Sandoe, P. & Simonsen, H.P. (1992) Assessing animal welfare: where does science end and philosophy begin? *Animal Welfare*, **1**, 257–67.

UFAW (1972) *UFAW Handbook on the Care and Management of Farm Animals*. UFAW, London.

Animals in research

Baird, R.M. & Rosenbaum, S.E. (1991) *Animal Experimentation*. Prometheus Books, London.

Buxton, P.A. (1947) What animals owe to experimental research. *Stephen Paget Memorial Lecture*, RDS, London.

Carter, C.J. (1981) The law of the matter viewed in relation to its ethics. *Conquest*, No. 17, 1–11, RDS, London.

Cass, J. (ed.) (1971) *Laboratory Animals: Bibliography of Informational Resources*. Hafner Publishing, New York.

Forsman, B. (1993) *Research Ethics in Practice: the Animal Ethics Committees in Sweden 1979–1989*. Centre for Research Ethics, Brogotan 4, S-41301 Goteborg, Sweden.

Henshaw, D. (1989) *Animal Warfare: the Story of the Animal Liberation Front*. Fontana/Collins, London.

Howard, W.E. (1993) Animal research is defensible. *Journal of Mammalogy*, **74**, 234–5.

Jennings, M. & Bennett, L. (1993) *Ethics Committees Worldwide: A Summary of Information*. RSPCA, Horsham.

Lane-Petter, W. (ed.) (1963) *Animals for Research*. Academic Press, London.

Lane-Petter, W. (1976) The ethics of animal experimentation. *Journal of Medical Ethics*, **2**, 118–26.

Langley, G. (ed.) (1989) *Animal Experimentation: The Consensus Changes*. Macmillan Press, London.

Langley, G. (ed.) (1989) *Why Experiments on Animals?* Macmillan Press, London.

Leahy, T. (1991) *Against Liberation*. Routledge, New York.

Lembeck, F. (ed.) (1989) *Scientific Alternatives to Animal Experiments*. Ellis Horwood.

Littlewood Report (1965) *Report of the Departmental Committee on Experiments on Animals*. HMSO, London.

Marsh, N. & Haywood, S. (eds) (1985) *Animal Experimentation, Improvements and Alternatives*. FRAME, Nottingham.

National Antivivisection Society (1993) *The Good Science Guide*. NAVS, London.

Phillips, M.T. & Sechzer, J.A. (1989) *Animal Research and Ethical Conflict, an Analysis of the Scientific Literature*. Springer-Verlag, Berlin.

Orlans, F.B. (1993) *In the Name of Science: Issues in Responsible Animal Experimentation*. Oxford University Press, New York.

Russell, W. & Burch, R. (1959) *The Principles of Humane Experimental Technique*. Methuen, London.

Ryder, R.D. (1975) *Victims of Science: The Use of Animals in Research*. Davis-Poynter.

Singer, P. (1990) *Animal Liberation*, 2nd edn. New York Review of Books, New York.

Smith, J.A. & Boyd, K.M. (1991) *Lives in the Balance: The Ethics of Using Animals in Biomedical Research*. Oxford University Press, Oxford.

Smyth, D.H. (1978) *Alternatives to Animal Experimentation*. Scolar Press and RDS, London.

Theune, E.P. & de Cock Buning, T.J. (1993) Assessing interests. An operational approach. *Science and Human–Animal Relationships*, pp. 143–60. SISWO, Amsterdam.

UFAW The Universities Federation for Animal Welfare has published numerous books on all aspects of animal studies. Particularly useful is their *Handbook on the Care and Management of Laboratory Animals* which has been continually brought up to date.

Uvarov, O. (1984) Research with animals: requirements, responsibilities, welfare. *Laboratory Animals*, **19**, 51–75.

Vyvyan, J. (1971) *The Dark Side of Science*. Michael Joseph.

Animals: awareness and pain

Archer, J. (1979) *Animals under Stress*. Arnold.

Barclay, R.J., Herbert, W.J. & Poole, T.B. (1988) *The Disturbance Index: A Behavioural Method of Assessing the Severity of Common Laboratory Procedures on Rodents*. UFAW, London.

Dawkins, M.S. (1980) *Animal Suffering, The Science of Animal Welfare*. Chapman and Hall.

Flecknell, P. (1984) *The Relief of Pain in Laboratory Animals*, Vol. 18, pp. 147–60. Tamworth.

Griffin, D. (1976) *The Question of Animal Awareness: Evolutionary Continuity of Mental Experience*. Rockefeller University Press, New York.

Griffin, D. (1978) Prospects for a cognitive ethology. *Behavioral and Brain Sciences*, **4**, 527–38.

Griffin, D. (1984) *Animal Thinking*. Harvard University Press, Cambridge, Massachusetts.

Griffin, D. (1992) *Animal Minds*. University of Chicago Press, Chicago.

Harrison, P. (1991) Do animals feel pain? *Philosophy*, **66**, 25–40.

Lansdell, H. (1993) The three Rs: a restrictive and refutable rigmarole. *Ethics and Behaviour*, **3**(2), 177–85.

LASA Working Party (1990) The assessment and control of the severity of scientific procedures on laboratory animals. *Laboratory Animals*, **24**, 97–130.

Morton, D. & Griffiths, P. (1985) Guidelines on the recognition of pain, distress and discomfort in experimental animals and an hypothesis for assessment. *Veterinary Record*, **116**, 20 April, 431–6.

Pluhar, E.B. (1993) Arguing away suffering: the Neo-Cartesian revival. *Between the Species*, Issue 9, 27–41.

Porter, D.G. (1992) Ethical scores for animal experiments. *Nature*, **356**, 101–102.

Rollin, B.E. (1989) *The Unheeded Cry: Animal Consciousness, Animal Pain and Science*. Oxford University Press, New York.

Sorabji, R. (1993) *Animal Minds and Human Morals: The Origins of the Western Debate*. Cornell University Press, Ithaca.

UFAW (1989) *Guidelines for the Recognition and Assessment of Pain in Animals*. Association of Veterinary Teachers and Researcher Workers, UFAW, London.

Index

Abelard, 13, 40, 278
Aguinas, 12, 44, 73, 113, 124
Algorithm for ethical acceptability, 242, 243
Alternatives, 188–210
Anthropomorphism, 130–32
APC, 211, 244
Attitudes to different species, 274–6
Aristotle, 3, 12, 19, 40, 74, 108, 126, 167
Augustine, 12, 72, 113, 124
Austin, 50, 59
Ayers, 15, 16, 25, 32, 57, 113

Behaviourism, 17, 152
Benefits, 214–17
Beneficence, 52
Bentham, 44, 48–9, 52, 113, 117–18, 134,
  161
Bergson, 74
Butler (Bishop), 53, 54
Broad, C.D., 33
Buddha, 14

Canadian Council of Animal Care, 246–8
Casuistry, 213
Categorical Imperative, 54
Certainty, 16, 17, 40
Codes, 21, 50–52
Commons (Right to), 80–82
Companion animals, 275
Conduct, 5, 6, 8, 12, 50, 58
Confucius, 5, 14
Conscience, 22, 46, 52, 55–6, 67
Consensus, 5
Consequentialism, 13, 59, 67
Conservation, 147
Consciousness (Animal), 153
Contract, 46
Cost/benefit, 47, 67, 211–14
Cromwell, 73

Culture, 68, 100, 102, 264, 273
Custom, 98

Darwin, 18, 135, 153, 168, 216
Decision Cube, 218–20
Deontology, 44, 46
Descartes, 17, 126, 152
Determinism, 72–8
Dewey, 61
Diderot, 73
Domestication, 144–6
Dostoyevsky, 14
Double Effect, 13, 42
Draco, 68
Duns Scotus, 277
Dutch System, 224–33
Duty, 44, 46, 53, 58, 60

ECVAM, 202
Education, 102–103, 186
Einstein, 75
Emotivism, 56–8
Enculturation, 100–102, 273
Environmental Enrichment, 206
Entertainment (by animals), 268
Epistemology, 16, 19
Error Theory, 23, 33
Ethics Committees, 245, 251, 261–2
Ethical Evaluation, 239–41
Ethical Review Process, 251–62
Ethical Theories, 8, 13
Ethics (Definition of), 5
Ethos, 6
Epicurianism, 9, 12
Exhibition (of animals), 267
Existentialism, 78
Extrapolation, 201

Falsification, 16

Felicific Calculus, 49, 50
Feltham, 167
First Order Ethics, 6
Flew, A., 16
Frankena, 120
Freedom, 70–78
Freedoms (The Five), 137
Freud, 11

Generosity Paradigm, 8
Good (The), 27, 30, 58
Grades of Right and Wrong, 264–72, 276–8
Guilt, 6, 11, 15, 52

Haeckel, 75
Hall, Marshall, 168, 191
Hammurabi, 5, 14, 104
Hare, R.M., 27, 30, 57
Harvey, 170
Hedonism, 12, 50, 52, 161
Hobbes, 10, 11, 53, 96, 113, 151
Honesty, 9, 12
Hume, 17, 20, 25, 30–31, 48, 53, 67, 113, 126

Institutions (Ethical), 31–2
Intuitionism, 53, 54, 58–9

Janus Principle, 26
James, William, 61
Johnson, Samuel, 9, 74, 167
Justice, 9, 12, 107–108
Justification, 6, 212–14
Justinian, 84, 124

Kant, 17, 18, 44–6, 53–4, 74, 151
Killing animals, 268–9, 272–3
Kipling, 15, 47, 69
Kuhn, 19

Law, 68–9, 103–108
Lewis, C.S., 15
Liberty, 78–83
Linzey, 8
Locke, 24, 53, 154
Logic Positivists, 16
Lucretius, 53, 113

Machiavelli, 9, 13, 44, 47–8

Marcus Aurelius, 73
Mackie, 30, 33, 56
Medical Ethics (Institute of), 233–7
Mill, James, 49
Mill, John Stuart, 29, 44, 48, 63, 105, 113
Moore, G.E., 28–9, 58–9, 63, 76, 113
Moral Maxims, 13
Moral Systems, 13–14
Moral Theology, 7–8
Mores, 9, 44, 68, 97–102

Naturalistic Fallacy, 29, 58, 60–61
Natural Law, 24, 67, 104
Newman (Cardinal), 17, 40, 44
Nietzsche, 13, 14, 39, 97–8
Norm of Morality, 66–9
Nowell-Smith, 26

Objectivism, 22–5, 57
Oppenheimer, 20

Pain, 155–60, 176, 213
Pascal, 24, 73
Pleasure, 51 (*see also* Hedonism)
PETA, 264
Plato, 3, 5, 12, 40, 107, 113, 115
Pollution, 80–81
Popper, 16
Porter, D.J., 127, 220–24
Power, 78, 98
Pragmatism, 61
Promises, 31–2, 46
Protagoras, 10, 12, 13, 43
Public Relations, 181–6
Puritans, 7, 12, 20

Rs(3), 188–93, 208
Reduction★, 202–205
Refinement, 205–208
Replacement★, 193–201
Rapport, 207
Rawls (John), 9, 53, 67
Reflective Equilibrium, 10
Regan, 134–5
Religion, 7–8, 14–15, 69, 124
Relativism, 43–4, 61, 100–102
Rights, 82–3
Rights (Animal), 132–43
Rollin, 152

Ross, W.D., 32, 60
Rousseau, 5, 53, 97
Russell, 108, 113

Salmond, 107
Sartre, 78
Scepticism, 20, 53
Schopenhauer, 73, 126, 161
Schweitzer, 161
Scoring System, 220–24
Searle, J., 31
Second Order Ethics, 6
Sidgwick, 5, 10, 24, 30, 49, 52, 92
Singer, 40, 114–21
Situation Ethics, 61–3
Slavery, 15, 52, 83–6
Social Contract, 10, 44, 53, 96–7
Society, 94–5, 97–100
Socrates, 3, 12, 39, 40, 47
Solipsism, 18
Solzhenitsyn, 91
Sophists, 12, 53
Spinoza, 44, 53, 73
Stevenson, C.L., 57, 59
Stoicism, 9, 39, 88
Subjectivism, 22–3, 54, 57
Swiss Ethical Requirements, 238
Swedish System, 245–6

Taboo, 5, 11, 68, 95
Tennyson, 40, 115
Teleology, 44, 46
Terence (Publius Terentius), 3, 20
Thatcherism, 9, 177
Thought (Animal), 154
Totem, 122, 123
Transport, 9, 141, 146–7, 149
Two Evils (Principle of), 13, 214
Thrasymarchus, 12

Universalization, 21, 25–6, 54
Utilitarianism, 48, 53, 63, 67, 78–9, 85–6,
    161, 212–13

Validation, 201–202
Value Judgements, 16, 20–23, 57
Verification, 16
Vienna Circle, 16
Voltaire, 102, 126

Warnock, G.J., 10
Warnock, Mary, 114
Westermark, 43
Will (The), 70–72
Williams, Bernard, 33, 39–40, 43, 51–2
Wittgenstein, 59, 76

Zoroaster (Zarathustra), 14

★ Evidence of real progress in 'Replacement' and 'Reduction' is illustrated by the number of animals used in research in the UK, which dropped from approx. $5\frac{1}{2}$ million in experiments involving pain, in 1973 to 2 635 969 in regulated procedures (a wider milder category) in 1997.